KARLHEINZ RICHTER · SIEGFRIED MACH · GEORG LISEWSKI

DIE PNEUMOPELVIGRAPHIE

Eine röntgenologische Methode zur Untersuchung der weiblichen Genitalorgane

PNEUMOPELVIGRAPHY

Examination of the Female Genital Organs by a Radiological Method

PNEUMO PELVIGRAPHY

Examination of the Female Genital Organs by a Radiological Method

by

Prof. Dr. sc. med. KARLHEINZ RICHTER
Professor of Radiological Diagnostics
Humboldt-Universität zu Berlin
I. Med. Klinik und Med. Polikliniken (Charité)
Head of the Department of Roentgenology

Dr. sc. med. SIEGFRIED MACH
Bezirkskrankenhaus Neuruppin
Medical Superintendant of the
Department of Gynecology

Dr. med. GEORG LISEWSKI
Humboldt-Universität zu Berlin
I. Med. Klinik (Charité)
Head of the Department of Endoskopy

With 191 illustrations

DIE PNEUMO PELVIGRAPHIE

Eine röntgenologische Methode
zur Untersuchung der weiblichen Genitalorgane

von

Prof. Dr. sc. med. KARLHEINZ RICHTER
Ordentlicher Professor für Röntgendiagnostik
Humboldt-Universität zu Berlin
I. Med. Klinik und Med. Polikliniken (Charité)
Leiter der Abteilung für Röntgendiagnostik

Dr. sc. med. SIEGFRIED MACH
Bezirkskrankenhaus Neuruppin
Chefarzt
der Frauenklinik

Dr. med. GEORG LISEWSKI
Humboldt-Universität zu Berlin
I. Med. Klinik (Charité)
Leiter der Abteilung für Endoskopie

Mit 191 Abbildungen

AKADEMIE-VERLAG · BERLIN 1973

Übersetzt in die englische Sprache von W. GHANTUS, Berlin
Translated into the English language by W. GHANTUS, Berlin

Erschienen im Akademie-Verlag GmbH, 108 Berlin, Leipziger Str. 3—4

Lizenznummer 202 · 100/567/73
Schutzumschlag- und Einbandgestaltung: Rolf Kunze
Gesamtherstellung: VEB Druckhaus „Maxim Gorki", 74 Altenburg
Bestellnummer: 5690 · ES 17 N
EDV-Nummer: 7614843
Printed in the German Democratic Republic

Inhaltsverzeichnis

Content

Vorwort

Die Pneumopelvigraphie ermöglicht die Darstellung der inneren weiblichen Genitalorgane und unterrichtet bei zahlreichen pathologischen Prozessen sehr genau über die morphologischen Veränderungen im Beckenraum. Der Wert dieser Untersuchungsmethode für die gynäkologische Diagnostik ist nur wenig bekannt. Weder die Radiologen noch die Gynäkologen sind mit dem Verfahren genügend vertraut, obwohl die technische Handhabung relativ einfach ist und die Aussagekraft von erfahrenen Untersuchern hoch eingeschätzt wird. Eine zusammenfassende Veröffentlichung des Gebietes in deutscher oder englischer Sprache fehlte bisher.

In enger Zusammenarbeit zwischen der Röntgenabteilung der I. Medizinischen Universitätsklinik und der Universitäts-Frauenklinik der Charité Berlin entwickelten wir eine einfache Untersuchungstechnik, die sich mit allgemein gebräuchlichen Untersuchungsgeräten durchführen läßt und in der Praxis ausgezeichnet bewährt hat. Anhand von mehreren hundert Untersuchungen gewannen wir die Überzeugung, daß die Pneumopelvigraphie eine wertvolle Bereicherung der gynäkologischen Diagnostik darstellt und in vielen differentialdiagnostisch schwierigen Situationen unentbehrlich werden kann. Als Voraussetzung sind die gezielte Indikation mit spezieller klinischer Fragestellung, die Beherrschung der Technik und die richtige Bildinterpretation hervorzuheben. Unsere Erfahrungen darüber haben wir in dieser Schrift zusammengefaßt. Das Buch soll die Anwendungsmöglichkeiten der Pneumopelvigraphie umreißen, die sinnvolle Indikationsstellung erleichtern und dem Interessenten beim Erlernen der Methode, bei der Bildanalyse und der Befunddeutung eine Hilfe sein. Aus diesem Grunde legten wir auf ein umfangreiches, ausführlich erläutertes Bildmaterial besonderen Wert. Um die praktische Bedeutung und die Leistungsfähigkeit des Verfahrens zu zeigen, wurden die Röntgenbefunde nach Indikationsgebieten zusammengefaßt und im Rahmen der klinischen Problematik jedes Einzelfalles beschrieben. Denn neben der Qualitat der Röntgendiagnostik ist ihre Verflechtung mit der Klinik für die diagnostische Aussage entscheidend. Für die anatomischen Bezeichnungen verwendeten wir die Nomina anatomica, New York 1961.

Herrn Prof. Dr. KRAATZ, Direktor der Universitäts-Frauenklinik der Charité, sprechen wir für seine

Foreword

Pneumopelvigraphy is a procedure to represent the internal female genital organs and to yield high-accuracy information on morphological changes in the pelvic cavity for a considerable range of pathological processes. There is only limited knowledge about the value for gynecological diagnosis of this examination method. Neither the radiologists nor the gynecologists have been sufficiently familiar with the procedure, although its technical handling is comparatively easy and its informative value highly appreciated by experienced examiners. No summarising publication of the subject in German or English has thus far been available.

A simple diagnostic technique, which is feasible with common examination equipment and has proved to be highly efficient in clinical practice, has been developed by the authors in close cooperation between the radiological department of the I. Medical Clinic and the Gynecological Clinic of the Charité Univerity Hospitals, Berlin. After having conducted several hundreds of examinations the authors believe that pneumopelvigraphy is a most helpful supplementation to gynecological diagnosis which may be quite indispensable in many situations where problems are regarding differential diagnosis. Clear-cut indication oriented faced to specific clinical questions, complete control of the technical processes involved, and adequate interpretation of the radiograph should be emphasised as the major prerequisites for success. The experience related to the subject and so far gained by the authors has been summarised in this book intended to outline the possible applications of pneumopelvigraphy, to facilitate consistent indication, and to help all those interested learn the method, analyse the radiographs, and interpret the findings. This is why a great number of illustrations has been added together with detailed explanations. The radiological findings are compiled by indications and described with reference to the clinical aspects of each case, with the view of demonstrating both the practical importance and the efficiency of the method and because it is not only the standard of radiological diagnosis as such but rather its coordination with the clinical findings which counts decisively for diagnostic information and consistency. The anatomic designations used in this publication are based on Nomina anatomica, New York 1961.

großzügige Unterstützung und wertvolle Beratung unseren tiefen Dank aus. Die Grafiken gestaltete Herr Dipl.-Grafiker H. LINK. Seiner schöpferischen Mitarbeit gebührt besonderes Lob. Herrn GHANTUS verdanken wir die Übersetzung des Manuskriptes ins Englische. Unser Dank gilt weiterhin der Fotografin, Frau D. HUHND, von der Zentralen Fotoabteilung der Charité und der Röntgenassistentin, Frau T. SCHRÖDER, in deren Händen die umfangreichen fototechnischen Arbeiten lagen, Frau E. ADAM für die gewissenhafte Durchsicht des Manuskriptes, Schwester E. BRANDT und den Röntgenassistentinnen der I. Medizinischen Universitätsklinik der Charité für ihren unermüdlichen Einsatz bei der Durchführung der zahlreichen Untersuchungen, sowie Frau Dipl.-Ing. GOLLY, Staatliche Zentrale für Strahlenschutz, Berlin, und Herrn Dipl.-Ing. KRÜGER, Strahlenphysikalische Abteilung der Geschwulstklinik der Charité, für die vorgenommenen Dosismessungen.

Ein besonderes Anliegen ist es uns, dem Akademie-Verlag für die Herausgabe und großzügige Ausstattung des Buches zu danken.

K. RICHTER
S. MACH
G. LISEWSKI

The authors should like to express their debt of gratitude to Prof. Dr. KRAATZ, Medical Superintendant of the Gynecological Clinic at the Charité University Hospitals of Berlin, for his generous support and valuable advice. The schematic drawings and anatomic sketches added to the reproduced radiographs were made by H. LINK, graduate draughtsman, whose creative cooperation was highly recognised. The translation into the English language of this book is owed to W. GHANTUS. Our appreciation includes also Mrs. D. HUHND, photographer in the Central Photo Section of the Charité, Mrs. T. SCHRÖDER, X-ray assistant, who had to deal with the tremendous amount of phototechnical work involved, Mrs. E. ADAM for her careful checking of the manuscript, nurse E. BRANDT and the X-ray assistants of the I. Medical Clinic at the Charité University Hospitals of Berlin for their untiring cooperation in tackling the large number of tests involved, as well as Mrs. GOLLY, diplomaed engineer in the National Radiation Shielding Centre of Berlin, and Mr. KRÜGER, diplomaed engineer in the radiation physics department of the Tumor Clinic at the Charité University Hospitals of Berlin, for the dosimetric work done by them.

The authors feel particularly obliged to extend their debt of gratitude and recognition to Akademie-Verlag für the publication and generous makeup of this book.

K. RICHTER
S. MACH
G. LISEWSKI

1. Einleitung

Die Gasfüllung des intraperitonealen Beckenraumes zur röntgenologischen Darstellung der inneren weiblichen Genitalorgane wird als *Pelvopneumoperitoneum, pelvine Pneumographie, Pneumogynäkographie* oder *pelvigraphie gazeuse* bezeichnet. In der modernen Literatur findet vorwiegend der Ausdruck Pneumopelvigraphie Verwendung. Nachdem LOREY die intraperitoneale Gasfüllung erstmalig zur Kontrasterzeugung bei Röntgenuntersuchungen des Abdomens anwandte (1912), wurde die Bedeutung dieses Verfahrens für die klinische Diagnostik rasch erkannt (WEBER, MEYERBETZ, RAUTENBERG). GOETZE gelang 1918 die erste Darstellung der weiblichen Beckenorgane. STEIN u. Mitarb. am Michael-Reese-Hospital in Chicago erwarben sich um die Entwicklung und Einführung der Methode in die Diagnostik gynäkologischer Erkrankungen ein besonderes Verdienst (1918—1935). In Deutschland erschien 1923 ein Röntgenatlas von WINTZ und DYROFF „Das Pneumoperitoneum in der Gynäkologie", in dem Fragen der Methodik, Indikationsstellung, Bildinterpretation und klinischen Bewertung eingehend besprochen wurden. Gemessen am damaligen Entwicklungsstand der Röntgentechnik enthalten die Ausführungen bemerkenswerte diagnostische Erkenntnisse. Weitere Berichte aus dieser Zeit stammen von ORNDORFF, CALIEZ, ZWALUWENBURG, CASE, PETERSON, JUNG u. SCHIRMER, BECLERE, POLAND u. DIETL (1919—1928). Im italienischen Schrifttum wurden erste Arbeiten von VALLEBONA u. DOGLIOTTI (1937) veröffentlicht. Seitdem fand die Pneumopelvigraphie in einigen europäischen Ländern zunehmend Verbreitung, vor allem in Frankreich und Italien. Dagegen hat sich das Verfahren in deutschen Kliniken nicht eingebürgert.

Bis heute liegen im Schrifttum etwa 150 Mitteilungen vor. Nach übereinstimmendem Urteil fast aller Autoren besitzt die Methode für bestimmte klinische Fragestellungen einen großen differentialdiagnostischen Aussagewert. Unsere eigenen Erfahrungen haben gezeigt, daß die Information der Pneumopelvigraphie in vielen Situationen mit keiner anderen Untersuchungsmethode außer der Probelaparotomie erreicht werden kann. Der Vorteil des Verfahrens liegt in der Möglichkeit, durch eine visuelle Orientierung den Palpationsbefund zu präzisieren, in wichtigen Details zu ergänzen und eine Reihe von Schwierigkeiten in der gynäkologischen Diagnostik

1. Introduction

The filling of gas into the intraperitoneal pelvic cavity for a radiological representation of the internal female genital organs is known under the names of *pelvopneumoperitoneum, pelvine pneumography, pneumogynecography,* or *pelvigraphie gazeuse.* In modern literature *pneumopelvigraphy* has been adopted as the most common term. The importance of this method to clinical diagnosis was understood rather soon (WEBER, MEYERBETZ, RAUTENBERG), after intraperitoneal gas filling had been used for diagnostic contrast radiography of the abdomen for the first time by LOREY (1912). In 1918, GOETZE was the first to succeed in a representation of the female pelvic organs. A particular contribution to the development and to the introduction of the method to gynecological diagnosis was made by STEIN and co-workers at the Michael-Reese Hospital of Chicago (1918—1935). In Germany, WINTZ and DYROFF published in 1923 a radiological atlas under the title "Das Pneumoperitoneum in der Gynäkologie" (Pneumoperitoneum in Gynecology) which provided a detailed coverage of problems related to the methods involved as well as to indication, radiographic interpretation, and clinical assessment. The diagnostic findings presented in that publication were of remarkable consistency when measured against the technological standards achieved in radiology by then. Other reports in that period were published by ORNDORFF, CALIEZ, ZWALUWENBURG, CASE, PETERSON, JUNG and SCHIRMER, as well as by POLAND and DIETL (1919—1928). The first reports in Italian literature were published by VALLEBONA and DOGLIOTTI (1937). Ever since, pneumopelvigraphy has gained increasing ground in some European countries, mainly in France and Italy, whereas the method failed to catch on German clinics.

Some 150 communications have become available in the literature by today. There is unanimous agreement between almost all the authors to the effect that for differential diagnosis of certain clinical problems the method is of a considerable consistency. Our own experience has shown that in many situations the amount of information obtainable from pneumopelvigraphy could not be matched by any other diagnostic approach, except for exploratory laparotomy. The possibility of scrutinising the accuracy of the palpation findings by visual orientation is a major advantage offered by

zu überwinden. Durch Kombination der Pneumopelvigraphie mit positiv kontrastgebenden Methoden, der Hysterosalpingographie und der Lymphographie, läßt sich die Informationsgewinnung in manchen Fragen weiter verbessern.

Die *Technik* wird unterschiedlich gehandhabt. Die Mehrzahl der Untersucher bevorzugt die abdominale *Anlage des Pneumoperitoneum.* Einzelne Autoren nehmen eine DOUGLAS-Punktion vor (DECKER, HENZL). Bei durchgängigen Eileitern besteht auch die Möglichkeit, das Gas durch die Tuben einzublasen (PETERSON). Zur Kontrasterzeugung finden vorwiegend Sauerstoff, CO_2 und N_2O Verwendung. Die Insufflation von Luft ist wegen der längeren Resorptionszeit verlassen worden. Die röntgenologische Aufnahmetechnik hat eine möglichst überlagerungsfreie Darstellung des vom Gas umflossenen Uterus und der Adnexe zum Ziel. Voraussetzungen dafür sind eine Hochlagerung des Beckens und ein geeigneter Strahlengang. Als Untersuchungsgeräte werden vorwiegend kippbare Buckytische verwendet, auf denen die Patientin Bauchlage einnimmt. Die Untersuchung kann auch in Rückenlage (LE GENISELL u. Mitarb.). oder in Knie-Ellenbogenlage an einem Durchleuchtungsgerät (SILINKOVA-MALKOVA) erfolgen. STEIN hat für Aufnahmen in Knie-Ellenbogenlage eine spezielle Gerätekonstruktion angegeben.

Die *Einstelltechnik für die Röntgenaufnahmen* ist ebenfalls verschieden. Günstige Projektionen ergeben sich durch Kippung der Röhre in kaudokranialer Richtung bei dorsoventralem Strahlengang. Dadurch können umständliche, für die Patientin sehr unbequeme Beckenlagerungen (HOFMANN) vermieden werden. Die empfohlenen Röhrenneigungen führen je nach dem Grad der Tischkippung zu senkrechter oder schräger Projektion. Der Winkel des Zentralstrahles mit der Bildebene liegt bei den verschiedenen Techniken zwischen 50° und 90°. Mit Hilfe von Stereoaufnahmen, mehrfachen Einstellungen mit verschiedener Röhren- und Beckenneigung und durch schräge Positionen versuchten manche Autoren, eine genaue Lagebestimmung pathologischer Verschattungen zu erreichen (WINTZ und DYROFF, ABRAMS u. HUGHES, LE GENISELL, AUBRY u. BARGES). Über Schichtuntersuchungen liegen nur wenige Berichte vor (BRAIBANTI; VALLEBONA u. DOGLIOTTI; BUSINGO; OLIVA; SILINKOVA-MALKOVA). Der Wert dieser Methode war bisher umstritten. Von verschiedenen Arbeitsgruppen wurde das Pelvopneumoperitoneum mit der Hysterosalpingographie (JUNG u. SCHIRMER, STEIN, BECLERE, VALLEBONA u. DOGLIOTTI, MAGENDIE u. Mitarb., LAGARDE, BOMPIANI u. Mitarb. u. a.), der Lymphographie (LAGARDE) oder der Laparoskopie

the method under review. In the same context, certain important details may be added to the result obtained from palpation and a number of problems eliminated faced otherwise in gynecological diagnosis. An even further improvement of certain aspects of information may be achieved by combining pneumopelvigraphy with positive contrast methods, i.e. hysterosalpingography and lymphography.

There are several ways in handling the *technique.* Abdominal *application of the pneumoperitoneum* is preferred by the majority of examiners and puncture of the pouch of Douglas by others (DECKER, HENZL). If the oviducts are permeable, the gas may be introduced also through the tubes (PETERSON). Oxygen, CO_2, and N_2O are the most common contrast media. Insufflation of air has been abandoned because of the excessive absorption time involved. The radiographic technique should be such that overshadowing is widely avoided in representing the uterus and adnexa flown round by the gas. This is best achieved by elevating the pelvis and choosing an appropriate path of rays. Tilting Bucky tables are preferred, with the patient lying in prone position. The examination may be carried out also with the patient in supine position (LE GENISELL and co-workers) or in genucubital position, using a fluoroscope (SILINKOVA-MALKOVA). A special apparatus design has been suggested by STEIN for radiography with the patient in genucubital position.

There are also different possibilities of apparatus adjustment. Favourable radiographs may be obtained by caudo-cranial tilting of the X-ray tube and dorsoventral ray path, an approach by which pelvis positions very uncomfortable to the patient (HOFMANN) can be avoided. The recommended X-ray tube inclinations would result alternatively in vertical or oblique projections, depending on the degree of table tilting. With these alternative techniques, the angles formed by the central ray with the radiographic plane would be from 50 to 90 degrees. Attempts were made by several authors to achieve precise location of pathological shadows by stereography, repetitive adjustment using different X-ray tube and pelvis inclinations, and oblique positioning (WINTZ and DYROFF, ABRAMS and HUGHES, LE GENISELL, AUBRY and BARGES). Only few reports are available about diagnostic tomography (BRAIBANTI, VALLEBONA and DOGLIOTTI; BUSINGO; OLIVA; SILINKOVA-MALKOVA). The value of this method has so far been a controversial subject. Several groups of authors combined polvopneumoperitoneum with hysterosalpingography (JUNG and SCHIRMER, STEIN, BECLERE, VALLEBONA and DOGLIOTTI, MAGENDIE and co-workers, LAGARDE, BOMPIANI and co-workers, et al.), lymphography

(Durando u. Faccini, Lenzi, Tenti u. Mitarb., Giudici u. Mitarb.) kombiniert. Neuerdings wiesen Radberg u. Wickbom darauf hin, daß sich die Beckenangiographie und das Pelvopneumoperitoneum bei bestimmten diagnostischen Fragen sinnvoll ergänzen können.

Unsere eigene Methodik gestalteten wir so einfach wie möglich, um von speziellen Gerätekonstruktionen unabhängig zu sein. Die Untersuchung kann in verschiedenen Varianten durchgeführt werden, deren Wahl nach der klinischen Fragestellung und dem Informationsinhalt der Aufnahme getroffen wird. Als besonders vorteilhaft erwies sich die Luftfüllung der Harnblase, die wir prinzipiell anwenden. An weiteren Maßnahmen können in die Untersuchung einbezogen werden: Lufteinblasung in das Rectum, Tomographie, Hysterosalpingographie, Lymphographie. Besondere Beachtung schenkten wir der Strahlenbelastung der Gonaden, die durch zweckmäßige Wahl der Belichtung, spezielle Entwicklungsverfahren, hochverstärkende Folien und hochempfindliche Filme ohne Verlust an Bildinformation niedrig gehalten werden kann. Die in unserem Arbeitskreis unter Anlegen eines strengen Maßstabes gewonnenen Erkenntnisse zeigten, daß der diagnostische Gewinn sowohl zur Strahlenbelastung als auch zum technischen Aufwand der Pneumopelvigraphie in einer durchaus angemessenen Relation steht. In der im folgenden beschriebenen Form eignet sich das Verfahren für viele Bereiche der gynäkologischen Diagnostik und ist anderen einfachen Methoden bei einer ganzen Reihe klinischer Fragen eindeutig überlegen.

(Lagarde) or laparoscopy (Durando and Faccini, Lenzi, Tenti and co-workers, Giudici and co-workers). Radberg and Wickbom suggested recently that in certain diagnostic situations pelviangiography with pelvopneumoperitoneum would prove to be a favourable combination.

The authors designed their own methods with the highest possible degree of simplicity, in order to be independent of sophisticated special equipment. Different variants are possible for the examination and adopted alternatively according to the clinical problem and depending on the information provided by the radiograph. Basically, they use air insufflation of the urinary bladder which proved to be very efficient. Other possible variants are rectal air insufflation, tomography, hysterosalpingography, and lymphography. Particular attention has been paid by the authors to gonadal exposure to radiation which can be kept low with no loss of radiographic information, by appropriate exposure, special developing processes, highly amplifying screens, and high-speed films. The results achieved by our own working group on the basis of scrupulous criteria have shown an adequate and justifiable relationship to exist between the diagnostic benefit, on the one hand, and the radiation exposure as well as technical effort implied in pneumopelvigraphy, on the other. The applications described in the following sections suggest the method to be applicable to many fields of gynecological diagnosis and to be clearly superior to other simple methods for quite a number of clinical problems.

2. Methodik

2.1. Vorbereitung

Vorbedingung ist der Ausschluß einer intrauterinen Schwangerschaft. Als Zeitpunkt für die Untersuchung wählt man bei Frauen im geschlechtsreifen Alter die erste Zyklushälfte. Die vorbereitenden Maßnahmen sind einfach. Die Patientin erhält am Vortage morgens ein Abführmittel. An diesem Tage wird nur flüssige Kost verabreicht. Am Untersuchungstage selbst bleibt die Patientin nüchtern. Eine medikamentöse Vorbereitung ist in der Regel nicht erforderlich. Bei Tumorpatientinnen mit Schmerzen sollte jedoch für eine ausreichende schmerzstillende Vorbehandlung Sorge getragen werden. Für ängstliche und nervöse Frauen ist die Applikation eines Sedativums zweckmäßig. Die Untersuchung erfolgt während eines stationären Aufenthaltes der Patientin in der Klinik.

2.2. Pneumoperitoneum

Zu Beginn der Untersuchung wird die Harnblase katheterisiert. Der Blasenkatheter bleibt danach liegen und wird durch eine Klemme verschlossen. Die Punktion der Bauchhöhle erfolgt ohne Lokalanästhesie mit einer Pneumothoraxnadel an typischer Stelle im linken Unterbauch. Bei sehr adipösen Bauchdecken sind entsprechend lange Kanülen zu benützen. Je nach Körpergröße und Konstitution werden 800 bis 1000 ml Gas insuffliert. Wir verwenden Sauerstoff oder CO_2. Von anderen Untersuchern wird auch Stickoxydul N_2O als geeignet empfohlen. Die Einblasung erfolgt am zweckmäßigsten mit speziellen Geräten, die eine Regulierung des Füllungsdruckes ermöglichen. Man kann jedoch auch mit einem einfachen, aus zwei 5 l-Flaschen bestehenden Füllsystem arbeiten, das sich bei Verwendung von Sauerstoff als Füllgas und Aqua destillata als Druckflüssigkeit gut eignet. Danach wird die Harnblase über den liegenden Katheter mit 60 ml Luft aus einer Spritze gefüllt.

Erfolgt die Pneumopelvigraphie zur Klärung pathologischer Tastbefunde oder zur Feststellung eines Tumorrezidivs, so erhält die Patientin zusätzlich über ein Darmrohr eine Luftfüllung des Rectum und Colon sigmoideum. Es ist zu empfehlen, die Lufteinblasung in die Harnblase und das Rectum erst auf dem Aufnahmetisch vorzunehmen, da während der zur Lagerung notwendigen Bewegung die Luft aus diesen Organen leicht wieder entweichen kann.

2. Methods

2.1. Preparation

The first codition is to rule out safely the presence of an intra-uterine pregnancy. For sexually mature women, examination should be dated in the first half of the cycle. The perparatory requirements are quite simple. A purgative is administered to the patient in the morning of the day preceding the examination. The diet allowed on this day has to be in liquid form, while on the day of examination the patient has to be kept fasting. Usually no premedication is required. Sufficient analgesic premedication, however, should be applied to patients afflicted with painful tumors. Application of a sedative is recommended for anxious and nervous women. The examination requires hospitalisation of the patient.

2.2. Pneumoperitoneum

The examination is initiated by catheterisation of the urinary bladder. The catheter is clamp-sealed and allowed to stay in its position. The peritoneal cavity is punctured by applying a pneumothorax needle to a typical site in the left part of the hypogastric region, with no local anaesthesia being required. Longer syringes should be used for highly adipose abdominal walls. Some 800 ml to 1000 ml gas are insufflated, depending on body size and constitution. The media used by the authors are oxygen or CO_2. Other examiners have recommended also N_2O nitrous oxide. Insufflation should best be carried out by means of special equipment by which the fill pressure may be kept under control. However, it is possible also by means of a simple filling system, consisting of two 5-litre flasks, which was found to be quite suitable when oxygen was used as filling medium and distilled water as pressure fluid. The urinary bladder above the resting catheter is then filled with 60 ml air from a syringe.

If pneumopelvigraphy is used to elucidate pathological findings obtained from palpation or to identify a recurrent tumor, a rectal tube is introduced for additional air insufflation of both the rectum and colon sigmoideum. It is recommended to start insufflation of the urinary bladder and rectum not until the patient is in proper position on the X-ray table, in order to avoid undue leakage of air from these organs likely to be caused by the movements of positioning.

Nach Beendigung der Untersuchung wird zunächst der Blasenkatheter geöffnet, damit die Luft ausströmen kann. Eine zweite Punktion des Abdomens zur Gasentfernung erweist sich auch bei Verwendung von Sauerstoff (wegen der relativ kleinen Volumina) nicht als notwendig. Die Patientin hält einen Tag lang Bettruhe ein. CO_2 wird sehr rasch resorbiert. Ist außer der Übersichtsaufnahme noch eine Tomographie erforderlich, so muß die Untersuchung ohne Unterbrechung zügig ablaufen, damit die CO_2-Füllung des Beckenraumes noch ausreicht. Die Resorption von Sauerstoff nimmt längere Zeit in Anspruch und ist erst nach mehreren Tagen vollständig. Bei der Laparotomie, die in einigen Fällen drei bis fünf Tage nach der Pneumopelvigraphie vorgenommen wurde, war ein Ausströmen von Gasresten nicht mehr festzustellen.

2.3. Röntgenuntersuchung

2.3.1. *Übersichtsaufnahmen*

Für die Übersichtsaufnahme genügt ein einfacher Blendentisch, der durch Anheben des Fußendes um 15° gegen die Horizontale gekippt wird. Bei dieser Tischneigung sind keine zusätzlichen Hilfsmittel, nicht einmal Schulterstützen erforderlich. Während die Patientin auf dem Buckytisch Bauchlage einnimmt, strömt das Gas ins kleine Becken. Gleichzeitig gleiten die Darmschlingen nach kranial. Dieser Vorgang wird durch die Bewegungen der Patientin bei der Lagerung unterstützt. Eine Röhrenkippung von 15° (aus der Senkrechten) in kaudo-kranialer Richtung ergibt einen Strahlengang, der annähernd der Achse des kleinen Beckens entspricht. Tischneigung und Röhrenkippung addieren sich, so daß der Winkel des Strahlenbündels mit der Bildebene 60° beträgt und der Zentralstrahl vom Lot auf der Bildebene um 30° ausgelenkt wird (Abb. 1). Die Einstellung erfolgt auf die Region zwischen Steißbeinspitze und Anus (Abb. 2). Die Kassettenmitte steht in Höhe der Crista ilica, Fokus-Film-Abstand 1 m, Filmformat 24/30 cm, Universalfolien oder hochverstärkende Folien, Streustrahlenraster (Schachtverhältnisse 15:1 oder 7:1).
Stehen Kippgeräte zur Verfügung, so ist eine Tischneigung von 25° bis 30° zu empfehlen (Abb. 3 und 4). Stärkere Schräglagen sind unnötig und werden von der Patientin unangenehm empfunden. Bei der Festlegung der Röhrenkippung aus der Senkrechten ist die jeweilige Tischneigung, welche gleichfalls zur Auslenkung des Strahlenkegels führt, zu berücksichtigen. Der Winkel zwischen Zentralstrahl und Bildebene soll stets etwa 60° betragen.

The catheter inserted into the bladder is opened for air discharge as soon as the examination is ended. In view of the relatively small volumes involved, another abdominal puncture for gas discharge is not even required in cases where oxygen is used. The patient should rest in bed one full day. CO_2 is absorbed quite readily. In cases where tomography is required in addition to general radiography, the examination should be carried out smoothly without any interruption to make use of the full CO_2 fill of the pelvic cavity. Absorption of oxygen takes more time and usually is complete only after several days. No leakage of residual gas was noted when in some cases laparotomy was performed three to five days after pneumopelvigraphy.

2.3. Radiography

2.3.1. *Standard radiography*

A simple Roentgen table tilted 15 degrees to the horizontal by foot-end lifting is quite sufficient for standard radiography. Such angle would eliminate the need for any additional devices, not even shoulder rests being required. Gas flows into the minor pelvis, the patient lying prone on a Bucky table, while the intestinal loops will slide cranially. This process is promoted by the positioning movements of the patient. The tube is tilted 15 degrees (from the vertical) caudo-cranially to achieve a path of rays that is almost identical with the axis of the minor pelvis. The summation of the table and tube gradients will give an angle of 60 degrees between the bundle of rays and the image plane, with the central beam being deflected by 30 degrees from the vertical of the image plane (Fig. 1). The apparatus is adjusted to the region between the tip of the coccyx and the anus (Fig. 2). The cassette should be with its centre aligned with the level of the crista ilica, focus-film distance being one metre and film size 24/30 cm. Needed are universal type or other highly amplifying screens and a scattered radiation grid, the grid ratio being 15:1 or 7:1.
The inclination of the table should be 25 to 30 degrees if tilting devices are available (Figs. 3 and 4). More oblique positions are unnecessary and would entail a feeling of discomfort in the patient. The inclination of the table which adds to the deflection of the cone of rays should be taken into account in any case when the tube is to be tilted from the vertical. The angle formed by the central beam with the image plane should always be about 60 degrees.

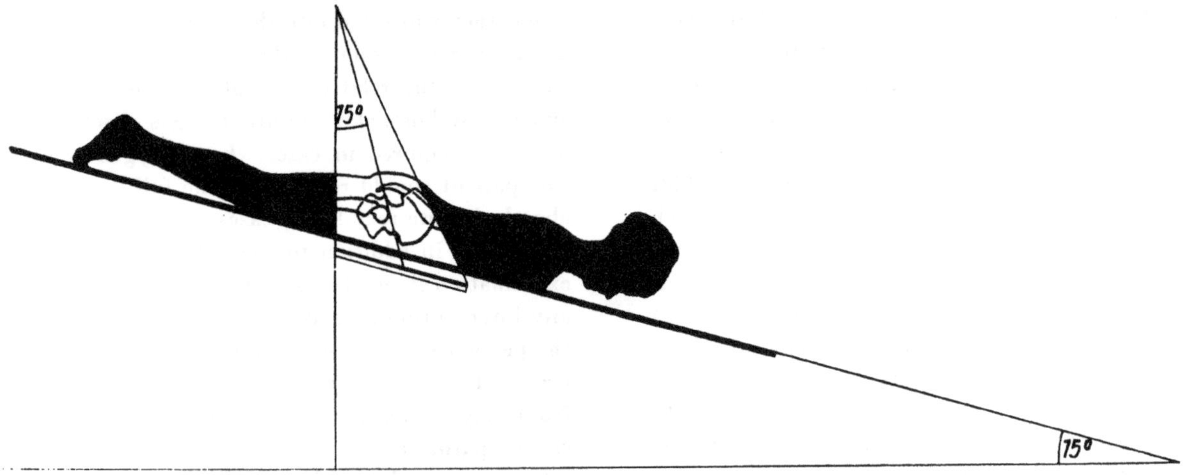

Abb. 1
Lagerung der Patientin und Röhreneinstellung zur *Übersichtsaufnahme*. Auslenkung des Zentralstrahls vom Lot auf der Bildebene = 30° (15° Tischneigung + 15° Röhrenkippung)

Fig. 1
Positioning of the patient and tube adjustment for *standard radiography*; vertical-image plane deflection of the central beam = 30 degrees (15 deg. table inclination + 15 deg. tube tilting)

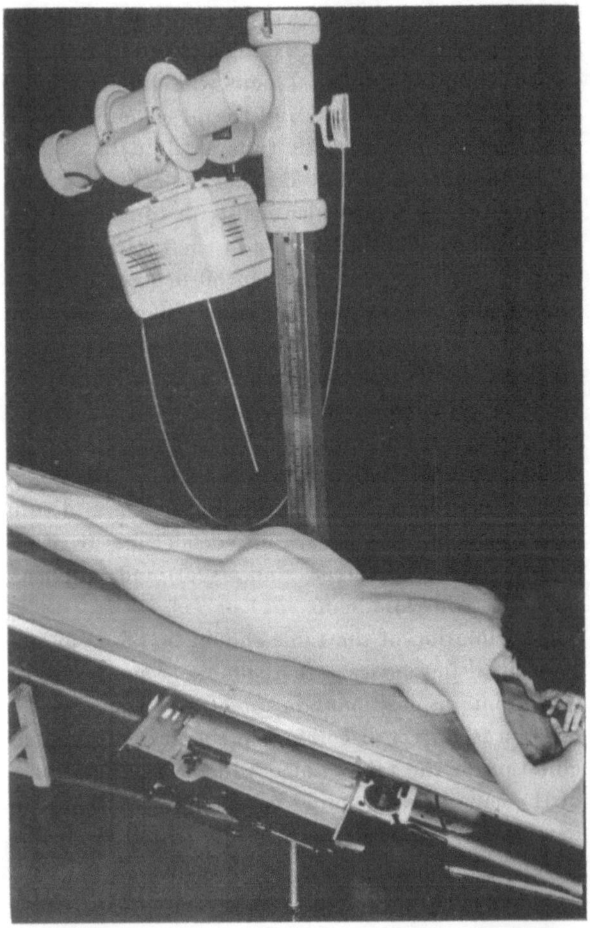

Abb. 2
Lagerung und Einstellung zur *Übersichtsaufnahme*. Der Flachblendentisch ist am Fußende durch einen untergestellten Bock angehoben. Die Neigung gegen die Horizontale beträgt 15°. Weitere Hilfsmittel sind bei dieser Technik nicht erforderlich

Fig. 2
Positioning and adjustment for *standard radiography*; the foot end of the flat diaphragm table supported for elevation; 15 deg. inclination to the horizontal; no additional auxiliaries needed for this technique

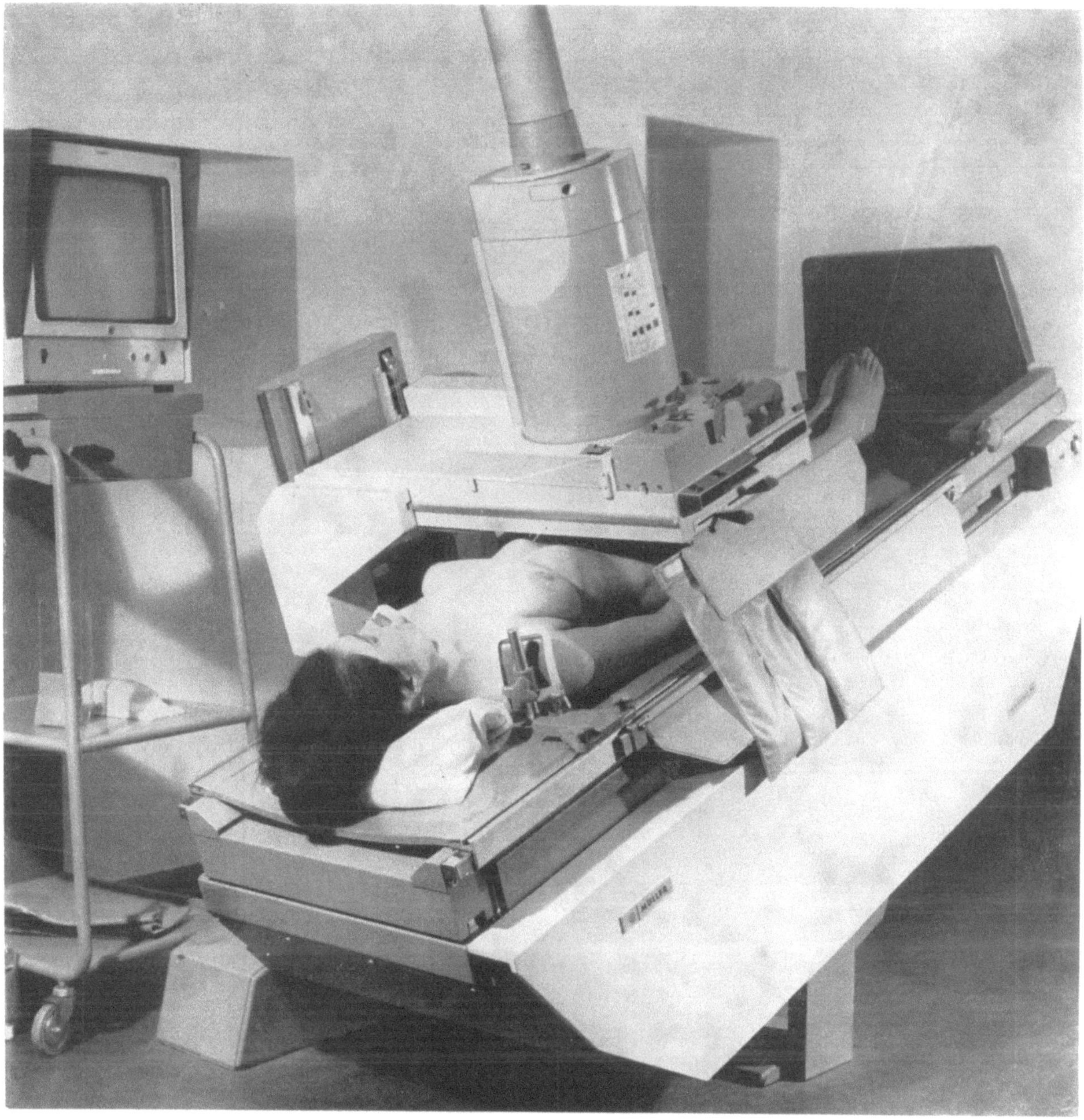

Abb. 3
Lagerung der Patientin auf einem Durchleuchtungsgerät (Diagnost 70, Firma Müller, Hamburg). Diese Technik ist für die *Kombination von Pneumopelvigraphie und Hysterosalpingographie* zu empfehlen, da der Füllungsvorgang beobachtet werden kann

Fig. 3
Positioning of patient on a fluoroscope (Type Diagnost 70, manufactured by Messrs. Müller, Hamburg); the technique is recommended for a *combination of pneumopelvigraphy with hysterosalpingography* for its possibility to observe the filling process

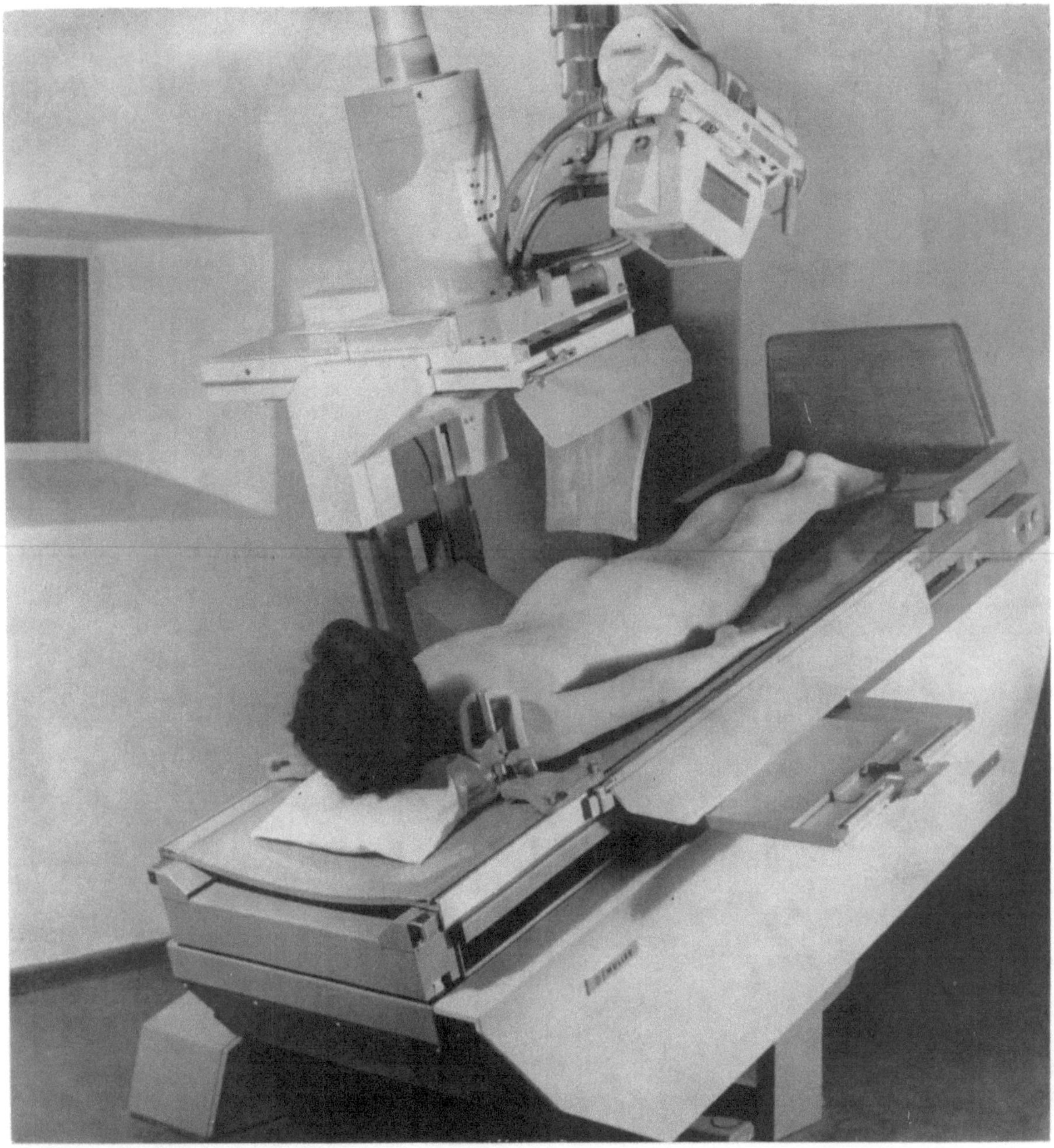

Abb. 4
Einstellung zur Übersichtsaufnahme. Läßt sich das Durchleuchtungsgerät in Verbindung mit einer zusätzlichen Obertischröhre gleichzeitig als Buckytisch verwenden, so ist lediglich die Umlagerung der Patientin auf den Bauch erforderlich. Das Zielgerät mit Röntgenbildverstärker und Fernsehkamera befindet sich seitlich in Parkstellung

Fig. 4
Adjustment for standard radiography: if the fluoroscope used allows coupling with an additional overhead tube for use as a Bucky table, prone re-positioning of the patient will be sufficient

2.3.2. *Schichtaufnahmen*

Schichtaufnahmen sind sehr aufschlußreich und erweitern in vielen Fällen die diagnostische Aussage. Wir haben deshalb die Tomographie in den Untersuchungsgang einbezogen. Bei jungen Patientinnen sind wir allerdings zurückhaltend und versuchen zunächst, mit der Übersichtsaufnahme auszukommen. Bleibt der Befund mehrdeutig, so wird in jedem Fall eine Schichtuntersuchung angeschlossen. Zur Beckenhochlagerung ist ein kippbares Schichtgerät erforderlich. Die Tischneigung soll 25° bis 30° betragen. Die Einstellung erfolgt in Bauchlage auf den unteren Punkt der MICHAELISschen Raute (Abb. 5, 6 und 7). Durch eine untergeschobene Kissenrolle werden die Oberschenkel um 5 bis 10 cm von der Tischplatte abgehoben, damit der Winkel zwischen Strahlenrichtung und Beckenachse möglichst klein bleibt (Abb. 6). Die besten Bilder ergibt nach unseren Erfahrungen die Linearverwischung in Richtung der Körperlängsachse. Ist der Pendelwinkel des Aufnahmesystems wählbar, so sind Einstellungen von 10° bis 30° zu empfehlen. Bei der Wahl der Schichttiefen muß man berücksichtigen, daß der Raum von der Symphyse bis zum Rectum darzustellen ist. Neben dem Einzelschichtverfahren kann die Simultanschichtung mit 4 oder 7 Filmen Anwendung finden.

Wir erprobten auch andere Lagerungen und Schnittführungen, z. B. im dextrosinistralen oder sinistrodextralen Strahlengang bei Seitenlage der Patientin. Ein entscheidender Informationsgewinn läßt sich dadurch jedoch nicht erreichen.

2.3.3. *Belichtung*

Für die Belichtung der Übersichts- und Schichtaufnahmen sind Strahlungen von 65—75 kV zu empfehlen. Diese Technik macht kleine Details innerhalb des gasgefüllten Beckenraumes durch ausreichende Kontraste sichtbar. Die Verwendung von Filmen höchster Empfindlichkeit, hochverstärkenden Folien, Spezialentwicklern und fotochemischen Verstärkungsverfahren ermöglicht es, das mAs-Produkt (und dementsprechend die Strahlenbelastung) niedrig zu halten, ohne daß ein nennenswerter Informationsverlust eintritt (BÖCK; BÖCK, RICHTER, KANKELWITZ u. KRUG; KANKELWITZ, TESCH u. BÖCK). Wird nach Tumorrezidiven gefahndet und weist das Becken infolge postoperativer und radiogener Fibrose intensive Verschattungen auf, so erzielt man mit Hilfe der Hartstrahltechnik besonders informative Bilder. Das gilt auch für die Kombination der Pneumopelvigraphie mit der Lymphographie.

2.3.2. *Tomography*

Much information is provided by tomograms which add considerably to the diagnostic finding in many cases. We have, therefore, decided to include tomography into the process of examination. However, some reservation is usually observed when it comes to young patients in which cases we try to do with standard radiography. Yet, tomography is added in every case where the finding obtained from standard radiography is ambiguous. For elevation of the pelvis a tiltable tomograph is required. Table inclination should then be between 25 and 30 degrees. The apparatus has to be focused to the lower point of the MICHAELIS rhomboid, with the patient lying prone (Figs. 5, 6, and 7). The thighs are propped up five to ten centimetres from the top of the table by means of a cushion to keep the angle formed by the direction of rays with the pelvic axis as small as possible (Fig. 6). It has been the authors' experience that the best tomograms are obtained from linear blurring towards the longitudinal body axis. Adjustment between 10 and 30 degrees is recommended when a system with selective pendulum angle is used. Representation has to include the whole region from the symphysis to the rectum, which should be considered in selecting the tomographic depths. Both single-layer and simultaneous tomography, using four or seven films, may be used.

The authors have also tried additional positions and sections, such as the dextrosinistral or sinistrodextral paths of rays, with the patient positioned laterally, but no essential additional information was gained.

2.3.3. *Radiation*

Radiation recommended to expose both standard radiographs and tomograms should be in the range of 65 to 75 kV, as such technique would produce sufficient blackening differences to render visible even smaller details in the gas-filled pelvic cavity. The mAs-product (and the corresponding radiation exposure) may be kept low, with no remarkable loss of information, by using films of highest speed, highly amplifying screens, special developers, and photochemical methods of amplification (BÖCK; BÖCK, RICHTER, KANKELWITZ and KRUG; TESCH and BÖCK). Highly informative radiographs may be obtained by means of the hard-ray technique if a recurrent tumor is the subject of search, with intensive shadows being found in the pelvis as a result of postoperative and radiogenic fibrosis. The same applies to cases where pneumopelvigraphy is combined with lymphography.

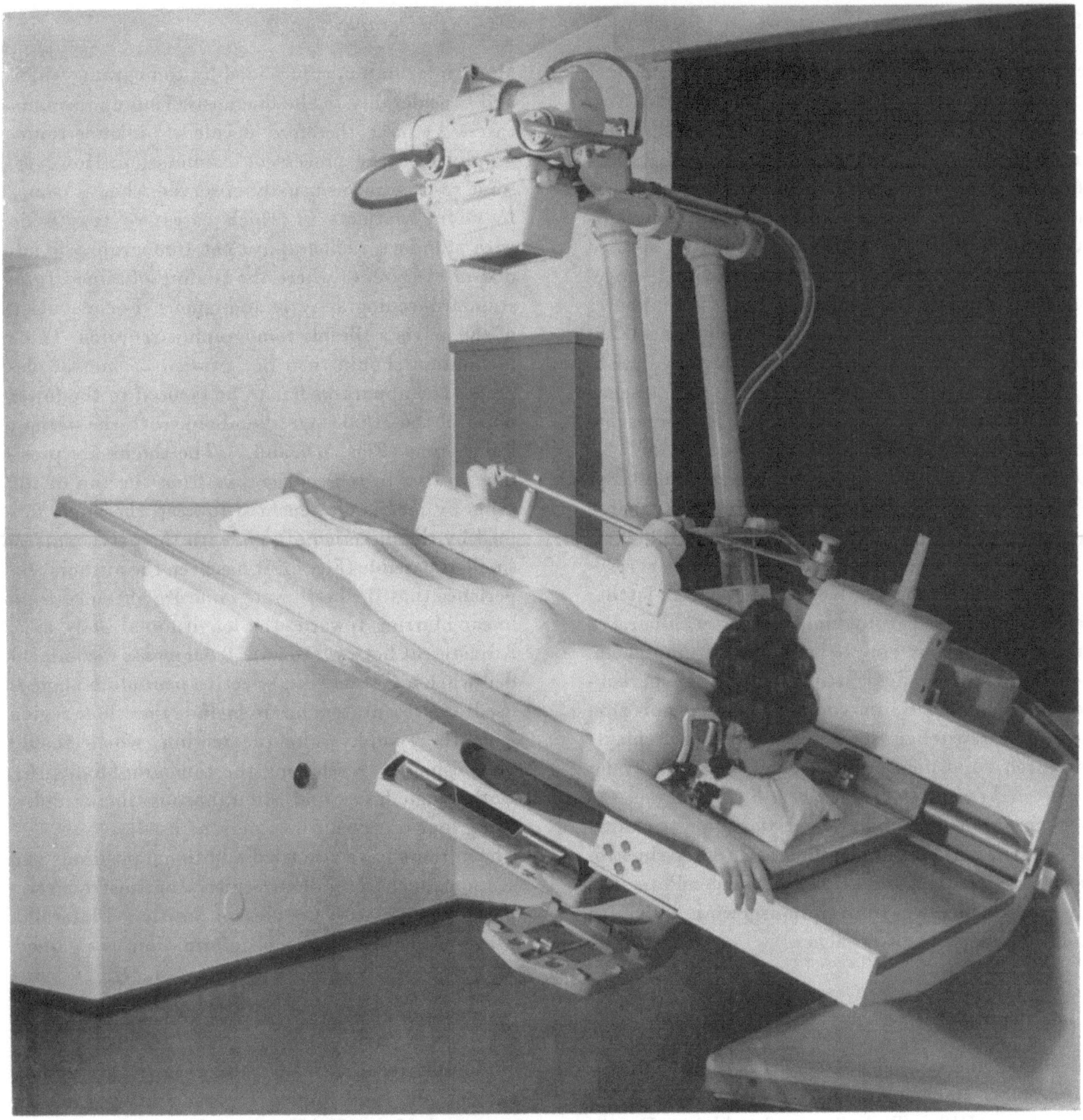

5

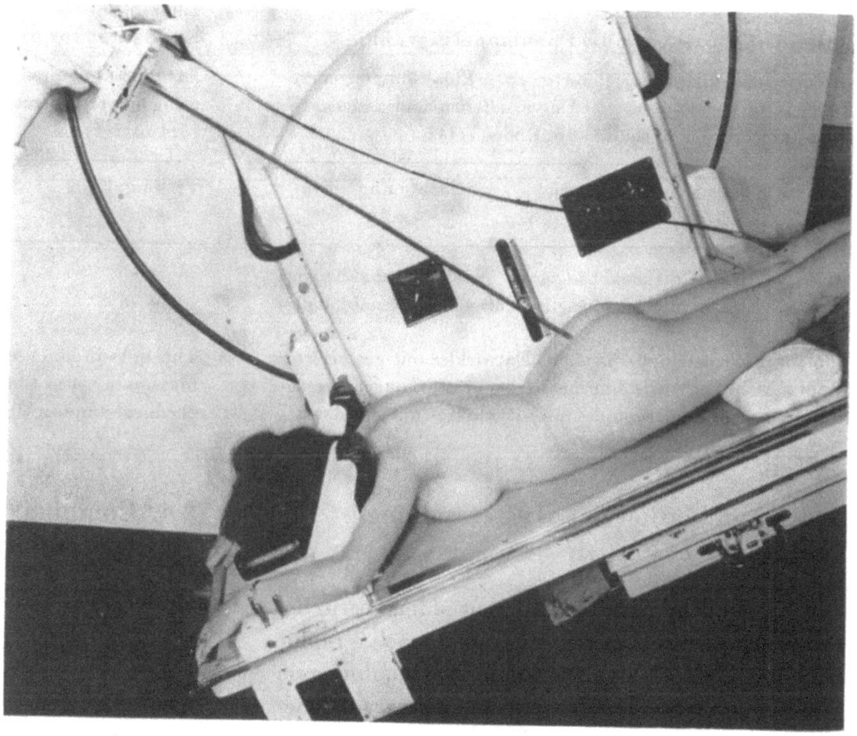

6

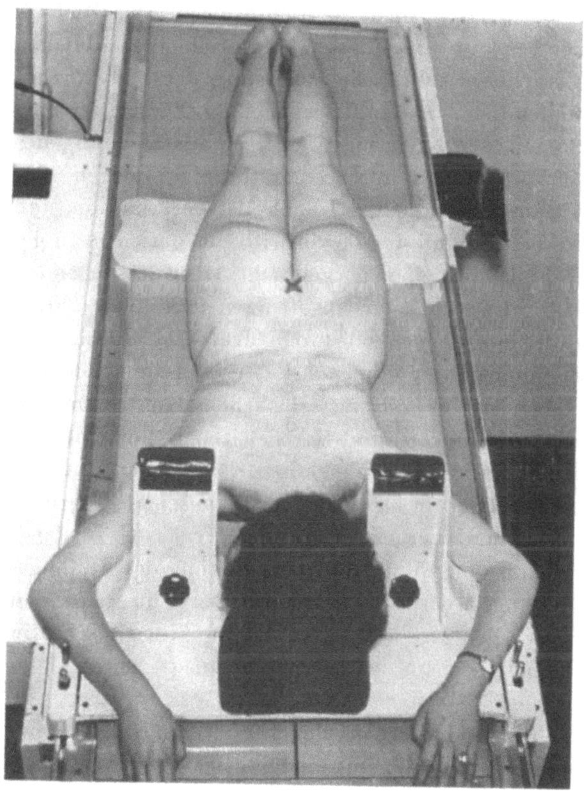

7

Abb. 5–7
Lagerung zur Schichtuntersuchung

Abb. 5: Tomographie mit dem Universal-Polytome (Firma Massiot, Paris)

Abb. 6 und 7: Tomographie mit dem Universal-Tomograph (Firma TuR Dresden). Die Einstellung erfolgt in jedem Fall auf den unteren Punkt der MICHAELISschen Raute (×)

Figs. 5–7
Positioning for tomography

Fig. 5: Tomography, using Universal-Polytome (Messrs. Massiot, Paris)

Figs. 6 and 7: Tomography, using Universal-Tomograph (TuR Dresden); focusing must always be adjusted to the lower point of the MICHAELIS rhomboid (×)

Tabelle 1
Belichtungswerte für die Pneumopelvigraphie

Orientierung über Einstellwerte an 6-Puls-Röntgengeneratoren unter Verwendung von Universalfolien und Streustrahlenrastern (Schachtverhältnis 15:1 oder 7:1)

Technik kV	Übersichtsaufnahmen mAs	Schichtaufnahmen mAs
120	10—20 (dickenabhängig)	7—15 (dickenabhängig)
65—75	50—90 (dickenabhängig)	30—50 (dickenabhängig)

Filme mit Höchstempfindlichkeit, Entwickler mit gesteigerter Empfindlichkeit, sowie fotochemische Verstärkungen ermöglichen eine Verminderung des mAs-Produktes um jeweils 50%

2.4. Kombination mit Hysterosalpingographie

Zur Klärung bestimmter differentialdiagnostischer Fragen ist es zweckmäßig, die Pneumopelvigraphie mit der Hysterosalpingographie zu kombinieren. Für diese Untersuchung ist ein Reinheitsgrad I oder mindestens II der Scheidenflora zu fordern. Nach Vorbereitung der Patientin und Katheterisierung der Harnblase erfolgt zunächst die Anlage des Pneumoperitoneum. Zur Einführung des Füllungsinstrumentes für die Hysterosalpingographie lagert man die Patienten am besten am Fußende des Aufnahmetisches in Steißrückenlage mit halbflektierten Ober- und Unterschenkeln. An den meisten Untersuchungstischen lassen sich dafür entsprechende Fußstützen seitlich leicht anbringen. Die Technik der Instrumenteinführung entspricht dem üblichen Vorgehen: Äußerliche Reinigung der Vulva, Einstellen der Portio mit zwei Spekula, Fassen der Portio mit der Kugelzange, nötigenfalls Dehnung des Zervikalkanals mit Hegarstiften, Einlegen des Füllungsinstrumentes. Nach dessen Fixation und Abdichtung an der Portio wird die Patientin in gewöhnliche Rückenlage gebracht. Über den liegenden Harnblasenkatheter insufflieren wir jetzt 60 ml Luft und verschließen den Katheter durch eine Klemme. Die Füllung des Uteruscavums und der Tuben erfolgt mit wasserlöslichem Kontrastmittel. Die Injektion ist mit der gebotenen Vorsicht von Hand langsam vorzunehmen. Die Kontrastmittelmenge liegt je nach den anatomischen Gegebenheiten und der diagnostischen Fragestellung zwischen 5 und 15 ml. Nach Beendigung des Füllungsvorganges wird die Patientin vorsichtig auf den Bauch gelagert und durch Kippung des Tisches in die beschriebene Aufnahmeposition (s. Seite 13) gebracht.

Stehen moderne Durchleuchtungs- und Aufnahmegeräte zur Verfügung, so läßt sich die Hysterosal-

Table 1
Exposures for pneumopelvigraphy

Exposures required for the use of six-pulse X-ray generators, using universal screens and scattered radiation grids (grid ratio: 15:1 or 7:1)

Technique kV	Standard radiography mAs	Tomography mAs
120	10—20	7—15
65—75	50—90	30—50

The mAs-product may be reduced by 50 per cent by using maximum-speed films, high-sensitivity developers and photochemical amplification

2.4. Combination with hysterosalpingography

If certain problems related to differential diagnosis are to be elucidated, a combination of pneumopelvigraphy with hysterosalpingography may be commendable. For such examinations the degree of purity of the vaginal flora should be I or at least II. The perparation of the patient and catheterisation of the urinary bladder are followed first by the application of the pneumoperitoneum. The filling instrument for hysterosalpingography is best introduced with the patient positioned in breech position at the foot-end of the X-ray table, her thighs and lower legs semiflexed. Appropriate foot supports may be attached easily to the sides of most types of examination tables. The technique to introduce the instrument is identical with the common procedure, including external cleaning of the vulva, cervical adjustment by means of two vaginal specula, gripping of the portio by means of a bullet forceps, if necessary insertion of Hegar's dilators to dilate the cervical canal, and insertion of the filling instrument. The fixation and sealing of the filling instrument at the portio is followed by moving the patient into common dorsal position. 60 ml air are then insufflated above the resting urinary bladder catheter which is sealed by clamping. A water-soluble contrast medium is used as fill of the unterine cavity and the tubes and should be injected slowly, carefully, and manually. The quantity to be injected should be in the range from five to 15 millilitres, depending on the given anatomic conditions and on the kind of diagnostic information desired. After filling the patient is carefully moved prone and brought into the position required for examination and described on page 13 by tilting the table.

In cases where modern fluoroscopes and X-ray equipment are available, hysterosalpingography

pingographie unter Durchleuchtung vornehmen und die Pneumopelvigraphie unmittelbar anschließen, ohne daß umständliche Umlagerungen der Patientin von einem Gerät auf das andere notwendig sind. Eine solche Kombination von zwei Untersuchungsgängen wird durch kippbare Durchleuchtungsgeräte ermöglicht, die sich in Verbindung mit einer zusätzlichen Obertischröhre gleichzeitig als Blendentische verwenden lassen (Abb. 3 und 4). Zunächst wird der Füllungsvorgang während der Hysterosalpingographie im Durchleuchtungsbild beobachtet. Nach Drehung der Patientin auf den Bauch erfolgt danach die Aufnahmeexposition für die Pneumopelvigraphie. Im allgemeinen verzichten wir jedoch auf die Durchleuchtung, um die Gonadendosis niedrig zu halten. Eine andere Möglichkeit besteht darin, die Hysterosalpingographie mit der Schichtuntersuchung zu kombinieren. In diesem Fall werden die Einführung des Instrumentes und die Kontrastmittelfüllung nach Lagerung der Patientin auf dem Schichtgerät vorgenommen.

2.5. Kombination mit Lymphographie

Für die Diagnostik von Metastasen und Rezidiven maligner Geschwülste ist die Kombination der Pneumopelvigraphie mit der Lymphographie zu empfehlen. Beide Untersuchungen werden an aufeinanderfolgenden Tagen oder mit wenigen Tagen Zwischenraum durchgeführt. Die Lymphographie geht voran. Bezüglich ihrer Technik und der röntgenanatomischen Grundlagen verweisen wir auf ausführliche Darlegungen in der Literatur (Dolan, Fuchs, Hahn u. Mitarb., Herman u. Mitarb., Kaindl u. Mitarb., Koehler u. Mitarb., Moulonguet-Doleris u. Mitarb., Rüttimann u. Mitarb., Sieber). Die Füllungs- und Speicherphase des Lymphsystems werden in ventrodorsalen und Schrägaufnahmen festgehalten. Die fortdauernde Speicherung des instillierten öligen Kontrastmittels in den Lymphknoten gibt uns die Möglichkeit, diese bei der Pneumopelvigraphie einen oder wenige Tage danach mit darzustellen. Wegen der auftretenden hohen Kontraste zwischen Lymphographie und Pneumoperitoneum erscheint es zweckmäßig, mit Hartstrahltechnik (120 kV) zu arbeiten. Sollen neben dem Beckenraum auch die paraaortalen Lymphknoten auf der gleichen Aufnahme mit abgebildet werden, so ist das Filmformat 30/40 cm oder 35/43 cm zu wählen.

may be conducted under fluoroscopy followed immediately by pneumopelvigraphy, with no tedious repositioning of the patient from one apparatus to another being required. Such combination of the two examinations is possible, if tiltable fluoroscopes are available which may be used also as diaphragm tables in combination with an additional overhead tube (Figs. 3 and 4). The process of filling for hysterosalpingography is kept under fluoroscopic control. The patient is then repositioned prone for pneumopelvigraphic exposure. In general, however, fluoroscopy is abandoned by the authors to minimise gonadal exposure. Hysterosalpingography may be combined also with tomography, with the introduction of the filling instrument and injection of contrast medium being conducted after positioning of the patient on the tomograph.

2.5. Combination with lymphography

Combination of pneumopelvigraphy with lymphography is recommended for the diagnosis of metastases and recurrent malignant tumors. The two examinations should be conducted an two successive days or with an interval of a few days. Lymphography has to be performed first. For more details of the lymphographic technique and the relevant fundamentals of X-ray anatomy the reader is referred to the detailed descriptions available in the literature (Dolan; Fuchs; Hahn and co-workers; Herman and co-workers; Kaindl and co-workers; Koehler and co-workers; Moulonguet-Doleris and co-workers; Rüttimann and co-workers; Sieber). The filling and storage phases of the lymphatic system are recorded by ventro-dorsal and oblique radiography. The lymphatic nodes may be represented, too, by pneumopelvigraphy performed one or few days after lymphography, since the instilled oily contrast medium will remain present in them. The hard-ray technique is recommended to account for the high contrasts likely to occur between lymphography and pneumoperitoneum. The film sizes should be 30/40 cm or 35/43 cm, if the para-aortic lymphatic nodes are to be represented in addition to the pelvic cavity in one and the same lymphogram.

3. Röntgenanatomische Grundlagen und Darstellung normaler Befunde

3.1. Übersichtsaufnahmen

Es wird eine möglichst überlagerungsfreie Darstellung der Beckeneingeweide, insbesondere der inneren weiblichen Genitalorgane, angestrebt. Durch die Gasfüllung des Cavum peritonei werden überall dort Röntgenkontraste erzeugt, wo das Bauchfell die Beckenhöhle auskleidet oder Eingeweide überzieht. Die zwischen Mastdarm und Harnblase in einer Bauchfellfalte, dem Lig. latum uteri, gelegenen Teile, der Uterus und die Adnexe, werden nach Hochlagerung des Beckens vom Gas umflossen und können schattengebend abgebildet werden. Die beste anatomische Übersicht läßt sich durch einen Einblick ins kleine Becken von kranial-ventral gewinnen (Abb. 8). Das Knochengerüst des Beckens und der Wirbelsäule wirkt bei dieser Blickrichtung am wenigsten störend. Dementsprechend erhalten wir ein gut brauchbares Röntgenbild, wenn die Richtung des Strahlenbündels etwa der Beckenachse entspricht.

Günstige Abbildungsbedingungen entstehen in Bauchlage der Patientin bei schräg von dorsal-kaudal nach kranial-ventral verlaufendem Strahlengang, dessen Richtung ungefähr mit der Beckenachse übereinstimmt. Die dafür notwendige Röhreneinstellung (Abb. 1) führt in Verbindung mit der Kippung des Buckytisches zu schräger Projektion der zu beurteilenden Objekte. Abb. 9 veranschaulicht die Strahlenrichtung und die Abbildungsverhältnisse der Beckeneingeweide. Der mit Gas gefüllte intraperitoneale Beckenraum stellt sich als großes Oval dar, das vom knöchernen Becken und einem mantelförmigen Weichteilschatten begrenzt wird. Dieser erscheint lateral breiter (Muskulatur, Bänder, Gefäße, Lymphknoten, Ureter). Die luftgefüllte Harnblase und die Symphyse projizieren sich in den unteren, das Rectum, Colon sigmoideum und Kreuzbein in den oberen Teil. Dazwischen werden die von Gas umgebenen Genitalorgane, der Uterus, die Ovarien und die Tuben, abgebildet. Außerdem gelingt es, verschiedene Ligamente als Teile des Befestigungsapparates zu differenzieren (Abb. 10—14).

Der normale *Uterus* liegt mitten im Becken. Seine Längsachse verläuft annähernd in der Beckenachse und entspricht dem Strahlengang. Demzufolge wird das Corpus uteri als querliegendes Schattenoval dargestellt, dessen Konturen auf beiden Seiten in das Ligamentum latum und die Tuba uterina auslaufen. Corpus uteri und Cervix uteri sind durch verschiedene Dichte gekennzeichnet. Bei normaler Ante-

3. Anatomic foundations in radiology and representation of normal findings

3.1. Standard radiography

The representation of the pelvic viscera, particularly the internal female genital organs, is desired to be essentially free of overshadowing. Radiographic contrasts are produced by gas insufflation of the peritoneal cavity at any site where the pelvic cavity is lined or viscera are covered by the peritoneum. Those parts situated between the rectum and urinary bladder in a peritoneal fold, the lig. latum uteri, the uterus, and the adnexa are flown round by gas, with the pelvis in elevated position, and may be represented in a radio-opaque manner. The best anatomic representation may be obtained from cranioventral introspection of the minor pelvis (Fig. 8). With such approach, obstruction likely to be caused by both the pelvic skeleton and the vertebral column may be reduced to a minimum. A suitable radiograph is thus obtained when the direction of the beam is somewhat equal to that of the pelvic axis.

Favourable conditions for representation may be achieved with the patient in prone position and the path of rays being oblique from dorsocaudal to cranioventral, its direction aligned to some extent with the pelvic axis. The tube adjustment required to that purpose (Fig. 1) together with the inclination of the Bucky table will lead to an oblique projection of the objects to be assessed. Both the direction of rays and the conditions for representation of the pelvic viscera are shown in Fig. 9. The gas-filled intraperitoneal pelvic space is represented as a large oval space limited by the bony pelvis and a mantle-shaped soft-tissue shadow, the lateral part of the latter appearing more broadly (muscles, ligaments, vessels, lymphatic nodes, ureter). The air-filled urinary bladder and the symphysis are projected in the lower and the rectum, colon sigmoideum, and sacrum in the upper part. The gas-enclosed genital organs, including the uterus, ovaries, and tubes, are projected in-between. In addition, some of the ligaments may be identified as parts of the fixing system (Figs. 10—14).

The *uterus* in normal condition is situated centrally in the pelvis, its longitudinal axis being almost identical with the pelvic axis and in line with the path of rays. Consequently, the corpus uteri is represented as a transverse oval shadow, its contours fading on either side into the ligamentum latum and the tuba uterina. The density of the corpus uteri differs from that of the cervix uteri. The oval shadow of the cervix will come to be located in the shadow of the

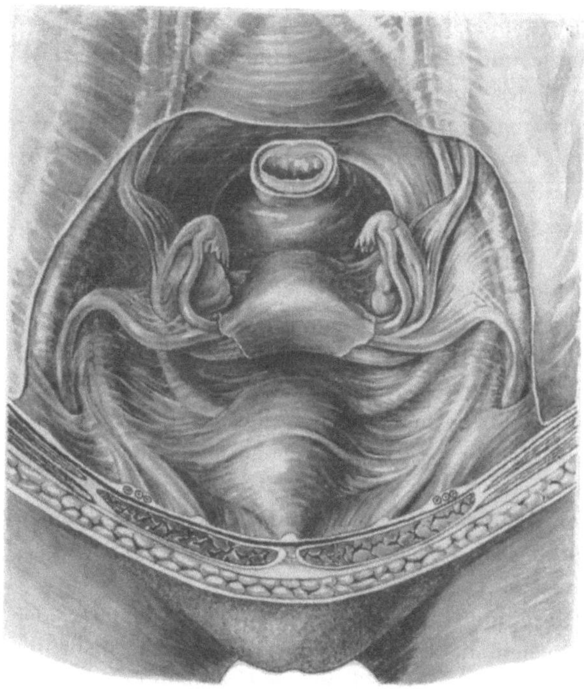

Abb. 8
Anatomischer Situs bei Blick ins Cavum peritonei pelvis von cranial-ventral

Fig. 8
Anatomical site viewed by cranioventral introspection of the cavum peritonei pelvis

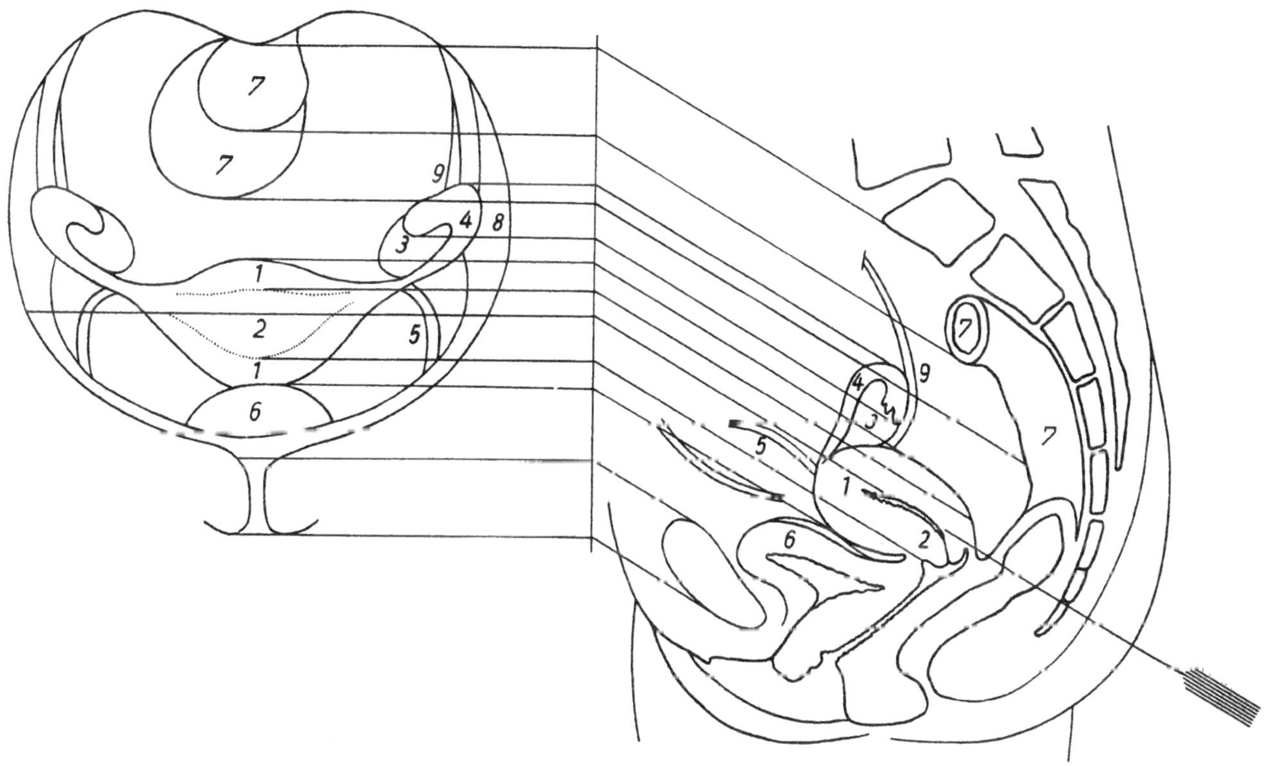

Abb. 9
Projektion der Beckenorgane auf der *Übersichtsaufnahme*
1 = Corpus uteri 2 = Cervix uteri; 3 = Ovarien; 4 = Tuba uterina; 5 = Lig. teres uteri; 6 = Harnblase; 7 = Rectum; 8 = innere Weichteilkonturen; 9 = Ureter

Fig. 9
Projection by *standard radiography* of the pelvic organs
1 = corpus uteri; 2 = cervix uteri; 3 = ovaries; 4 = tuba uterina; 5 = lig. teres uteri; 6 = urinary bladder; 7 = rectum 8 = inner soft tissue contours; 9 = ureter

flexio und Übereinstimmung zwischen Uteruslängsachse und Strahlengang ordnet sich das Schattenoval des Gebärmutterhalses innerhalb des Uterusschattens an. Pathologische Uteruslagen und Abweichungen der Strahlenrichtung führen zu Konturverschiebungen mit exzentrischer Darstellung oder ungenügender Abbildung des Zervixschattens.

Die Topographie der normalen *Adnexe* ist variabel. Dadurch werden unterschiedliche Projektionsbilder hervorgerufen. Form und Größe der Keimdrüsen differieren individuell. Die Anordnung und Stellung der Ovarien umfaßt zahlreiche Varianten, auch ohne daß pathologische Verhältnisse zugrunde liegen. In der Regel besteht eine mehr oder weniger deutliche Lageasymmetrie. Unterschiedliche Achsenstellungen des linken und rechten Ovars können auf der Übersichtsaufnahme Größendifferenzen vortäuschen.

Tuben und *Ovarien* projizieren sich aufeinander oder nebeneinander. Auf Grund der Projektionsbedingungen und je nach Lage des Uterusfundus und der Adnexe können sowohl der isthmische als auch der ampulläre Tubenabschnitt mehr oder weniger verkürzt erscheinen. In der Regel stellt sich ein leicht gewundener Tubenverlauf dar. Die dem Ovar benachbarte Tubenampulle und der Fimbrientrichter lassen sich häufig differenzieren.

Genitalligamente werden sichtbar, wenn sie Duplikaturen des Peritoneums abheben, so daß sie zwischen gasgefüllten Bauchfelltaschen als schattengebende Aussparungen stehen bleiben. Das gilt für das Lig. teres uteri, das Lig. ovarii proprium und das Lig. suspensorium ovarii. Das Lig. teres uteri gehört zu den regelmäßig nachweisbaren Bilddetails. Die ungefähr frontal gestellte, quer durch das Bekken ziehende Bauchfellduplikatur (Lig. latum) hebt sich in ihren lateralen Teilen mit dem Lig. teres uteri als Inhalt von der Excavatio vesicouterina und der Excavatio rectouterina als scharf begrenzter, streifenförmiger Schatten ab. Sein Verlauf richtet sich bogenförmig nach lateral und ventral. Das vom Seitenrand der Gebärmutter zum Ovar ziehende Lig. ovarii proprium ist gelegentlich, besonders bei veränderter Achsenstellung des Ovars, sichtbar. Das gleiche trifft für das Lig. suspensorium ovarii und die Plica vesicouterina zu.

Die über einen Katheter mit Luft gefüllte *Harnblase* stellt sich mit ihrer Wand als bogenförmig verlaufender schmaler Schatten dar. Das in der Kreuzbeinhöhle gelegene *Rectum* wird gewöhnlich rechts vor dem Os cacrum abgebildet. Im entleerten Zustand ruft es glatt begrenzte rundliche Verschattungen hervor, deren Konturen aufeinander projiziert werden. Ist es mit Gas gefüllt, so kann man die Darmwand unterscheiden. Dieselben Kriterien gel-

uterus, if anteflexion is normal and if the longitudinal axis of the uterus is in agreement with the path of rays. Pathological uterine locations and deviations of the path of rays would result in a displacement of contours entailing excentric or unsatisfactory representation of the cervical shadow.

The *topography* of normal *adnexa* is subject to variation, which will cause differing projections. In addition, differences in shape and size are found to exist between the gonads. Numerous arrangements and locations of the ovaries are possible even without the presence of a pathological condition. A more or less pronounced asymmetry in location is quite common. Different sizes may be simulated in a standard radiograph as a result of differences between the axial location of the left ovary and that of the right one.

Tubes and *ovaries* are projected superimposed or adjacent. Both the isthmic and the ampullar tubal sections may appear in more or less shortened projection, depending on the given conditions of projection as well as on the locations of both the fundus uteri and adnexa. Generally, the tube is represented slightly curved. Both the ampulla of the uterine tube, next to the ovary, and the fimbrial funnel may be differentiated in many cases.

Genital ligaments will become visible if they contrast with peritoneal duplicatures, so that they remain present as radio-opaque recesses between gas-filled peritoneal pouches. This applies to the lig. teres uteri, lig. ovarii proprium, and lig. suspensorium ovarii. The lig. teres uteri is one of those details that are always detectable. The lateral parts of the peritoneal duplicature (lig. latum), being in a somewhat intrapelvic fronto-transverse location and including the lig. teres uteri, will contrast as a sharply defined striped shadow with the excavatio vesicouterina and excavatio rectouterina. The arciform course of the peritoneal duplicature is lateral and ventral. The lig. ovarii proprium extending from the lateral margin of the uterus to the ovary will occasionally become visible, in particular when the axis of the ovary is changed. The same applies to the lig. suspensorium ovarii and plica vesicouterina.

The wall of the *urinary bladder* into which air was insufflated through a catheter is projected as a small arciform shadow. The *rectum* situated in the hollow of the sacrum usually is projected on the right in front of the sacrum. In evacuated condition the rectum will produce smoothly deliminated round shadows, the contours of which being projected upon one another. However, the intestinal wall can be differentiated when the rectum is filled with gas. The same criteria apply to the *colon sigmoideum*

10

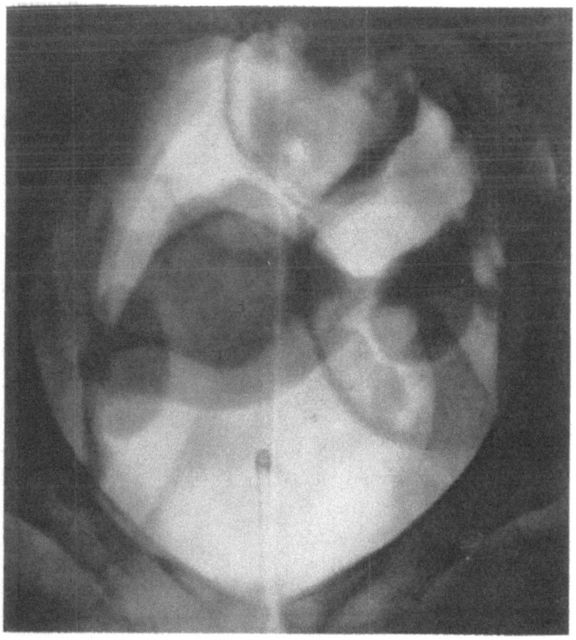

10 a

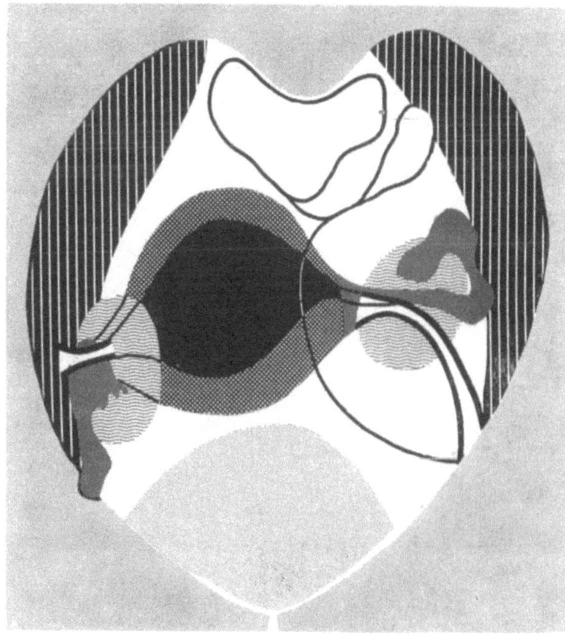

Abb. 10
Normale Genitalorgane
Dextropositio uteri

25jähr. Patientin mit sekundärer Amenorrhoe und primärer Sterilität

Indikation: Bestimmung der Ovariengröße wegen Verdachtes auf Stein-LEVENTHAL-Syndrom

Abb. 10: *Übersichtsaufnahme*

Fig. 10
Normal genital organs
Dextropositio uteri

Age of patient 25, afflicted with secondary amenorrhea and primary sterility

Indication: Determination of ovarian size for suspicion of STEIN-LEVENTHAL's syndrome

Fig. 10: *Standard radiograph*

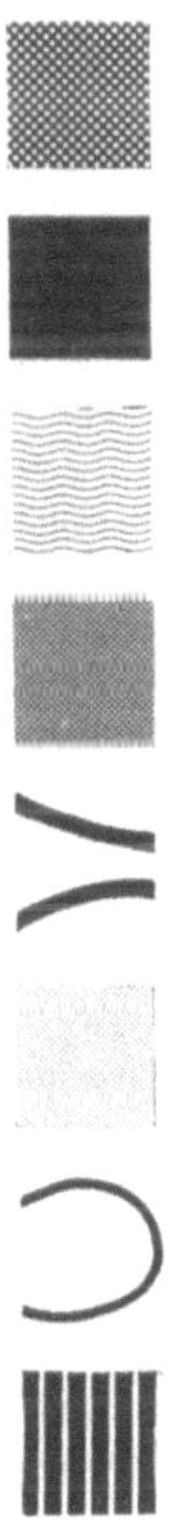

Corpus uteri	corpus uteri
Cervix uteri	cervix uteri
Ovarien	ovaries
Tuben	tuba uterina
Lig. teres uteri	lig. teres uteri
Harnblase	urinary bladder
Rectum und Colon sigmoideum	rectum and colon sigmoideum
Laterale innere Weichteile des Beckens	lateral inner soft tissue contours of the pelvis

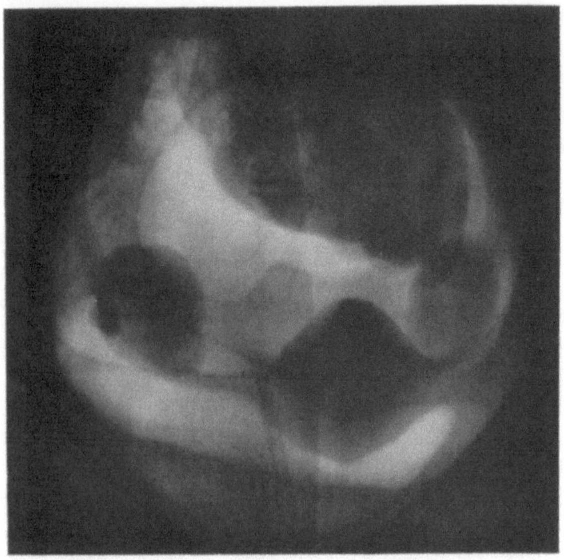

11

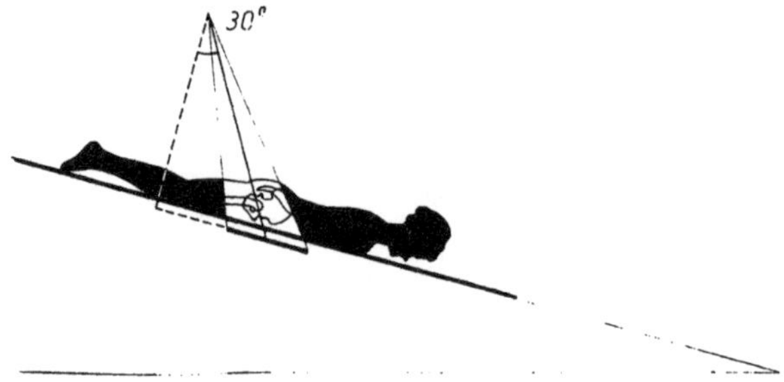

11 a

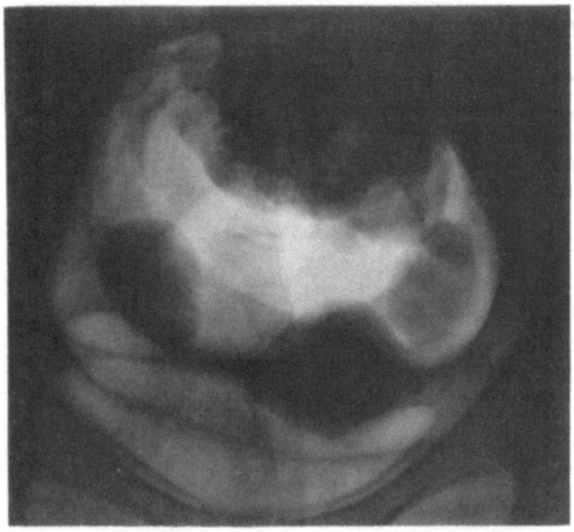

12

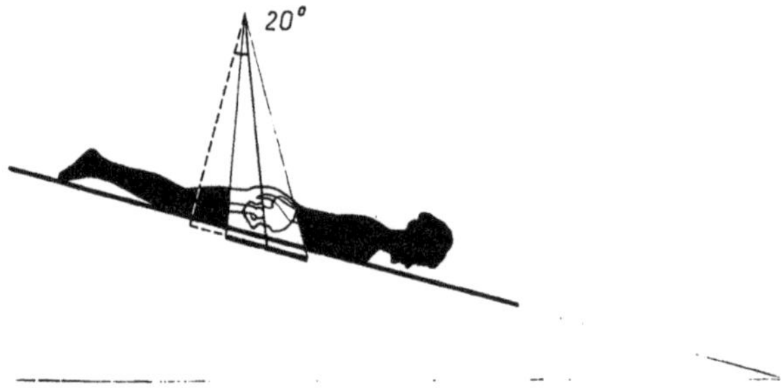

12 b

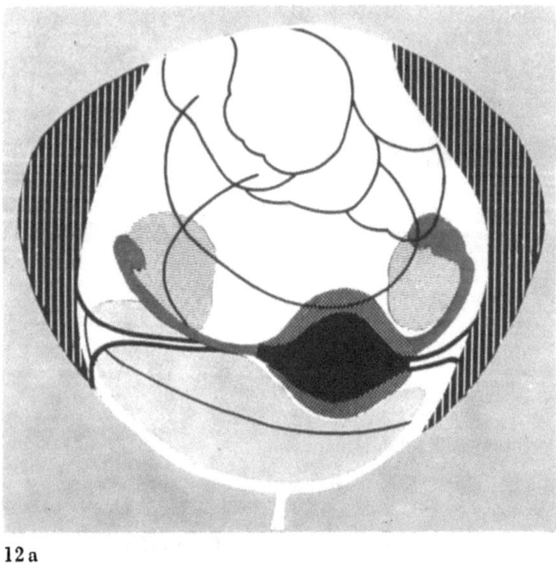

12 a

Abb. 11 u. 12

Normale Genitalorgane

Sinistropositio uteri

27jähr. Patientin mit sekundärer Amenorrhoe und Hirsutismus

Indikation: Bestimmung der Ovariengröße wegen Verdachtes auf STEIN-LEVENTHAL-Syndrom

Übersichtsaufnahmen bei verschiedener Einstellung (Röhrenkippung). Auslenkung des Zentralstrahles aus dem Lot auf der Bildebene 30° (Abb. 11) und 20° (Abb. 12). Die projektionsbedingten Differenzen sind erkennbar, bleiben jedoch für die Befundinterpretation ohne wesentliche Bedeutung

Figs. 11 and 12

Normal genital organs

Sinistropositio uteri

Age of patient, 27, afflicted with secondary amenhorrhea and hirsutism

Indication: Determination of ovarian size for suspicion of STEIN-LEVENTHAL's syndrome

Standard radiographs made with different adjustments (tube gradients); vertical-image plane defelctions of central beam 30 deg. (Fig. 11) and 20 deg. (Fig. 12); projection-dependent differences are descernible but without essential relevance to interpretation

13

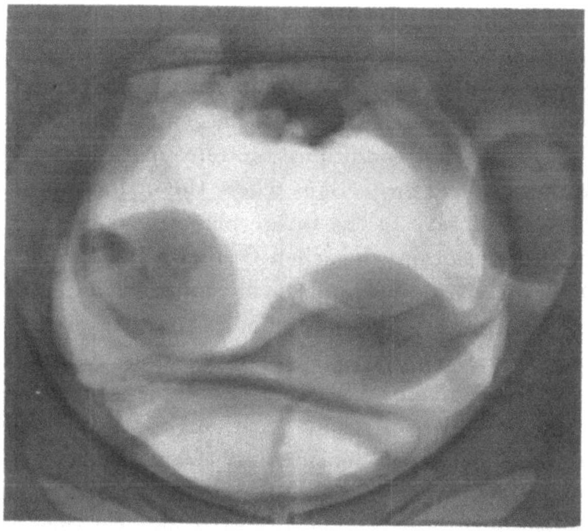

13a

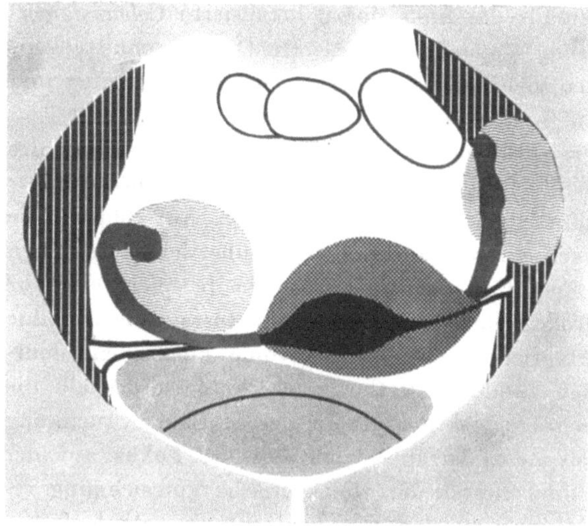

Abb. 13

Normale Genitalorgane

Sinistropositio uteri

31jähr. Patientin mit Oligomenorrhoe und Hirsutismus

Indikation: Bestimmung der Ovariengröße wegen Verdachtes auf STEIN-LEVENTHAL-Syndrom

Übersichtsaufnahme

Fig. 13

Normal genital organs

Sinistropositio uteri

Patient, 31, afflicted with oligomenorrhea and hirsutism

Indication: Determination of ovarian size for suspicion of STEIN-LEVENTHAL's syndrome; *standard radiograph*

14

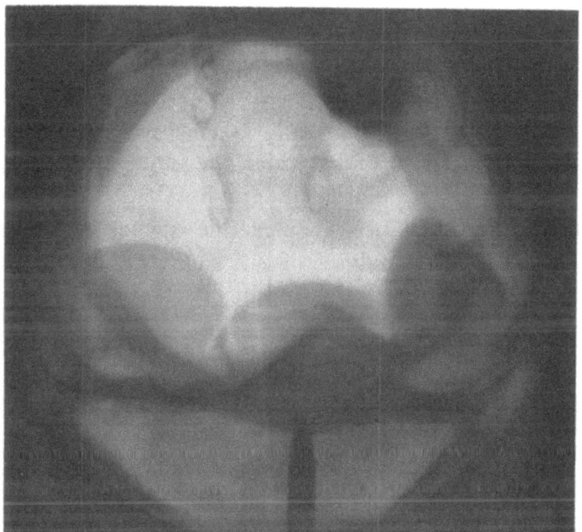

14a

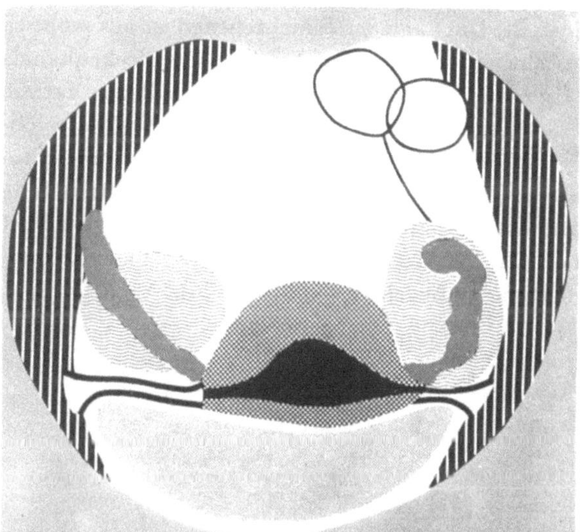

Abb. 14

Genitale mit infantilem Uterus

20jähr. Patientin mit primärer Amenorrhoe und starker Adipositas

Indikation: Darstellung der nicht tastbaren Adnexe

Übersichtsaufnahme

Fig. 14

Genital organ with infantile uterus

Patient, 20, afflicted with primary amenorrhea and severe adiposity

Indication: Visualisation of unpalpable adnexa; *standard radiograph*

ten für das links dorsal lokalisierte *Colon sigmoideum*. Ungenügend entleerte Darmabschnitte können vielgestaltige Verschattungen hervorrufen und die Genitalorgane störend überlagern.
Projektionen ohne die beschriebene Neigung des Strahlenkegels gegen die Bildebene ergeben weniger günstige Abbildungsbedingungen. Auf Bildern, die nach Art gewöhnlicher Beckenübersichtsaufnahmen angefertigt wurden, lassen sich beispielsweise nur große, aus dem Becken herausragende Gebilde (Ovarialkystome, Uterusmyome) ausreichend deutlich abbilden. Methode der Wahl ist deshalb die Schrägprojektion. Trotz der starken Auslenkung des Zentralstrahles vom Lot des Fokus auf der Bildebene ist die projektorische Verzeichnung relativ gering und für die Deutung pathologischer Verschattungen praktisch bedeutungslos (Abb. 11 und 12).

which is in left dorsal location. Insufficiently evacuated intestinal sections may produce most various shapes of shadows and, consequently, cause trouble by confusing overshadowing of the genital organs.
Less favourable conditions for representation will be the result of projections where the inclination of the cone of rays to the image plane deviates from the description given earlier. Ordinary radiography of the pelvis, for example, will render visible with sufficient clarity only large bodies that are protruding from the pelvis, such as ovarian cystomas or uterine myomas. Therefore, oblique projection is the method of choice. Although the central beam is deflected considerably from the vertical of the focus on the image plane, distortion of projection will be relatively small and practically negligible to the interpretation of pathological shadows (Figs. 11 and 12).

3.2. Schichtaufnahmen

Das Ziel der Schichtuntersuchung ist eine verbesserte Information über Einzelheiten, die auf Übersichtsaufnahmen nicht sicher beurteilt werden können. Bei der auf Seite 19 beschriebenen Lagerung der Patientin werden Frontalschichten dargestellt. Die Lage der Schichtebenen ist aus Abb. 15 ersichtlich. Infolge der Neigung des Beckenkanals liegen die frontalen Schnittebenen in Bezug auf die Beckenachse schräg im Beckenraum. Die tomographische Abbildung der Objekte erfolgt unter anderen Projektionsbedingungen als ihre Darstellung auf der Übersichtsaufnahme. Der Unterschied ist bei der vergleichenden Bildanalyse und Befunddeutung zu beachten (Abb. 16—26).

3.2. Tomography

Improved information about details not identifiable safely from the standard radiograph is the purpose of tomography. Positioning of the patient, as demonstrated on page 19, shows frontal layers. The positions taken by the layer planes may be seen from Fig. 15. Due to the inclination of the pelvic canal, the frontal sectional planes are situated obliquely to the pelvic axis in the pelvic cavity. The conditions of tomographic projection of the given objects are found differ from those under which the same objects are projected by standard radiography. This difference should be taken into consideration when it comes to a comparative analysis of the radiographs and to an interpretation of the findings (Figs. 16—26).

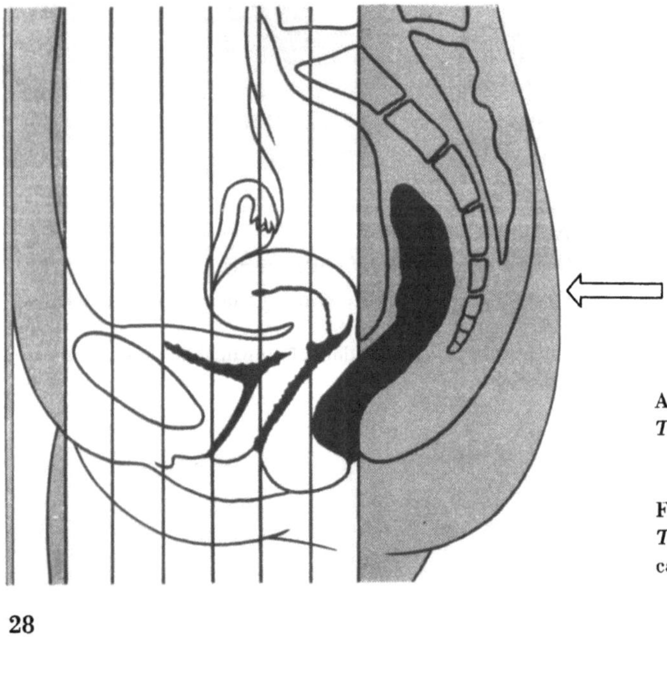

Abb. 15
Tomographie: Lage der Schichtebenen im Beckenraum

Fig. 15
Tomography: Position of tomographic planes in the pelvic cavity

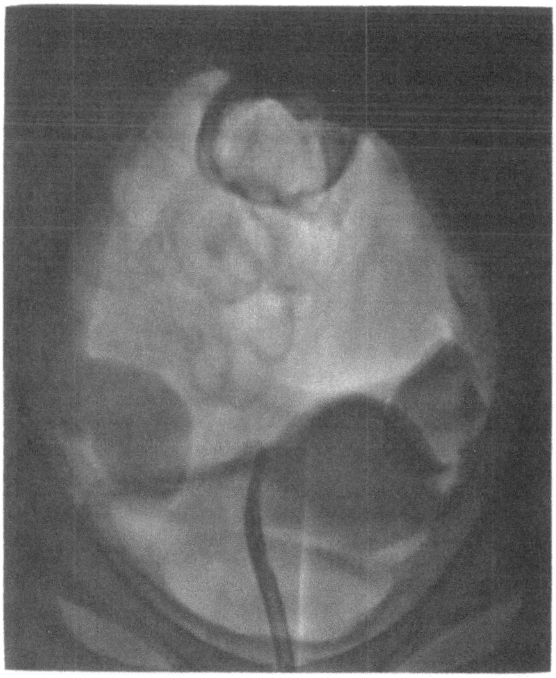

16

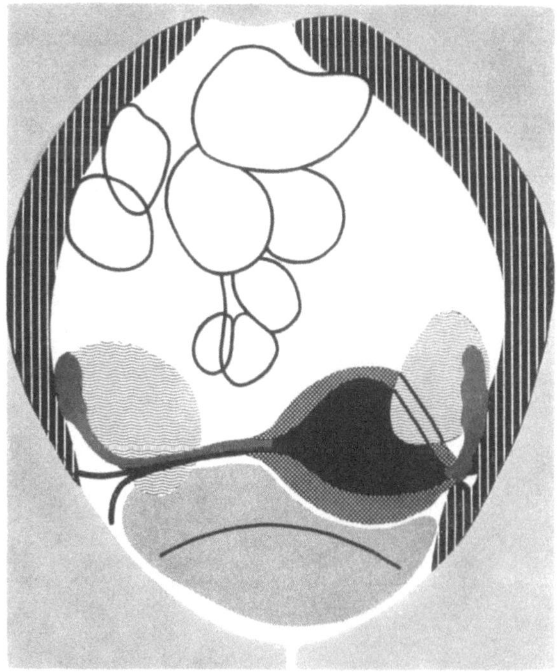

16a

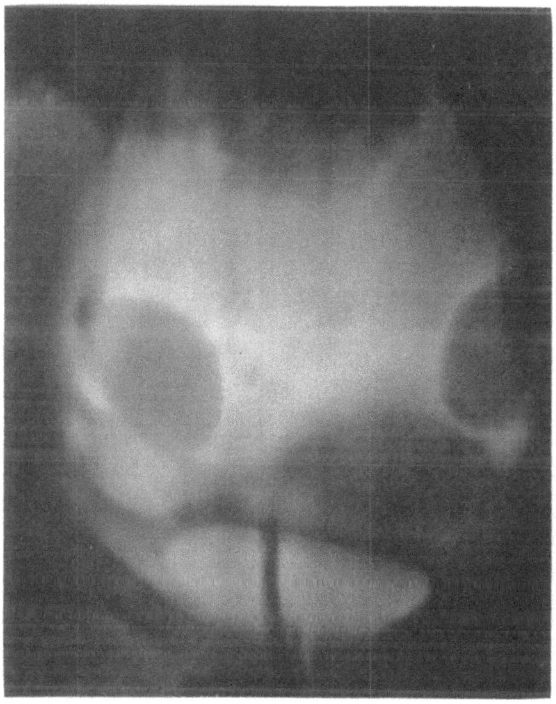

17

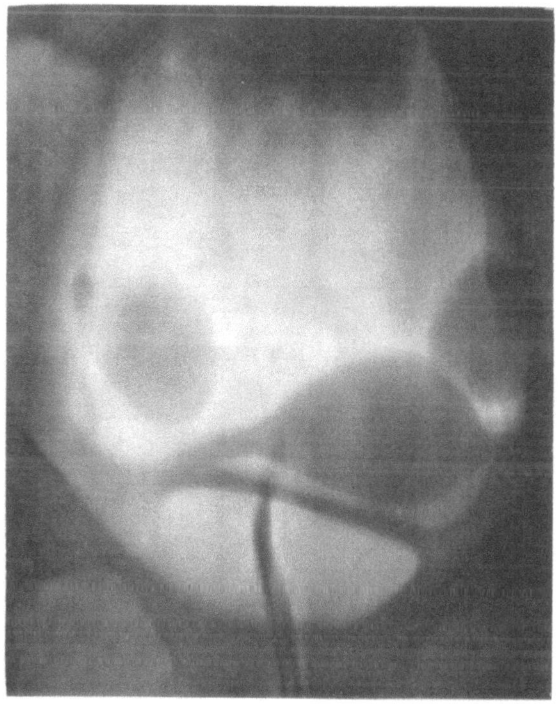

18

Abb. 16–18

Normale Genitalorgane

Sinistropositio uteri

22jähr. Patientin mit sekundärer Amenorrhoe, primärer Sterilität, Hirsutismus

Indikation: Darstellung der Ovarien wegen Verdachtes auf STEIN-LEVENTHAL-Syndrom

Abb. 16: *Übersichtsaufnahme*

Abb. 17 und 18: Die *Schichtaufnahmen* in 5 cm und 6 cm Tiefe zeigen die normalgroßen Ovarien, die Tuben, rechts mit der Anheftungsstelle am Uterus, den Harnblasenscheitel und das Rectum

Figs. 16–18

Normal genital organs

Sinistropositio uteri

Patient, 22, afflicted with secondary amenorrhea, primary sterility, and hirsutism

Indication: Visualisation of ovaries for suspicion of STEIN-LEVENTHAL's syndrome

Fig. 16: *Standard radiograph*

Figs. 17 and 18 are *tomograms*, 5 cm and 6 cm in depths, showing ovaries of normal size, tubes with insertion to uterus on the right, fundus of urinary bladder, and rectum

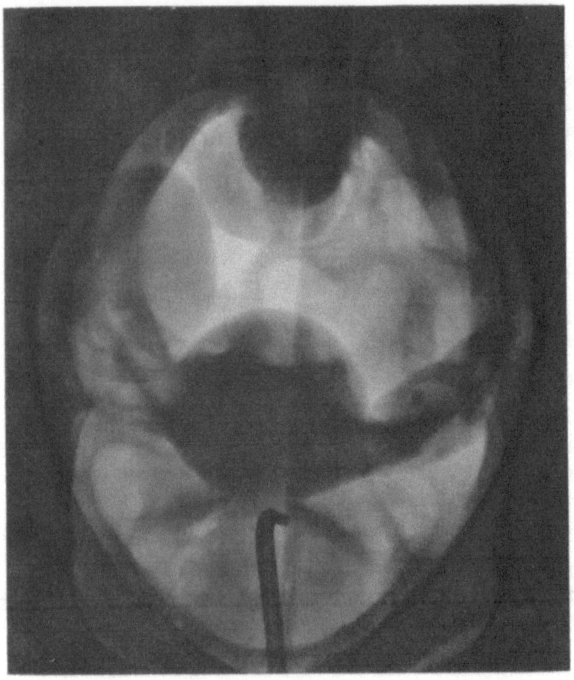

19

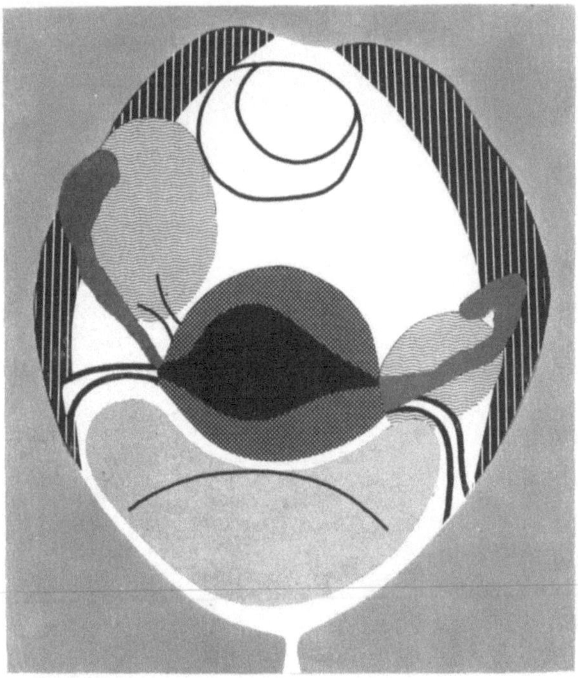

19 a

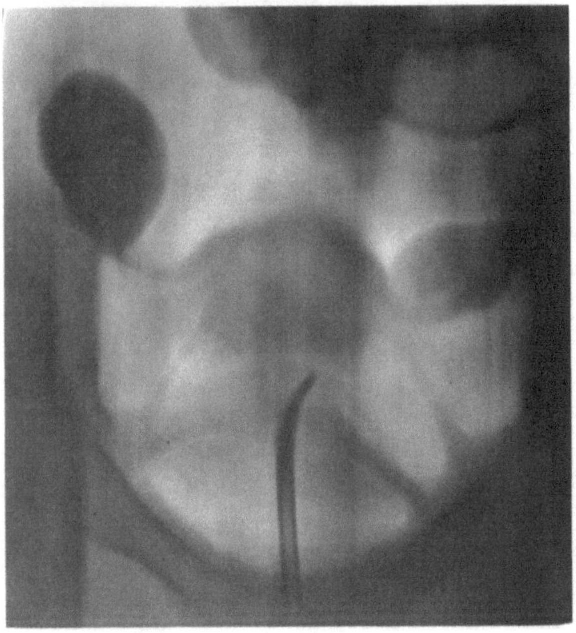

20

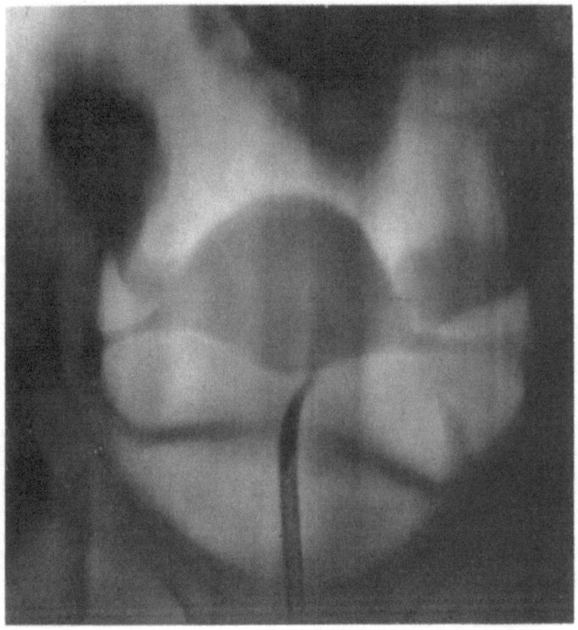

21

Abb. 19–21

Normale Genitalorgane

20jähr. Patientin mit primärer Amenorrhoe, hochgradiger Adipositas

Indikation: Beurteilung der nicht palpablen Adnexe

Abb. 19: *Übersichtsaufnahme.* Unterschiedliche Achsenstellung und geringe Größendifferenz der Ovarien

Abb. 20 und 21: Die *Tomogramme* in 5 cm und 6 cm Tiefe bestätigen den Größenunterschied der Ovarien. An weiteren Einzelheiten sind sichtbar: Corpus uteri, Tubenabgänge, Lig. teres uteri, Lig. ovarii proprium, Harnblasenwand

Figs. 19–21

Normal genital organs

Patient, 20, afflicted with primary amenorrhea and advanced adiposity

Indication: Assessment of unpalpable adnexa

Fig. 19 is a *standard radiograph* showing differing axial positions and slight difference between sizes of ovaries

Figs. 20 and 21 are *tomographs*, 5 cm and 6 cm in depths, to confirm difference between ovarian sizes; other visible details are corpus uteri, tubal insertions, lig. teres uteri, lig. ovarii proprium, wall of urinary bladder

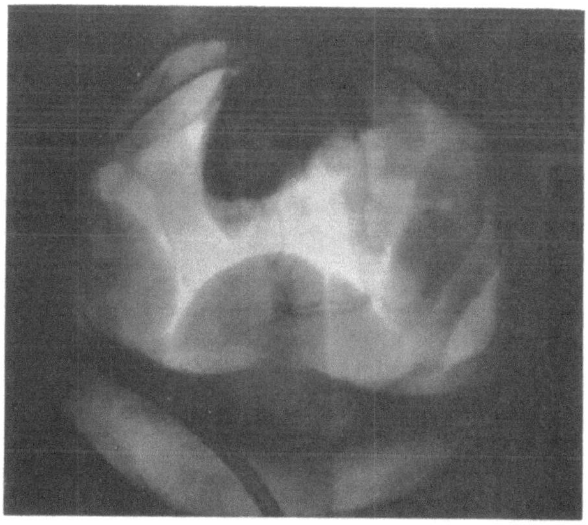

22

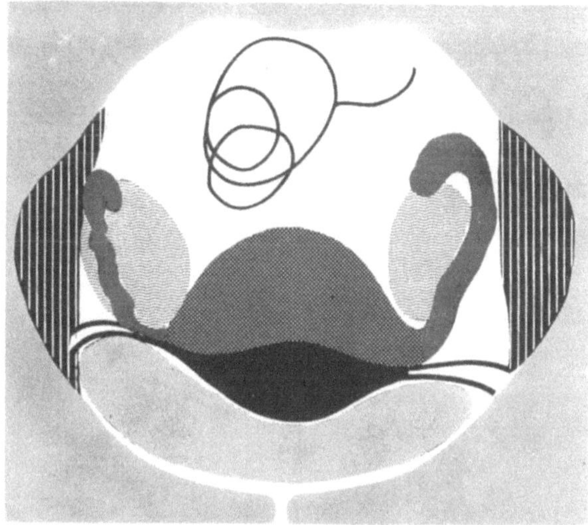

22 a

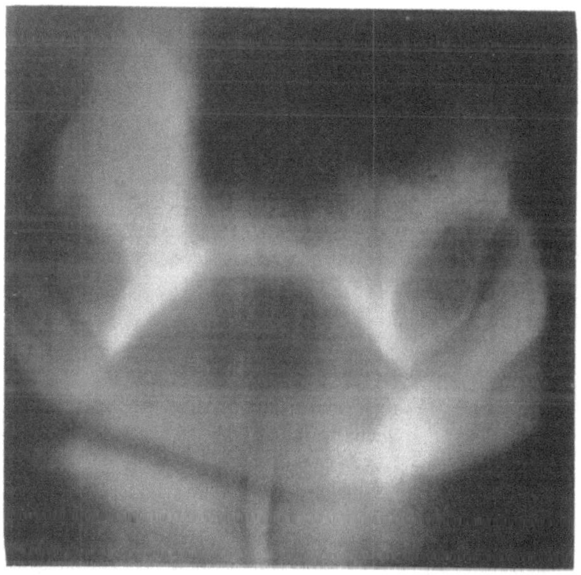

23

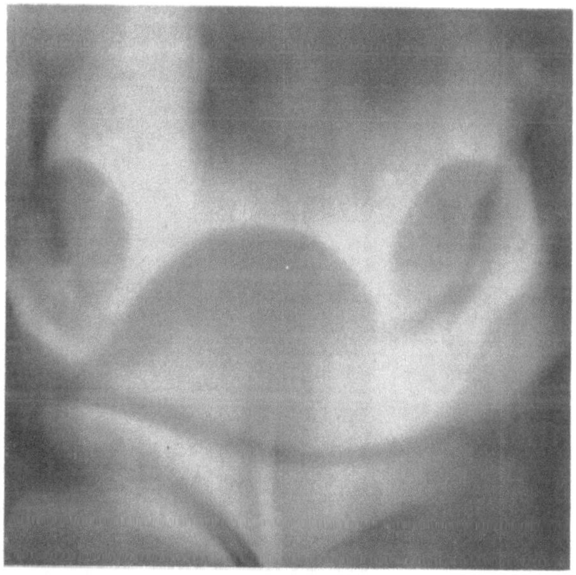

24

Abb. 22–24

Normale Genitalorgane

24jähr. Patientin mit Oligomenorrhoe, starker Adipositas

Tastbefund: Verdacht auf Ovarialzysten

Indikation: Darstellung der Ovarien zur Klärung des Befundes

Abb. 22: *Übersichtsaufnahme*

Abb. 23 und 24: Die *Schichtaufnahmen* in 6 cm und 7 cm Tiefe zeigen vor den normal geformten, nicht vergrößerten Ovarien die Tuben, an denen sich die Anheftung am Uteruskörper, der isthmische und ampulläre Teil differenzieren lassen

Figs. 22–24

Normal genital organs

Patient, 24, afflicted with oligomenorrhea and severe adiposity

Palpation finding: Suspicion of ovarian cysts

Indication: Visualisation of ovaries to elucidate finding

Fig. 22: *Standard radiograph*

Figs. 23 and 24 are *tomograms*, 6 cm and 7 cm in depths, showing, in front of normally shaped and unenlarged ovaries, the tubes, with the insertion to the uterus as well as the isthmic and ampullary parts differentiable

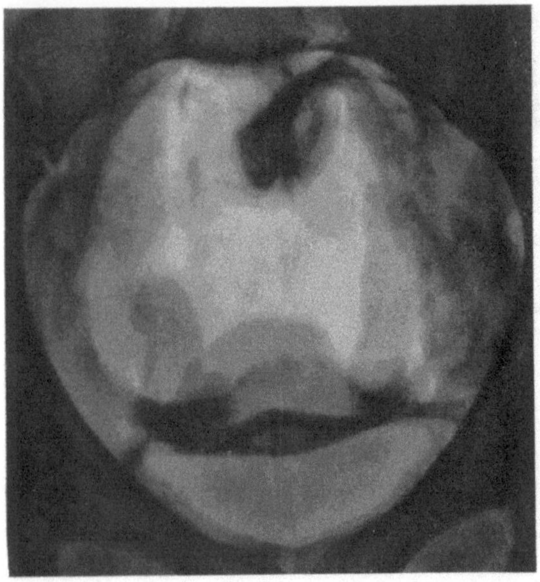

25

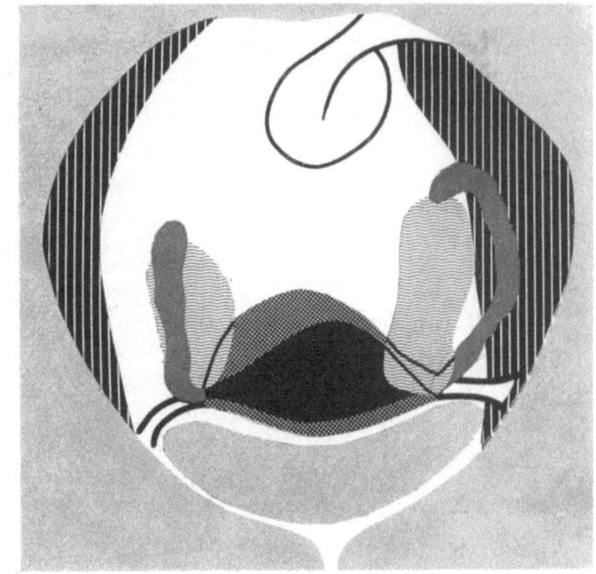

25 a

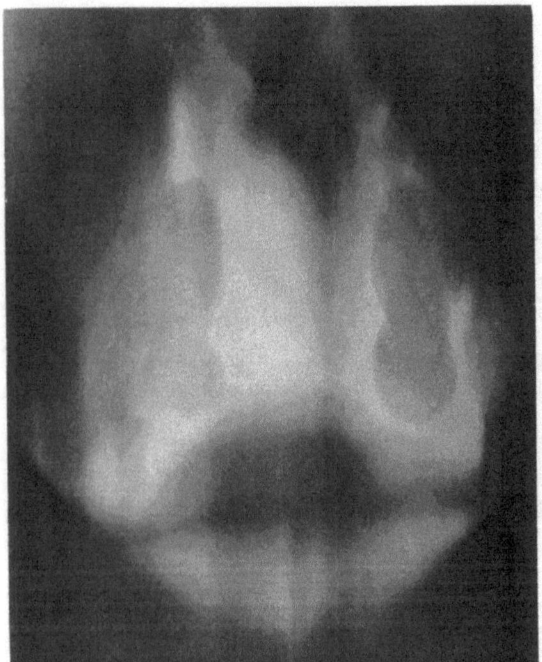

26

Abb. 25 und 26

Normale Genitalorgane

25jähr. Patientin mit primärer Amenorrhoe, Hirsutismus

Indikation: Größenbestimmung der Ovarien wegen Verdachtes auf STEIN-LEVENTHAL-Syndrom

Abb 25: *Übersichtsaufnahme*

Abb 26: *Schichtaufnahme* in 5 cm Tiefe. Die Keimdrüsen erscheinen schmal und langgestreckt, auf Grund der Messung nicht vergrößert. Rechts sind Ampulle und Infundibulum der Tube sichtbar. Unten stellt sich eine Verschattung des Harnblasenscheitels (Apex vesicae) mit „umgekehrtem" Flüssigkeitsspiegel infolge einer Harnansammlung dar

Figs. 25 and 26

Normal genital organs

Patient, 25, afflicted with primary amenorrhea and hirsutism

Indication: Determination of ovarian size for suspicion of STEIN-LEVENTHAL's syndrome

Fig. 25: *Standard radiograph*

Fig. 26: *Tomogram*, 5 cm in depth; the gonads appearing narrow and elongated and unenlarged on account of the measurement applied; visible on the right are ampulla and tubal infundibulum, shadow of fundus of the bladder visualised below, with fluid level appearing "reversed" due to accumulation of urine

Durch die Bauchlage der Patienten nähern sich die beweglichen *Ovarien* und die in der kranialen Kante des Lig. latum uteri verlaufenden Eileiter der vorderen Bauchwand und werden in ventralen Ebenen abgebildet. Geringe Differenzen der Achseneinstellung beider Ovarien sind regelmäßig nachweisbar und für die Interpretation ohne Bedeutung. Stärkere Abweichungen lassen sich durch die synoptische Analyse mehrerer benachbarter Schichten erkennen. Auf diese Weise kann eine Vortäuschung von Größenunterschieden beider Ovarien mit Hilfe der Tomographie leicht aufgeklärt werden. Unter Berücksichtigung des gerätegebundenen Vergrößerungsfaktors sind orientierende Messungen der Ovarien möglich. Zahlreiche Vergleiche mit dem Operationssitus ergaben eine große Genauigkeit dieser Maße. Lage und Verlauf der *Tuben* lassen sich in den einzelnen Abschnitten (Isthmus und Ampulle) genau erkennen.

Der *Uteruskörper* mit den Anheftungsstellen der Eileiter und den Ligg. ov. propria wird in mittleren Ebenen angeschnitten. Die Lage der Schichten entspricht bei physiologischer Anteflexio etwas schräg von der Hinterwand (Facies intestinalis) zur Vorderwand (Facies vesicalis) durch die Gebärmutter geführten Querschnitten. Bei Streckstellung des Uterus nähert sich die Schnittführung mehr einem frontalen Uteruslängsschnitt.

Dorsal in der Kreuzbeinhöhle kommt das *Rectum* zur Darstellung. Weitere Einzelheiten sind in verschiedenen Tiefen nachweisbar: *Harnblasenwand*, *Lig. teres uteri*, *Lig. suspensorium ovarii*, *Colon sigmoideum*, *Mesocolon sigmoideum*. Wenn zwischen der Luftfüllung der Harnblase und der Tomographie längere Zeit verstreicht, tritt in den ventralen Ebenen eine Verschattung des Harnblasenscheitels auf (Abb. 26). Die Ursache ist eine Harnansammlung. Infolge der Kopftieflage der Patientin füllt die insufflierte Luft den Harnblasenfundus aus, während sich die Harnpfütze im Blasenscheitel (Apex vesicae) bildet. Daraus resultiert bei Betrachtung des Bildes der Eindruck eines „umgekehrten" Flüssigkeitsspiegels. Diese Verschattung tritt nur in den ventralen Ebenen in Erscheinung und läßt sich durch die geradlinige Begrenzung von der weiter dorsal gelegenen Gebärmutter unterscheiden.

The prone position of the patient will bring the movable *ovaries* and the oviducts, that are accommodated in the cranial edge of the lig. latum uteri, closer to the anterior abdominal wall for representation in ventral planes. Slight deviations regarding the focal adjustment of the two ovarian axes are detected quite regularly, but these are unimportant to interpretation. If larger deviations occur, these may be identified by a synoptic analysis of several adjacent layers, so that a simulated difference between the sizes of the two ovaries may be elucidated readily by means of tomography. Orientation measurement of the ovaries is possible within the limits of the given magnifying factors that depend on the equipment available. High accuracy of such measurements was confirmed by numerous comparisons between the measured values, on the one hand, and the site of operation, on the other. Both the position and course of the *Fallopian tubes* can be identified most accurately by the various sections, such as isthmus and ampulla.

The *uterus* with the sites of attachment of the oviducts and the ligg. ov. propria is intersected in medium planes. In case of physiological anteflexion, the positions of the strata involved are somewhat equal to cross-sections running obliquely from the posterior wall (facies intestinalis) to the anterior wall (facies vesicalis) through the uterus. With the uterus in extended position, the section will come to be somewhat similar to a frontal logitudinal section through the uterus.

The *rectum* is represented dorsally in the hollow of the sacrum. Further details, such as the *wall of the bladder*, *lig. teres uteri*, *lig. suspensorium ovarii*, *colon sigmoideum*, *mesocolon sigmoideum*, are detectable in various depths. A shadowing of the fundus of the bladder will occur in the ventral planes, if a longer period of time is allowed to elapse between air insufflation of the urinary bladder and tomography (Fig. 26). This is caused by an accumulation of urine. Due to the lowered position of the patient's head the insufflated air will fill the base of the bladder, while residual urine is shifted to the fundus of the bladder (apex vesicae). The tomograph will, therefore, give the impression of a "reversed" fluid level. Such shadowing will occur only in the ventral planes and may be differentiated by its straight delimitation from the uterus which is situated further dorsally.

4. Klinische Bewertung

4.1. Indikationen

Mit der Pneumopelvigraphie steht eine Untersuchungsmethode zur Verfügung, die über die Morphologie der inneren weiblichen Genitalorgane detailliert Auskunft gibt und deren Aussagekraft zur Zeit nur von der Laparotomie oder in Detailfragen von der Laparoskopie erreicht wird. Andererseits ist zu berücksichtigen, daß eine Punktion und Gasfüllung der Bauchhöhle erforderlich sind und die Keimdrüsen der Röntgenstrahlung direkt ausgesetzt werden. Die Methode sollte deshalb nach Ausschöpfung der einfachen diagnostischen Verfahren Anwendung finden, und zwar dann, wenn von dem Resultat voraussichtlich therapeutische Konsequenzen abhängen. Für die Festlegung der Indikationen sind folgende Gesichtspunkte zu berücksichtigen:

a) Bei differentialdiagnostisch schwierigen Entscheidungen lassen sich mehrdeutige Palpationsbefunde mit Hilfe der Pneumopelvigraphie oftmals klären.

b) Zweifelhafte oder negative Palpationsergebnisse, die zum Krankheitsbild im Widerspruch stehen, können durch die visuelle Darstellung der inneren Genitalien zuverlässig überprüft werden.

c) Die Methode ermöglicht es, eine Reihe diagnostisch wichtiger Veränderungen im Beckenraum zu erfassen, die der manuellen Untersuchung und anderen einfachen Verfahren unzugänglich sind.

Dementsprechend betrachten wir folgende klinische Fragen als *Indikationen*:

1. Die Bestimmung der Organzugehörigkeit von Geschwülsten mit mehrdeutigem Palpationsbefund, insbesondere die Differentialdiagnose von Ovarialtumoren, Uterusmyomen und Adnexprozessen. Außer der Organabgrenzung ist in manchen Fällen durch die Röntgenuntersuchung auch eine Artdiagnose möglich, z. B. bei Adnextuberkulose durch den Nachweis von Verkalkungen oder bei Dermoiden durch die Abbildung von Knochen- und Zahnanlagen.

2. Die Erfassung und Lokalisation von Rezidiven maligner Geschwülste nach Radikaloperation oder Strahlentherapie. Durch die Kombination des Pneumoperitoneum mit der Lymphographie lassen sich gleichzeitig Lymphknotenmetastasen direkt darstellen.

4. Clinical assessment

4.1. Indications

Pneumopelvigraphy is an examination method by which detailed information may be achieved about the morphology of the internal female genital organs, with its positive evidence and consistency being comparable, for the time being, only with laparotomy or with laparoscopy, when its comes to details. Yet, it should also be borne in mind that puncture and gas insufflation of the peritoneal cavity are required and that the gonads are exposed directly to X-ray radiation. Therefore, the method should be used preferably when all the simple diagnostic procedures are exhausted and when the result would predictably have therapeutic consequences. The following aspects should be considered with regard to the indications:

a) Ambiguous palpation findings may often be elucidated by means of pneumopelvigraphy when a highly involved decision has to be taken in a differential diagnosis.

b) Dubious or negative palpation findings that are contradictory to the clinical picture may be scrutinised reliably by a visual representation of the internal genitals.

c) The method helps to identify in the pelvic cavity a number of changes which are important to diagnosis but usually not detectable by palpation or other simple procedures.

The following clinical problems are, therefore, accepted as *indications*:

1. Organ-oriented localisation of tumors that produce ambiguous palpation findings, in particular the differential diagnosis of ovarian tumors, hysteromyomas, and adnexal processes. In certain cases, diagnostic radiography will not only help the examiner to differentiate the affected organ, but also to perform a differential diagnosis, for example, by identifying clacifications in cases of adnexal tuberculosis or by achieving a representation of osseous and dental germs in cases of dermoids.

2. Detection and localisation of recurrent malignant tumors after radical surgery or radiotherapy. In addition, metastasation at lymphatic nodes may be represented directly by a combination of the pneumoperitoneum with lymphography.

3. Die genaue Bestimmung der Ovariengröße, vor allem bei Verdacht auf STEIN-LEVENTHAL-Syndrom.
4. Die Exploration des Beckenraumes nach rudimentären und auf fehlende Keimdrüsen bei Gonadendysgenesie und- agenesie.
5. Die Darstellung der inneren Genitalstrukturen bei uterovaginalen Mißbildungen.

Bei den unter 1. und 5. genannten Indikationen kann eine Kombination mit der Hysterosalpingographie die Aussage verbessern. Diese Modifikation erweist sich als vorteilhaft,

- wenn zur Sterilitätsdiagnostik gleichzeitig die Tubendurchgängigkeit geprüft werden soll;
- wenn zur Klärung von Mißbildungen die Darstellung des Uteruskavums und der Tubenlichtungen von Interesse ist;
- wenn man trotz guter Gasfüllung des Beckens auf der Übersichtsaufnahme den Uterus, die Tuben und Ovarien innerhalb pathologischer Schattenstrukturen nicht ausreichend sicher unterscheiden kann.

Die Indikation zur zusätzlichen Hysterosalpingographie ergibt sich dabei teilweise erst im Verlaufe der Untersuchung. Bei der Vorbereitung der Patientin (Keimgehalt des Vaginalsekretes) und des Instrumentariums sollte man mit dieser Situation rechnen, um eine Wiederholung der Untersuchung zu vermeiden.

4.2. Kontraindikationen und Komplikationen

Kontraindikationen sind: Akut entzündliche Erkrankungen des Bauchraumes, Peritonitis und Ileus. Auch ins Abdomen aufsteigende Riesenzysten der Ovarien sehen wir als Gegenindikation an, weil man die Zysten meistens anpunktiert und das Gas in das vom Kystom ausgefüllte kleine Becken nicht eindringen kann. Grundsätzlich gilt auch Schwangerschaft als Kontraindikation. Eine Ausnahme bilden manche Verdachtsfälle von Extrauteringravidität, bei denen das Pelvopneumoperiteneum vereinzelt schon mit gutem Erfolg zu Rate gezogen wurde (STEIN, STEIN und LEVENTHAL, STEIN und ARENS). Bei schlechtem Allgemeinzustand, respiratorischer Insuffizienz und Herzerkrankungen ist Zurückhaltung geboten. Für die Durchführung einer gleichzeitigen Hysterosalpingographie ist ein Reinheitsgrad des Vaginalsekretes über II als strikte Kontraindikation anzusehen.

Ernsthafte *Komplikationen* des Pelvopneumoperitoneums haben wir nicht beobachtet. Gefürchtet

3. Accurate determination of ovarian size, mainly when the presence of STEIN-LEVENTHAL's syndrome is suspicioned.
4. Exploration of the pelvic cavity for rudimentary or the absence of gonads in cases afflicted with gonodal dysgenesis or agenesis.
5. Representation of the internal genital structures in cases of uterovaginal malformation.

With reference to the indications enlisted under 1. and 5., information may be improved by a combination with hysterosalpingography. Such modification has been found to be favourable,

if at the same time tubal patency is to be tested for sterility diagnosis;

if the cavity of the uterus and the tubal lumena are to be represented to elucidate malformation;

if in spite of adequate gas insufflation of the pelvis, a standard radiograph fails to provide a picture by which the uterus, the tubes, and the ovaries within pathological shadow structures could be differentiated with sufficient safety.

An indication in favour of additional hysterosalpingography will often arise only in the course of an examination. In order to avoid the need for repeated examination, such situation should be reckoned with when the patient (microbial content of vaginal secretion) and the instruments are prepared.

4.2. Contraindications and complications

Contraindications are acute inflammatory diseases of the abdominal cavity, peritonitis, and ileus. Giant cysts of the ovaries ascending into the abdominal space are also considered to be a contraindication by the authors, since a puncturing of such cysts will usually not be avoidable and the gas will be obstructed from penetrating into the minor pelvis filled with the cystoma. Basically, pregnancy is considered to be another contraindication. An exception may be allowed for certain suspicious cases of extrauterine gravidity where sometimes adequate information was obtained from the use of the pelvopneumoperitoneum (STEIN, STEIN and LEVENTHAL, STEIN and ARENS). Caution should be observed when it comes to patients who are in a poor general condition or afflicted with respiratory insufficiency and cardiac diseases. When hysterosalpingography is to be applied simultaneously, any purity degree above II of the vaginal secretion has to be considered as a stringent contraindication.

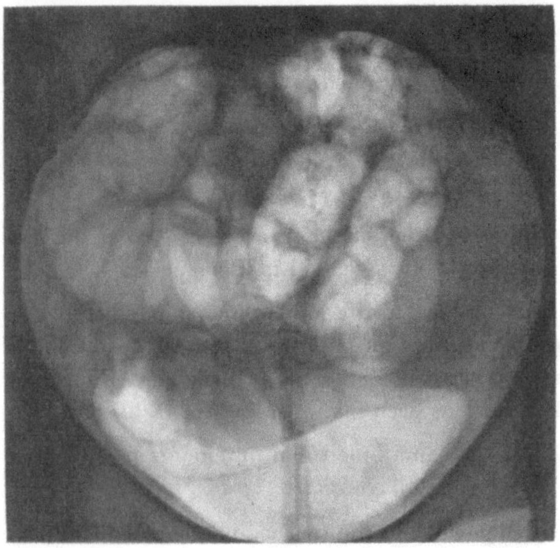

27

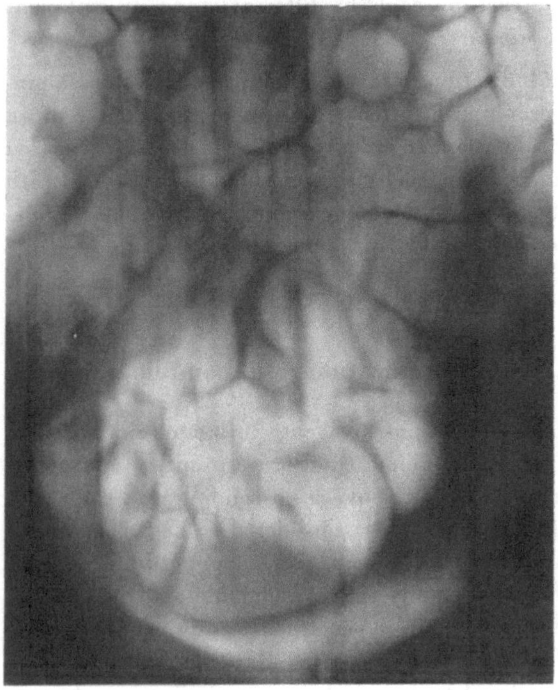

28

Abb. 27 und 28

Komplikation des Pneumoperitoneum

Punktion und Gasfüllung des Dünndarms

21jähr. Patientin mit Oligomenorrhoe und Verdacht auf STEIN-LEVENTHAL-Syndrom

Indikation: Beurteilung der Ovariengröße

Abb. 27: *Übersichtsaufnahme*

Abb. 28: *Schichtaufnahme*

Starker Meteorismus infolge Punktion einer Dünndarmschlinge. Im Cavum peritonei nur geringe Gasfüllung und demzufolge mangelhafte Darstellung des Uterus und der Adnexe, die für eine diagnostische Beurteilung nicht ausreicht

Figs. 27 and 28

Complication of the pneumoperitoneum

Puncturing and gas insufflation of the small intestine

Patient, 21, afflicted with oligomenorrhea, suspicion of STEIN-LEVENTHAL's syndrome

Indication: Assessment of ovarian size

Fig. 27: *Standard radiograph*

Fig. 28 is a *tomogram*, displaying severe meteorism caused by puncture of a loop of the small intestine; poor visualisation of uterus and adnexa, not sufficient for diagnosis, due to poor gas insufflation of the peritoneal cavity

wird die Gasembolie, die aber glücklicherweise nur selten auftritt (DASHER u. Mitarb., BELBENOIT u. LOUISON). Die Patientin ist dabei sofort auf die linke Seite zu lagern.
Bei sehr adipösen Patientinnen kann sich ein praeperitoneales Emphysem bilden, wenn die Länge der Punktionsnadel nicht ausreicht. Verwachsungen des Darmes mit der vorderen Bauchwand haben manchmal zur Folge, daß man den Darm anpunktiert. Bei diesen Patientinnen läßt sich wegen der mangelhaften oder ausbleibenden Gasfüllung des Cavum peritonei ein diagnostisches Resultat in der Regel nicht erzielen (Abb. 27 und 28). Meistens geben die Frauen jedoch keine Beschwerden an. Auf den Röntgenbildern zeigt sich dann ein starker Meteorismus des Dünndarms.

4.3. Strahlenbelastung

Nicht selten ist die Pneumopelvigraphie bei Frauen im generationsfähigen Alter oder jugendlichen Patientinnen durchzuführen. Es erscheint daher notwendig, die Gonadendosis zu kennen. Mit Hilfe von Dosimetern (Kondiometern), die ins seitliche Scheidengewölbe eingeführt wurden, ermittelten wir die aus Tabelle 2 ersichtlichen Werte.

Tabelle 2.
Gonadendosis

	Übersichtsaufnahme mR	Schichtuntersuchung[1]) mR
Strahlung mit 120 kV	20— 40	nicht gemessen
Strahlung mit 65—75 kV	60—100	320—370

[1]) Tomographie mit 5 Einzelschichten oder Simultantomographie mit 7 Filmen

Im Vergleich zu anderen Untersuchungen (z. B. retrograde Colondarstellung, Urographie, Hysterosalpingographie), die oft zu höheren Belastungen führen, sind die Dosen durchaus vertretbar. Wenn die Hartstrahltechnik Anwendung findet, liegen die Werte besonders niedrig. Mit Hilfe von Filmen höchster Empfindlichkeit, hochverstärkenden Folien, Spezialentwicklern und fotochemischen Verstärkungsverfahren läßt sich eine Herabsetzung der angegebenen Gonadendosis um 50% und mehr erzielen (BÖCK; BÖCK und Mitarb., KANKELWITZ und Mitarb.).

Serious *complications* of the pelvopneumoperitoneum were not observed by the authors. Aeroembolism constitutes a severe risk but, fortunately, occurs rarely (DASHER and co-workers, BELBENOIT and LOUISON). In such case, the patient has to be positioned immediately to the left side.
A preperitoneal emphysema may develop in highly adipose patients when the length of the puncture needle is insufficient. Intestinal adhesions with the anterior abdominal wall may sometimes entail puncturing of the intestine, so that, generally, no diagnostic result will be obtainable from such patients because of an insufficient or missing gas insufflation of the peritoneal cavity (Figs. 27 and 28). However, most of the patients would not report any complaint. The radiograph will then exhibit strong meteorism of the small intestine.

4.3. Radiation exposure

Pneumopelvigraphy has to be performed quite often with puberal women or juvenile patients, which seems to call for the need to know the gonadal dose. The values given in Table 2 were determined by the authors by introducing dosimeters (condiometers) into the lateral vaginal fornix.

Table 2
Gonadal dosage

	Standard radiography mR	Tomography[1]) mR
Radiation with 120 kV	20— 40	not measured
Radiation with 65—75 kV	60—100	320—370

[1]) Tomography with five single layers or similtaneous tomography, using seven films

These doses are quite moderate and justifiable when compared with those often used for other types of examinations which imply much higher exposure, for example, retrograde colonography, urography, hysterosalpingography. The values may be kept particularly low when the hard ray technique is used. The gonadal dosage given in Table 2 may be reduced by 50 per cent or even more by using films of maximum sensitivity, highly amplifying screens, special developers, and photochemical amplification (BÖCK; BÖCK and co-workers; KANKELWITZ and co-workers).

5. Darstellung pathologischer Befunde

5.1. Tastbare Tumoren des Uterus und der Adnexe

Die Differentialdiagnose tastbarer Tumoren des Uterus und der Adnexe kann manche Schwierigkeiten bereiten. Bei der Bestimmung der Organzugehörigkeit gibt es Täuschungsmöglichkeiten in vielfacher Hinsicht. Besonders bei Stielbildungen oder intraligamentärer Ausbreitung von Ovarialtumoren und Uterusmyomen, bei Tumorkombinationen und Vergesellschaftung mit entzündlichen Adnexprozessen kann die Eindeutigkeit des Tastbefundes mitunter völlig in Frage gestellt sein. Nach unseren Erfahrungen gibt die Pneumopelvigraphie in solchen Fällen diagnostisch wichtige Aufschlüsse. Wie Vergleiche mit dem Operationssitus zeigten, sind die Röntgenbefunde sehr zuverlässig. Bleibt die anatomische Situation auch nach Anlage des Pneumoperitoneum unübersichtlich, so helfen die zusätzliche Hysterosalpingographie und die Tomographie weiter.

5.1.1. *Uterusmyome*

Myome sind gut darzustellen, wenn sie die vom Peritoneum überzogene Oberfläche des Uterus vorwölben. Aus der Gebärmutterwand herausragende größere Knollen können meistens ohne weiteres differenziert werden (Abb. 29—31). Relativ häufig sind sie als Nebenbefund zu beobachten. Auch kleine Myomknollen lassen sich erkennen, sobald sie das Niveau der Serosafläche beeinflussen. Oftmals sind die Myome in diesem Stadium noch nicht palpabel. Der Nachweis kann jedoch wichtig sein, weil auf Grund ihrer Multiplizität die Differenzierung großer, subserös aus dem Uterus herausgewachsener Myome erleichtert wird.

Für die Diagnose *gestielter* und *intraligamentär entwickelter Myome* ist die Darstellung einer Stielverbindung mit der Gebärmutter entscheidend. Sie gelingt am zuverlässigsten mit Hilfe der Tomographie. Außerdem ist der Nachweis der Ovarien und Tuben neben dem Tumor zu fordern. Gerade in dieser Frage ist die Pneumopelvigraphie der manuellen Untersuchung überlegen (Abb. 32—38). Die Kombination mit Hydrosalpinx und/oder Ovarialtumoren macht mitunter eine zusätzliche Hysterosalpingographie notwendig. Sehr große Myome, die das kleine Becken ausfüllen und in den Bauchraum hineinragen, stellt man — falls erforderlich — zweckmäßiger im senkrechten p.a.-Strahlengang dar. Ihre

5. Representation of pathological findings

5.1. Palpable tumors of the uterus and adnexa

Many a problem may be faced when a differential diagnosis is to be made of palpable tumors of the uterus and adnexa. There are most various potential errors likely to crop up in organ-oriented localisation. The consistency of a palpation finding may sometimes be dubious at all mainly in cases of pediculation or intraligamentous propagation of ovarian tumors and hysteromyomas, tumor combinations, and association with inflammatory adnexal processes. It has been the experience of the authors that in such cases important diagnostic information may be obtained from pneumopelvigraphy. Evidence to a high reliability of the radiological findings has been produced by comparisons with the site of operation. If the anatomical situation remains to be unclarified even after the application of the pneumoperitoneum, further elucidation will be achieved by adding hysterosalpingography and tomography.

5.1.1. *Hysteromyoma*

Myomas may be represented readily, if they cause bulging of that part of the uterus surface which is covered by the peritoneum. Larger bulbs protruding from the wall of the uterus usually may be differentiated without any difficulty (Figs. 29—31). They are observed comparatively often as secondary findings. Even smaller myoma bulbs may be detected as soon as they affect the surface level of the serous membrane, although the myoma as such will often not be palpable yet in such early phase. Identification, however, may be of great importance, since it will facilitate, due to the phenomenon of multiplicity, the differentiation of larger myomas growing subserously beyond the uterus.

The diagnosis of *pediculated myomas* and those of *intraligamentous development* will depend decisively on radiological detection of a pediculated connection with the uterus. This may be done most reliably by means of tomography. The radiograph has to show also the ovaries and tubes next to the tumor. This is one of the very specific aspects where pneumopelvigraphy has proved its superiority to manual examination (Figs. 32—38). Sometimes addition of hysterosalpingography will become necessary to deal with a combination with sactosalpinx and/or ovarian tumors. Very large myomas filling the minor pelvis and protruding into the abdominal cavity may best

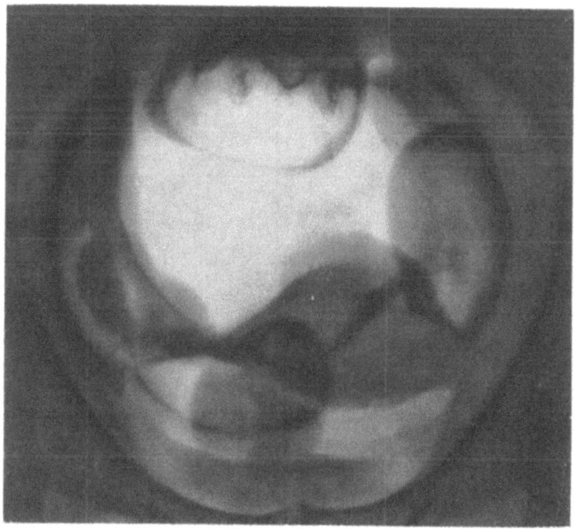

29

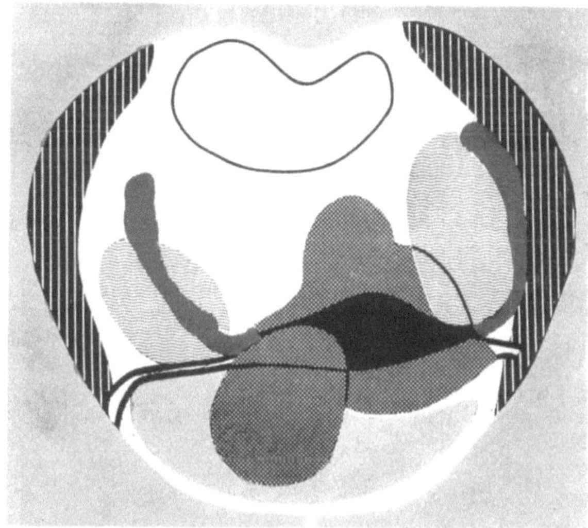

29 a

Abb. 29 und 30

Uterus myomatosus

Subseröse Myome

36jähr. Patientin mit primärer Sterilität und dringendem Kinderwunsch, Zustand 15 Jahre nach Sterilitätsoperation (Schlitzung beider Tuben)

Tastbefund:

Uterus normal groß, anteflektiert und mobil, am Fundus kleine knotenförmige Vorwölbung

Indikation: Ausschluß einer Mißbildung, Kombination mit Hysterosalpingographie zur Klärung der Tubendurchgängigkeit.

Abb. 29: *Übersichtsaufnahme*

Auf der Vorderwand und Hinterwand des Corpus uteri je eine subseröse Myomknolle.

Bei der anschließenden Hysterosalpingographie wird ein Tubenverschluß im Isthmus beiderseits nachgewiesen

Abb. 30: Das *Tomogramm* in 8 cm Schichttiefe zeigt die Myomknolle an der Hinterwand

Verlauf: Keine Therapie, weil die Patientin der vorgeschlagenen zweiten Sterilitätsoperation nicht zustimmt

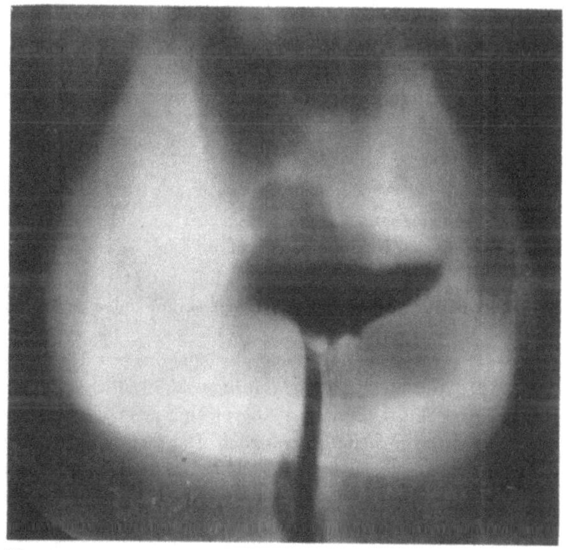

30

Figs. 29 and 30

Uterus myomatosus

Subserous myomas

Patient, 36, afflicted with primary sterility; urgent desire for children; condition 15 years after surgery to remedy sterility (lancing of either tube)

Palpation finding: Uterus of normal size, anteflexed and movable, small nodular bulging at fundus

Indication: ruling out of malformation, combination with hysterosalpingography to elucidate tubal patency

Fig. 29 is a *standard radiograph* displaying one subserous myoma bulb each on the anterior and posterior walls of the uterus; additional *hysterosalpingography* confirmed tubal occlusion on either side of isthmus

Fig. 30 is a *tomogram*, 8 cm in depth, showing myoma bulb at posterior wall

Course: No therapy, since the patient did not agree with the proposal to undergo a second operation to remedy her sterility

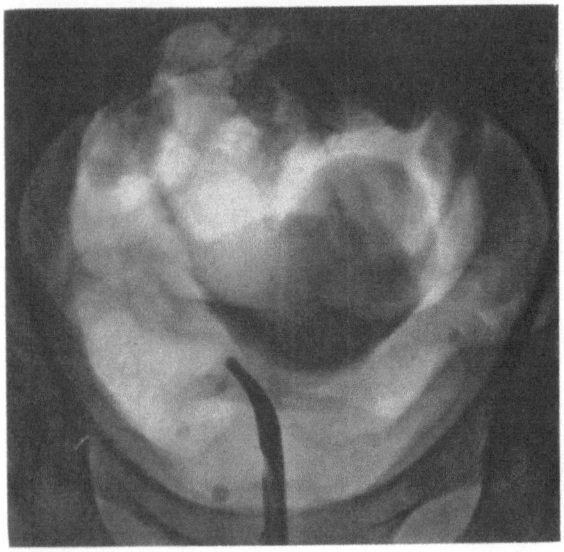

31

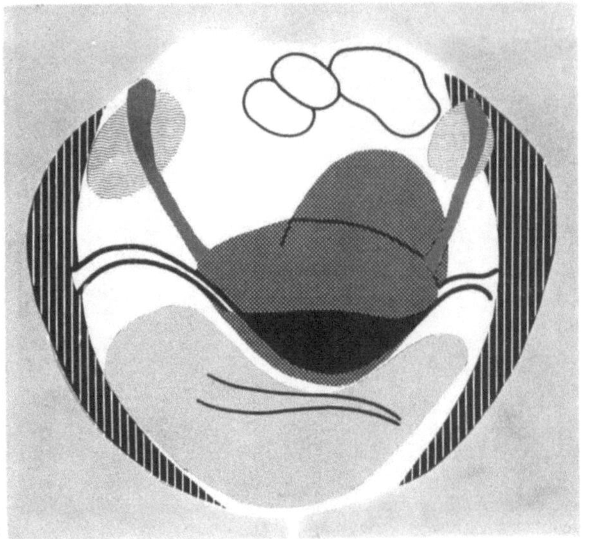

31 a

Abb. 31
Uterus myomatosus **Subseröses Myom**

64jähr. Patientin mit rezidivierenden Blutungen in der Menopause

Tastbefund: Uterus unauffällig, Adnexe wegen starker Adipositas nicht sicher zu beurteilen

Indikation: Ausschluß eines Ovarialtumors

Abb. 31: Subseröses Korpusmyom

Verlauf: Vaginale Totalexstirpation des Uterus unter Mitnahme beider Adnexe

Histologischer Befund: Fibromyom des Corpus uteri mit regressiven Veränderungen, fibroglanduläre Polypen der Korpusschleimhaut

Fig. 31
Uterus myomatosus **Subserous myoma**

Patient, 64, afflicted with recurrent menopausal bleeding

Palpation finding: Uterus not providing any pathological findings, while safe palpation of adnexa prevented by severe adiposity

Indication: Ruling out of ovarian tumor

Fig. 31 shows subserous corpus myoma

Course: Radical hysterectomy, vaginal approach, including removal of the two adnexa

Histological finding: Fibromyoma of the corpus uteri with regressive changes, fibroglandular polyps of fundus mucosa

Abb. 32—35
Uterus myomatosus
Subseröses Myom, intramurale Myome

42jähr. Patientin mit Schmerzen im linken Unterbauch

Tastbefund: Rechtsseitiger Ovarialtumor oder subseröses Myom

Indikation: Bestimmung der Organzugehörigkeit des Tumors

Abb. 32: Auf der *Übersichtsaufnahme* rundlicher Tumor rechts hinter dem Uterus. Die Abgrenzung des Ovars ist nicht mit ausreichender Sicherheit möglich. Der Befund wird durch eine gestielte subseröse Myomknolle hervorgerufen, gleicht jedoch auf der Summationsaufnahme dem Bild einer Ovarialzyste. Eine von der Hinterwand des Uterus nach kranial in den Tumorschatten hineinziehende Kontur (→) entspricht dem Stiel des Myoms (Deutung nach Kenntnis der Tomogramme)

Abb. 33 und 34: *Schichtaufnahmen* in 5 cm und 7 cm Tiefe zeigen den Unterusschatten, der im Fundusteil mehrere rundliche Verdichtungen durch intramurale Myomknollen aufweist. Die Eileiter erscheinen unauffällig, die Ovarien klein. Man erkennt die gewunden verlaufenden Tuben mit den Anheftungsstellen am Uterus und das rechte Ovar. Hinter dem Uterus, der die Harnblase flach eindellt, wird ein ovalärer Tumorschatten abgebildet, dem links die Tube und rechts der Eileiter und das Ovar benachbart sind. Ein schmaler Gasspalt trennt den Tumor von beiden Adnexen. Eine Stielverbindung zur Hinterwand des Corpus uteri ist sichtbar. Dadurch wird der Befund als gestielte Myomknolle gekennzeichnet

Verlauf: Abdominale Totalexstirpation des Uterus, Bestätigung der Diagnose

Abb. 35: Das Operationsfoto zeigt das subseröse Myom und den Stiel zum Corpus uteri

Figs. 32—35
Uterus myomatosus
Subserous myoma, intramural myomas

Patient, 42, complaining about pain in the lower abdomen, left

Palpation finding: Ovarian tumor or subserous myoma on the right

Indication: Identification of the tumor-afflicted organ

Fig. 32: *Standard radiograph* displaying rounded tumor on the right behind the uterus, no safe delimination of the ovary; the finding displayed by the standard radiograph gives the impression of an ovarian cyst, although it is caused by a pediculated subserous myoma bulb; a contour reaching cranially from the posterior wall of the uterus into the tumor shadow (→) appears as the myoma pedicle (interpretation based on tomograms)

Figs. 33 and 34 are *tomograms*, 5 cm and 7 cm in depths, displaying the uterus shadow with several rounded densifications in the fundus which are caused by intramural myoma bulbs; the oviducts appear unpathological and the ovaries small; discernible are the curved tubes with the uterus insertions and the right ovary; an oval tumor shadow neighboured by the tube, on the left, as well as oviduct and ovary, on the right, are displayed behind the uterus which slightly depresses the urinary bladder; the tumor is separated from the two adnexa by a narrow gas-filled gap; a pediculated connection with the posterior wall of the corpus uteri is visualised, so that the finding is identified as a pediculated myoma bulb

Course: Abdominal radical hysterectomy confirms diagnosis

Fig. 35 is a photograph taken of the operation and shows both the subserous myoma and its pediculated connection with the corpus uteri

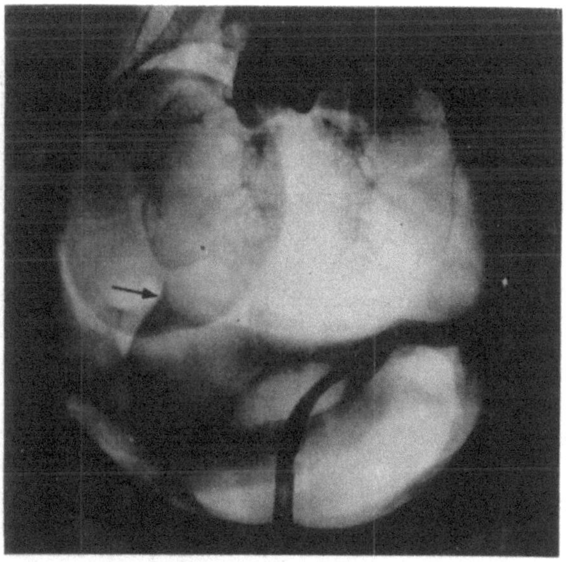

32

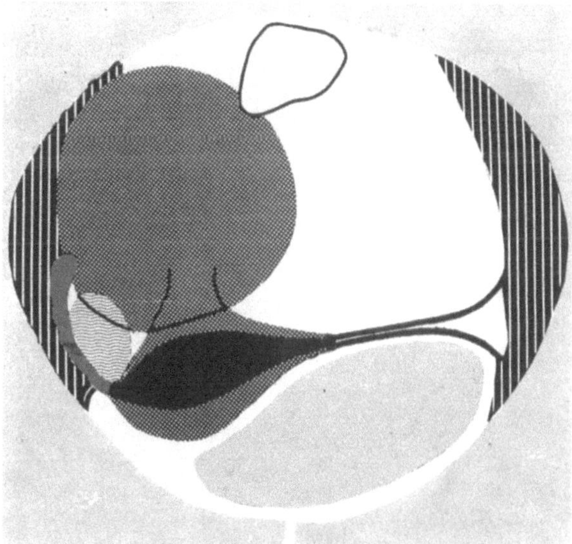

32 a

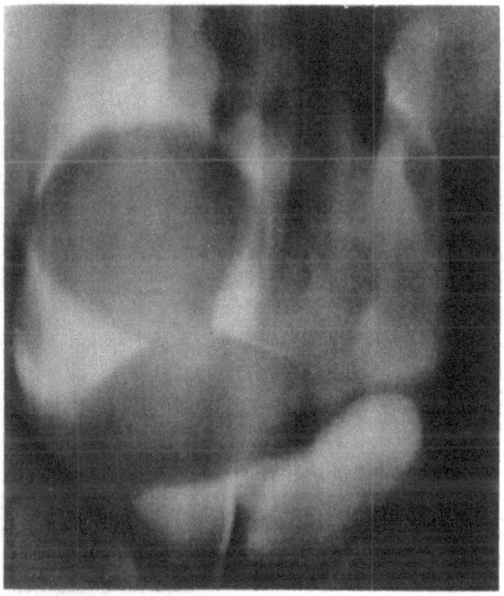

33

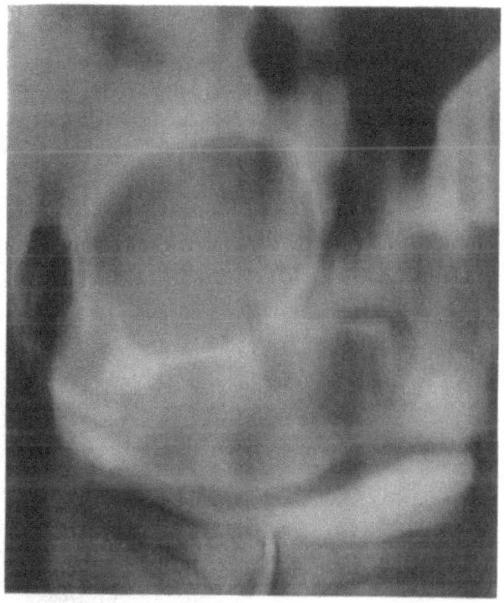

34

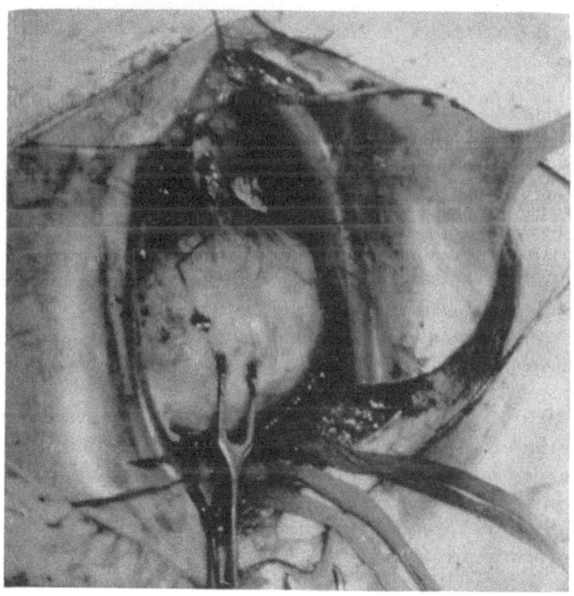

35

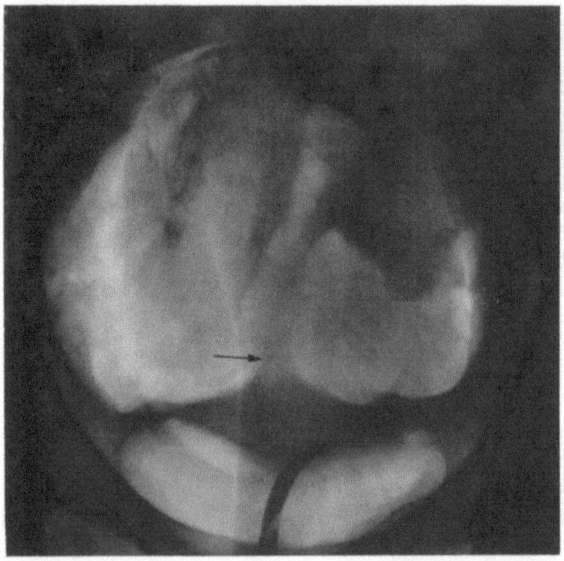

36

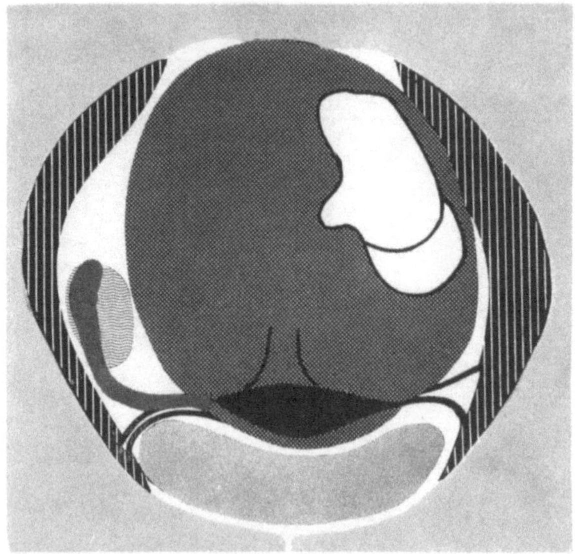

36a

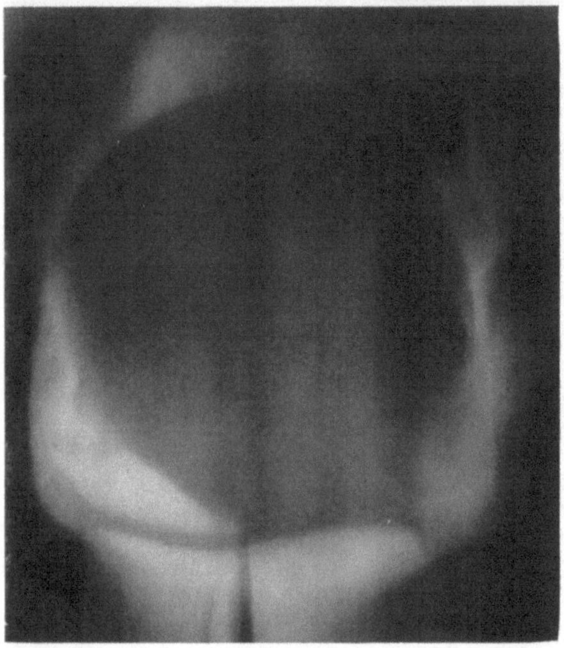

37

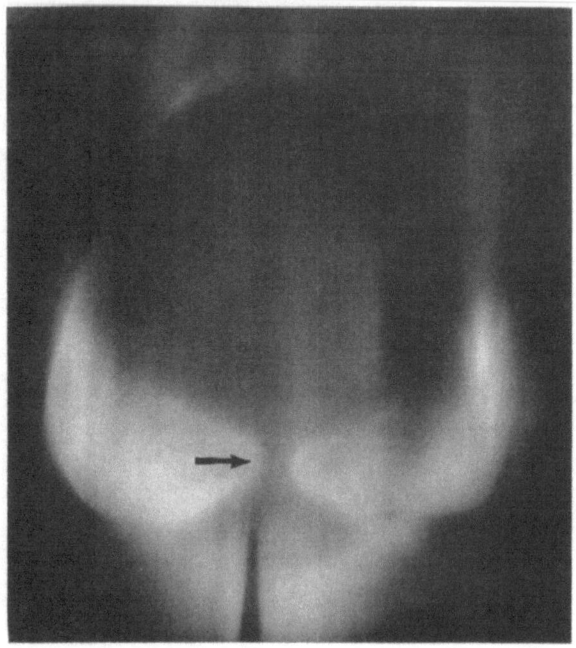

38

Abb. 36–38

Uterus myomatosus

Subseröses Myom

62jähr. Frau mit Schmerzen im Unterbauch und Fluor

Tastbefund: Uterus retroflektiert, rechts großer, prallelastischer Tumor, Adnexe nicht abzugrenzen

Indikation: Differenzierung zwischen Ovarialtumor und Uterus myomatosus

Abb. 36: Kindskopfgroßes, dünn gestieltes subseröses Korpusmyom. Auf der *Übersichtsaufnahme* sind Uterus, Stiel (→), Myom und rechte Tube erkennbar

Abb. 37 und 38: Die *Tomogramme* zeigen in einer ventralen Schichtebene die kugelige Myomgestalt, beide Ovarien und Teile beider Tuben. In einer mittleren Ebene ist der dünne Stiel des Myoms dargestellt (→)

Verlauf: Vaginale Totalexstirpation des Uterus unter Mitnahme beider Adnexe

Figs. 36–38

Uterus myomatosus

Subserous myoma

Patient, 62, complaining about pain in the lower abdomen and vaginal discharge

Palpation finding: Uterus retroflexed, large engorged and elastic tumor on the right, with adnexa not delimitable

Indication: Differentiation between ovarian tumor and uterus myomatosus

Fig. 36 shows thin pediculated subserous corpus myoma of child's head size; uterus, pedicle (→), myoma, and right tube are viualised by the *standard radiograph*

Figs. 37 and 38 are *tomograms* showing in a ventral tomographic plane the spherical shape of the myoma, the two ovaries, and parts of either tube; the thin pedicle of the myoma is displayed in a medium plane (→)

Course: Vaginal radical hysterectomy, including complete adnexectomy

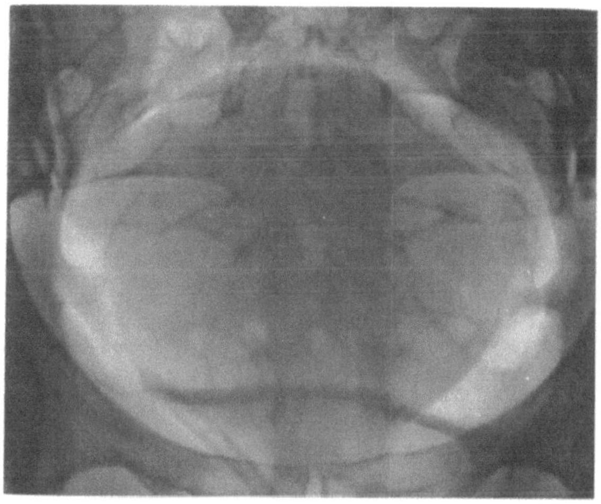

39

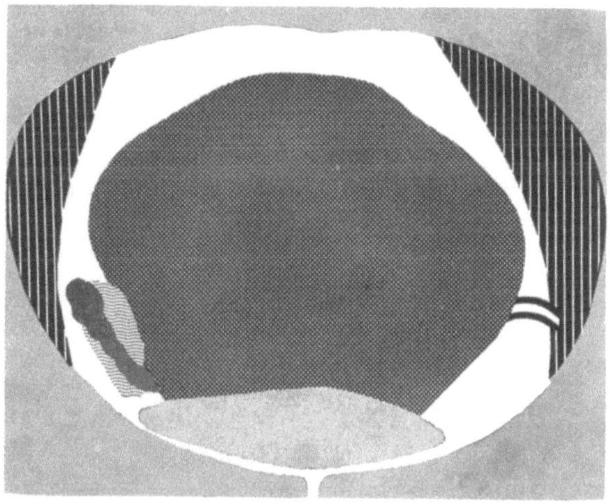

39 a

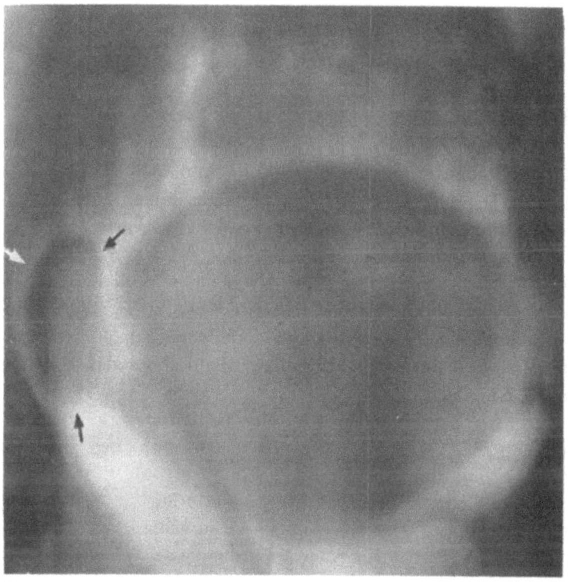

40

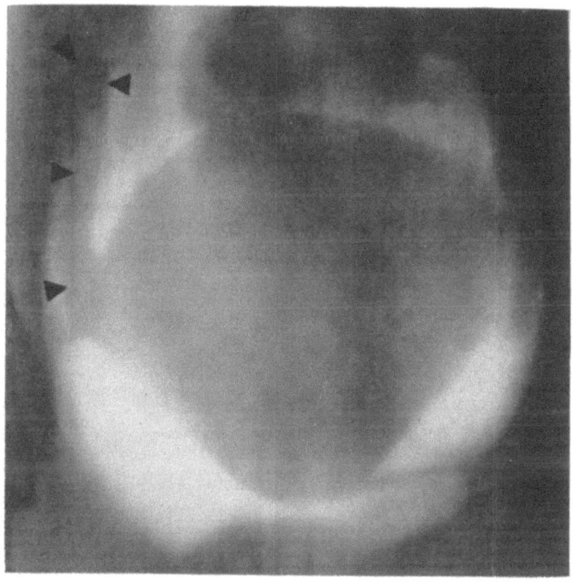

41

Abb. 39–42

Uterus myomatosus

Subseröses Myom

45jähr. Pat. mit Schmerzen im Unterbauch beim Sitzen
Tastbefund: Uterus etwas vergrößert, rechts großer derber Tumor, von dem die Adnexe nicht abgrenzbar sind
Indikation: Bestimmung der Organzugehörigkeit des Tumors
Abb. 39: Subseröses Fundusmyom. Die *Übersichtsaufnahme* im senkrechten pa-Strahlengang zeigt die kraniale und laterale Begrenzung des aus dem Becken etwas herausragenden Myoms
Abb. 40 und 41: Auf den *Schichtbildern* sind in 6 cm und 7 cm Tiefe die Adnexe und der Umfang des Myoms dargestellt
→ = Ovar ▶ = Tube
Verlauf: Abdominale Totalexstirpation des Uterus
Abb. 42: Operationspräparat

Figs. 39–42

Uterus myomatosus

Subserous myoma

Patient, 45, complaining about pain in the lower abdomen, when in seated position
Palpation finding: Uterus somewhat enlarged and large hard tumor on the right with no delimitability of adnexa
Indication: Identification of tumor-afflicted organ
Fig. 39 shows subserous fundus myoma; *standard radiograph*, taken with vertical posterior-anterior path of rays, displaying cranial and lateral demarcation of the myoma which is somewhat protruding from the pelvis
Figs. 40 and 41 are *tomograms*, 6 cm and 7 cm in dephts, demonstrating the adnexa and outline of myona
→ = ovary ▶ = tube
Course: Abdominal radical hysterectomy
Fig. 42: Surgical specimen

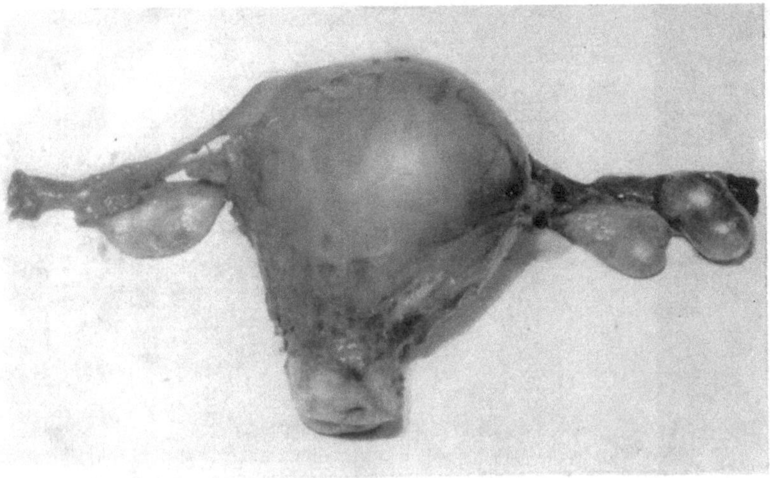

42

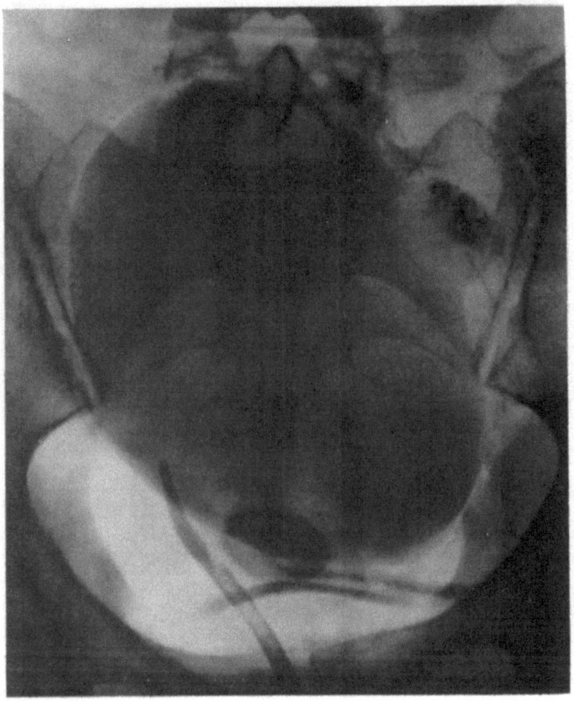

43

Abb. 43–46

Uterus myomatosus

39jähr. Patientin mit Druckgefühl im Abdomen

Tastbefund: Sehr großer, ins Abdomen hineinragender Tumor, wahrscheinlich Myom, Adnexe nicht tastbar

Indikation: Bestimmung der Organzugehörigkeit des Tumors

Abb. 43: Riesiger myomatöser Uterus mit vielhöckriger Gestalt. Die Myomknollen sind teilweise verkalkt. Die *Übersichtsaufnahme* ist im senkrechten pa-Strahlengang exponiert worden. Man erkennt ein enorm großes Myom und mehrere mittelgroße Knollen

Abb. 44: *Tomogramm* im frontalen (sinistrodextralen) Strahlengang.

A = Corpus uteri; B = riesiges Fundusmyom; C = einzelne Myomknollen; D = Excavatio rectouterina; E = Rectum; F = Harnblase; G = Excavatio vesicouterina

Abb. 45: Kalkstruktur einer Myomknolle im Schichtbild

Verlauf: Abdominale Totalexstirpation des Uterus

Abb. 46: Operationspräparat

Figs. 43–46

Uterus myomatosus

Patient, 39, feeling abdominal pressure

Palpation finding: Very large tumor reaching into abdomen and assumed to be a myoma, with adnexa not palpable

Indication: Identification of tumor-afflicted organ

Fig. 43: Giant myomatous uterus of polycyclic shape, with some of the myoma bulbs calcified; vertical postero-anterior path of rays was used for exposure of the *radiograph*; visualised are a very large myoma and several bulbs of medium size

Fig. 44 is a *tomogram* taken with frontal (sinistrodextral) path of rays:

A = corpus uteri; B = giant fundus myoma; C = singular myoma bulbs; D = excavatio rectouterina; E = rectum; F = urinary bladder; G = excavatio vesicouterina

Fig. 45 is a tomogram showing the calcareous structure of a myoma bulb

Course: Abdominal radical hysterectomy

Fig. 46: Surgical specimen

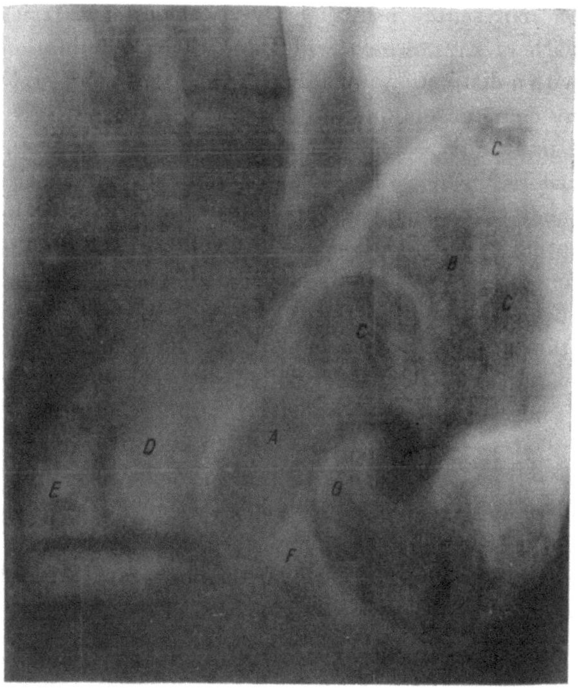

44

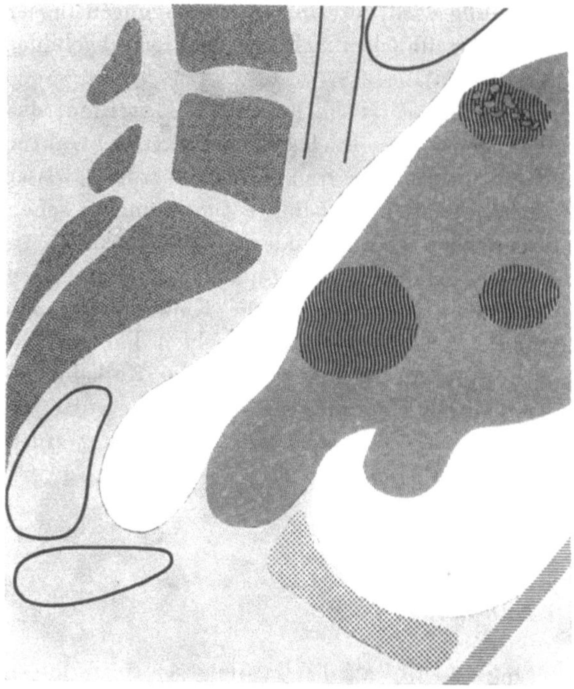

44 a

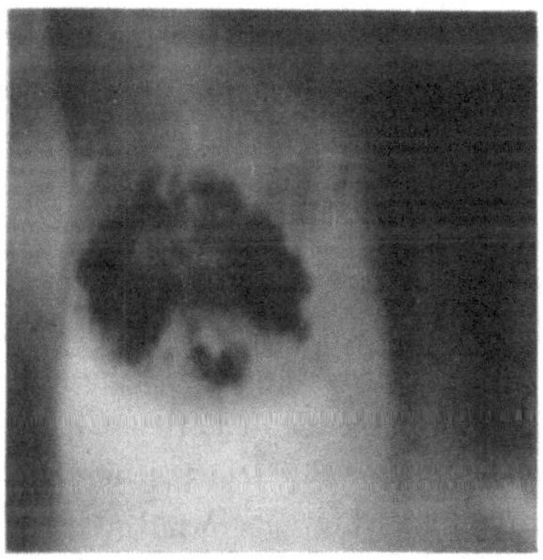

45

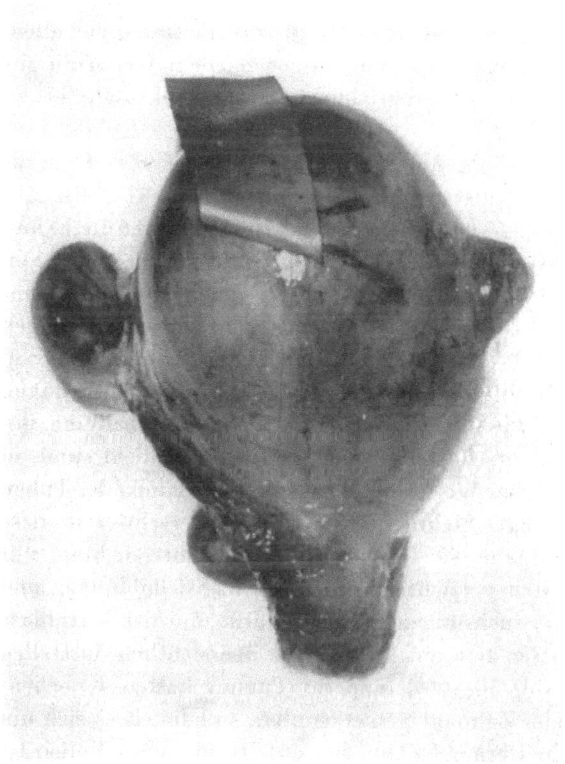

46

Begrenzung wird unter diesen Bedingungen besser als bei der üblichen Schrägprojektion abgebildet (Abb. 39—46).

Die *Verkalkung* ist ein bekanntes Kriterium, das zur Diagnose wesentlich beitragen kann. Struktur und Lokalisation der Kalkherde sind trotz gewisser Varianten typisch, so daß ihre Zuordnung oft schon auf einfachen Röntgenbildern (ohne Pneumoperitoneum) gelingt. Auf pneumopelvigraphischen Aufnahmen komplettieren die Kalkschatten den Befund (Abb. 43—46). In einzelnen Fällen können intramurale Myome auch ohne Kalkeinlagerungen durch höhere Schattendichte hervortreten und dadurch im Tomogramm erkennbar werden (Abb. 33 und 34).

5.1.2. *Ovarialtumoren*

Umfang und Gestalt der Ovarialgeschwülste lassen sich im Pneumopelvigramm gut erkennen, weil der größte Teil ihrer Oberfläche vom Gas umflossen wird. *Die Darstellung erfolgt hauptsächlich mit dem Ziel, bei mehrdeutigen Tastbefunden zu klären, ob der palpierte Tumor vom Ovar ausgeht.* An erster Stelle ist die Abgrenzung von der Gebärmutter durchzuführen, um einen Uterus myomatosus, vor allem ein gestieltes Myom, auszuschließen. Weiterhin gilt es, die Differentialdiagnose der Saktosalpinx zu stellen.

Die röntgenmorphologischen Bilder der Ovarialgeschwülste sind vielgestaltig (Abb. 47—76). Abhängig von der Größe der Tumoren, ihrer intra- und extraligamentären Wachstumsrichtung und von peritonealen Verwachsungen können Gebärmutter und Eileiter die verschiedensten Lageveränderungen durch Verdrängung oder Heranziehung erfahren. Die differentialdiagnostische Aussage hängt davon ab, ob das Röntgenbild eine Unterscheidung des Tumorschattens vom Uterus ermöglicht und in welcher Weise außerdem eine Beurteilung der Tuben gelingt. Mehrdeutige Strukturen erschweren diese Aufgabe, so daß auf die Schichtuntersuchung nur selten verzichtet werden kann. Stielbildungen und Verwachsungen mit dem Darm und der Harnblase lassen sich auf diese Weise übersichtlich darstellen (Abb. 50—66). Sind im Tumorschatten Knochen- oder Zahnanlagen erkennbar, so handelt es sich um ein Dermoid (Abb. 60—66). In manchen Fällen ist die Kombination mit der Hysterosalpingographie erforderlich (Abb. 67—76).

Auch bei kleinzystischer Degeneration der Ovarien mit zweifelhaftem Tastbefund kann man die Pneumopelvigraphie mit gutem Erfolg zu Rate ziehen.

be represented by using a vertical posteroanterior path of rays, which will show their delimination with a distinction much better than that achievable by common oblique projection (Figs. 39—46).

Calcification is known and generally accepted as a criterion which may add essentially to the consistency of a diagnosis. Both the structure and localisation of calcifications are of a typical pattern, although certain variants may possible occur, so that successful identification will often be possible even from ordinary radiographs (with no pneumoperitoneum). The picture provided by a pneumopelvigraph will then be completed by the presentation of calcareous patches (Figs. 43—46). In certain cases, it will be possible that visibility is achieved even of intramural myomas with no calcareous infiltration, due to their higher shadow density, which consequently become detectable in the tomogram (Figs. 33 and 34).

5.1.2. *Ovarian tumors*

Both the size and shape of ovarian tumors may be detected readily from the pneumopelvigram, since most to their surface will be flown round by gas. *Representation will be desirable mainly in the event of ambiguous palpation findings, with the view of deciding if the palpated tumor is originating from an ovary.* Its differentiation from the uterus has to be done first to rule out the presence of a hysteromyoma and, in particular, the presence of a pediculated myoma. Differential diagnosis of sactosalpinx should be the next step.

The radiographs showing the morphology of ovarian tumors may present a wide range of variants (Figs. 47—76). Both the uterus and oviducts may be found in most various positions as a result of displacement or approachment, depending on the given tumor size, the direction of intraligamentous and extraligamentous growth, and on the presence of peritoneal adhesions. The information obtainable from differential diagnosis will depend on whether a differentiation of the tumor shadow from the uterus is rendered possible by the quality of the radiograph as well as on the extent to which the tubes are assessed. Therefore, diagnostic tomography can be renounced only in rare cases, since it will help to elucidate in an uninvolved manner ambiguous structures, pediculations, and adhesions with both the intestine and the urinary bladder (Figs. 50—66). Visual appearance of osseous or dental germs in the tumor shadow indicates the presence of a dermoid (Figs. 60—66). Combination with hysterosalpingography will be necessary under certain circumstances (Figs. 67—76).

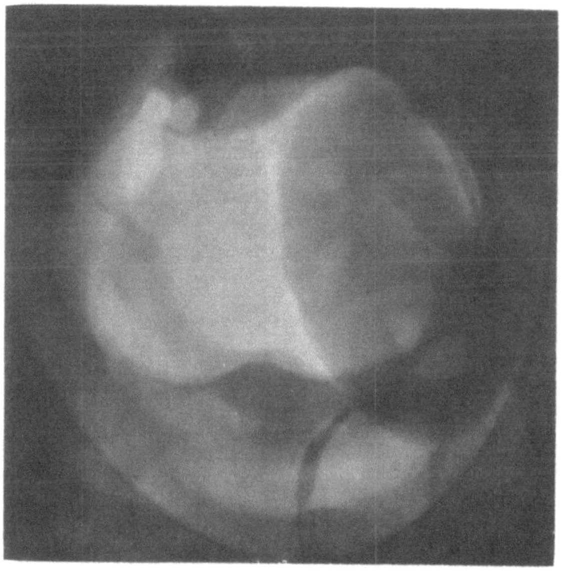

47

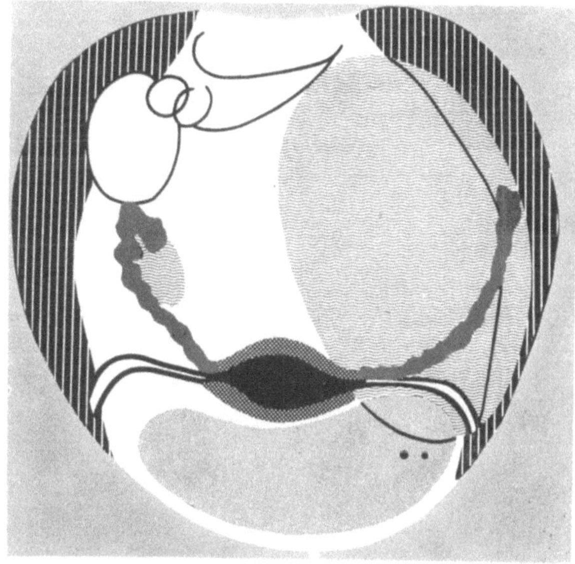

47a

Abb. 47 und 48

Ovarialzyste

Cystadenoma serosum simplex

58jähr. Patientin, bei der anläßlich einer Reihenuntersuchung der Verdacht auf eine pflaumengroße Zyste des linken Ovars erhoben wurde

Tastbefund: Bei Nachuntersuchungen im Verlaufe von 9 Monaten ergaben sich unterschiedliche Palpationsbefunde. Das Ovar wurde teils unauffällig, teils vergrößert getastet. Die Frage einer Größenzunahme ließ sich während der Beobachtungszeit nicht sicher entscheiden

Indikation: Beurteilung der Ovarien

Abb. 47: Auf der *Übersichtsaufnahme* faustgroße Zyste des linken Ovars mit glatter Oberfläche. Uterus atrophisch, rechtes Ovar atrophisch. Tuben unauffällig

Verlauf: Vaginale Totalexstirpation des Uterus unter Mitnahme beider Adnexe

Abb. 48: Operationsfoto

Figs. 47 and 48

Ovarian cyst

Cystadenoma serosum simplex

Patient, 58, suspect of the presence of a plum-size cyst at left ovary, with tentative diagnosis made in a routine examination

Palpation finding: Follow-up checks performed during twelve months gave different palpation findings, some of them suggesting unpathological and others enlarged ovaries; no safe assessment of growth was possible in the follow-up period

Indication: Assessment of ovaries

Fig. 47 is a *standard radiograph* showing a fist-size cyst with smooth surface in the left ovary; both the uterus and right ovary are atrophic, with the tubes being without pathological findings

Course: Vaginal radical hysterectomy, including removal of either adnexa

Fig. 48: Photograph of operation

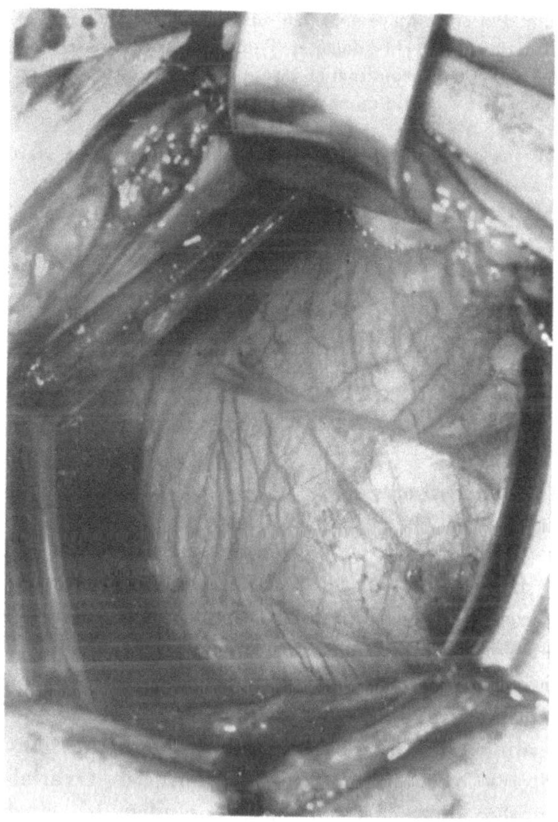

48

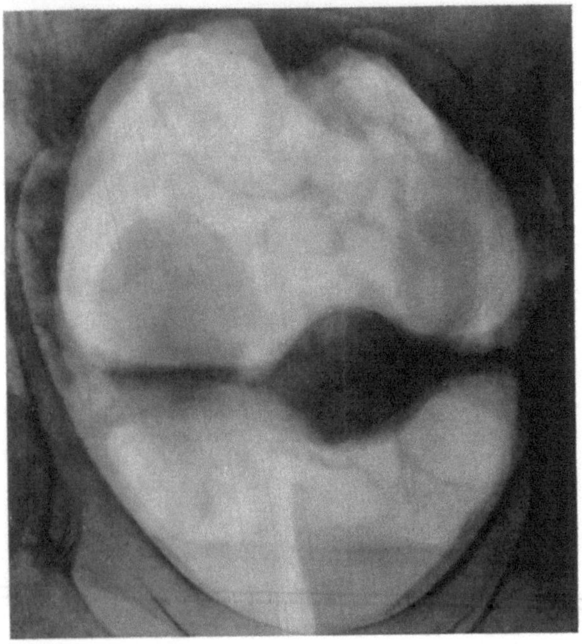

49

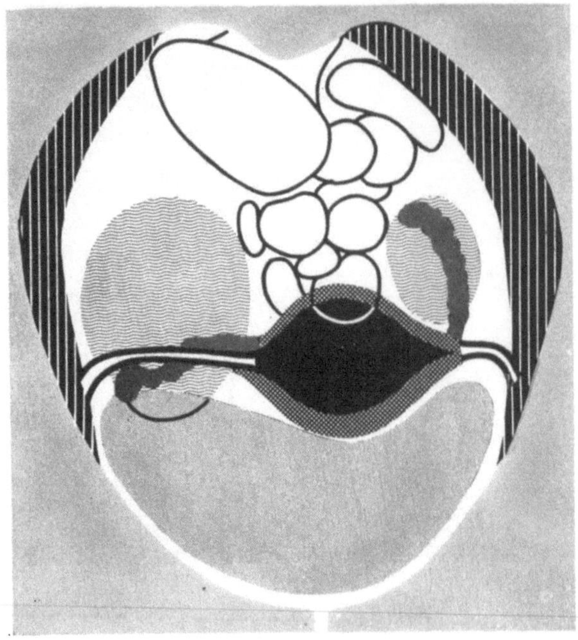

49 a

Abb. 49
Ovarialzyste
Kystadenoma pseudomucinosum glandulare

48jähr. Patientin mit Schmerzen im rechten Unterbauch.
Tastbefund: Rechts dolenter Tumor von der Größe eines Hühnereies, Uterus normal groß, anteflektiert, mittelständig
Indikation: Bestimmung der Organzugehörigkeit des Tumors
Abb. 49: Auf der *Übersichtsaufnahme* hühnereigroßer, glatt begrenzter Ovarialtumor rechts
Verlauf: Vaginale Totalexstirpation unter Mitnahme beider Adnexe

Fig. 49
Ovarian cyst
Kystadenoma pseudomucinosum glandulare

Patient, 48, complaining about pain in right lower abdomen
Palpation finding: Dolent tumor of hen-egg size on the right, uterus of normal size, anteflexed, and in central position
Indication: Identification of the tumor-afflicted organ
Fig. 49 is a *standard radiograph* showing, on the right, smoothly demarcated tumor of the ovary of hen-egg size
Course: Vaginal radical surgery, including removal of either adnexa

Bei Vorliegen multipler Zysten weisen die Ovarien auf dem Röntgenbild eine vielhöckrige Gestalt auf (Abb. 77—83).

5.1.3. *Tubenprozesse*

Aus dem Pneumopelvigramm sind Rückschlüsse auf Erkrankungen der Tuben möglich, wenn ihr äußeres Kaliber zunimmt, Versteifungen auftreten oder Verkalkungen und peritoneale Verwachsungen dargestellt werden. Verdickungen der Eileiter bei *Saktosalpinx* führen auf der Übersichtsaufnahme allerdings häufig zu Strukturen, die nicht ohne weiteres von unregelmäßig geformten Ovarialtumoren unterscheidbar sind. Vor allem bei einer Beteiligung des Ovars an entzündlichen Adnexprozessen und seiner Einbeziehung in eine *Pyosalpinx*, *Haematosalpinx* oder einen *Tubenhydrops* werden die verschiedensten Verschattungen hervorgerufen. Verziehungen durch Perisalpingitis erschweren die Bildanalyse zusätzlich. Eine bessere

Pneumopelvigraphy may be used quite successfully also for more information about *small-cyst degeneration of the ovaries* when the palpation findings are dubious. The presence of multiple cysts will be revealed radiographically by a poly-protuberant form of the ovaries (Figs. 77—83).

5.1.3. *Tubal processes*

Conclusions as to the presence of tubal diseases may be drawn from a pneumopelvigram, when the external calibers of the tubes are shown to be on a growing trend or when stiffening takes place or calcification and peritoneal adhesions are represented. However, thickening of the oviducts in cases of *sactosalpinx* often tends to produce in a standard radiograph structures that cannot be easily differentiated from irregularly shaped ovarian tumors. Most various shadows will be produced, for example, by participation of the ovaries in inflammatory adnexal processes and by their affection in cases of

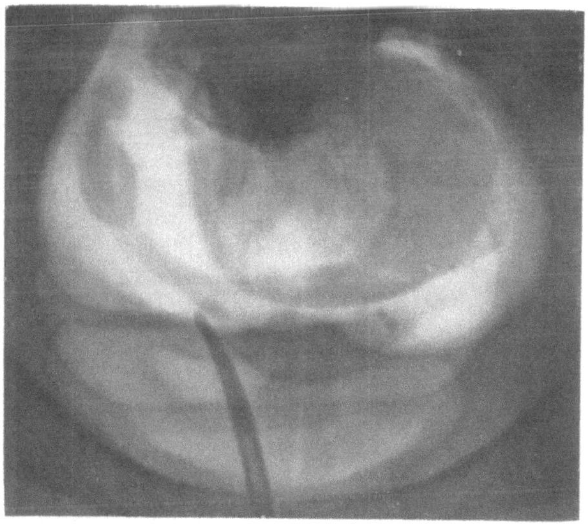

50

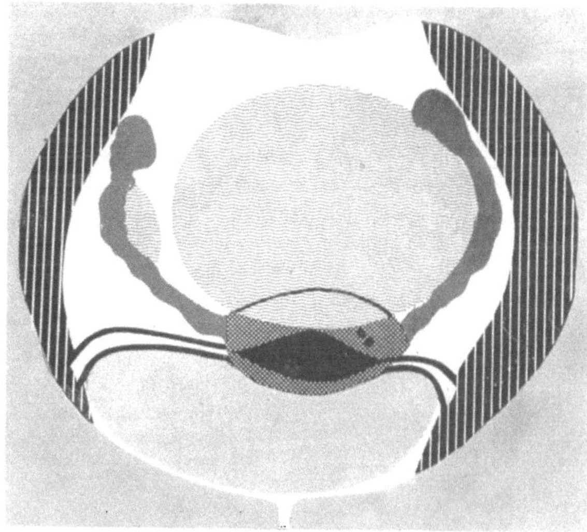

50 a

Abb. 50 und 51

Ovarialzyste

Cystadenoma papilliferum

63jähr. Patientin ohne Beschwerden

Tastbefund: Gänseeigroßer, vom Uterus nicht abgrenzbarer Tumor

Indikation: Bestimmung der Organzugehörigkeit des Tumors

Abb. 50: Auf dem *Übersichtsbild* projiziert sich der linksseitige ovaläre Tumorschatten teilweise auf den Uterus. Rechtes Ovar und rechte Tube sind gut zu unterscheiden

Abb. 51 zeigt ein *Tomogramm* in 6 cm Tiefe. Der Tumor geht vom linken Ovar aus, das rechte Ovar und die rechte Tube sind gut zu unterscheiden

Verlauf: Abdominale Totalexstirpation des Uterus unter Mitnahme beider Adnexe

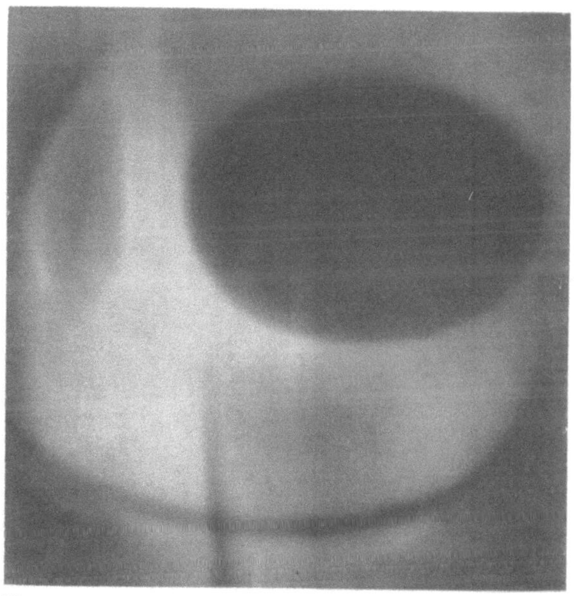

51

Figs. 50 and 51

Ovarian cyst

Cystadenoma papilliferum

Patient, 63, with no complaints

Palpation finding: Presence of tumor of goose-egg size, not delimitable from uterus

Indication: Identification of the tumor-afflicted organ

Fig. 50 is a *standard radiograph* where the left oval tumor shadow is projected to some extent to the uterus, with right ovary being easily and clearly differentiable from right tube

Fig. 51 is a *tomogram*, 6 cm in depth, showing the tumor to originate from the left ovary, with right ovary being clearly differentiable from right tube

Course: Abdominal radical hysterectomy, including removal of either adnexa

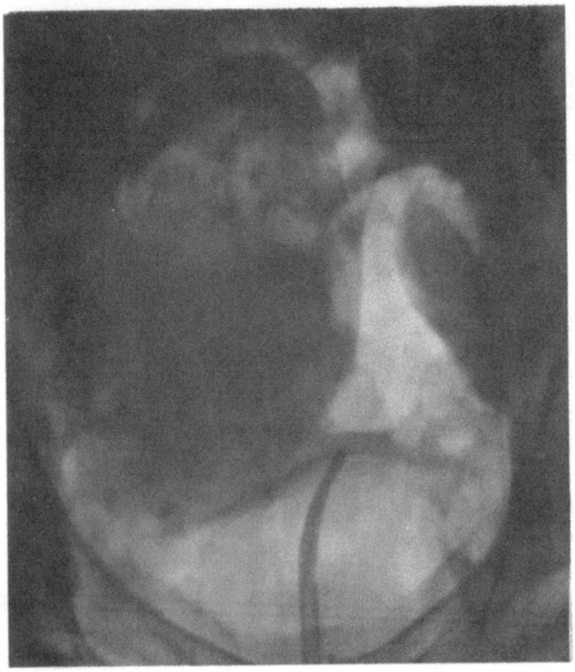

52

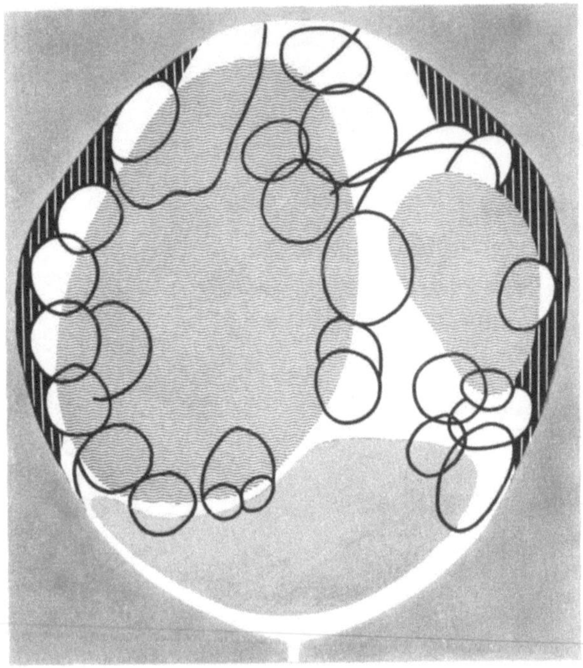

52a

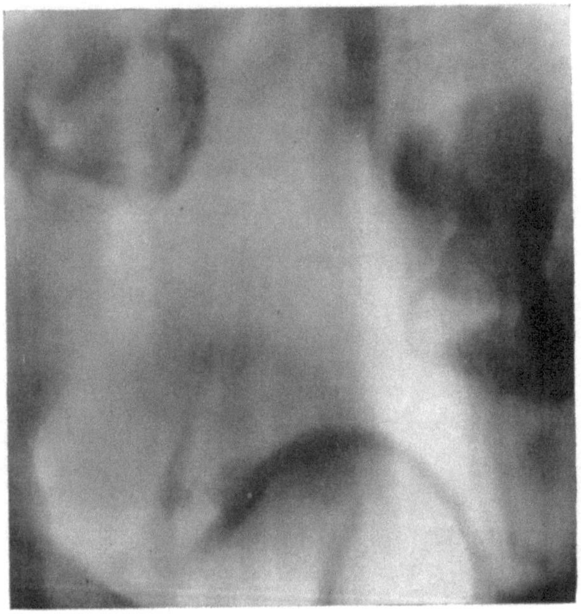

53

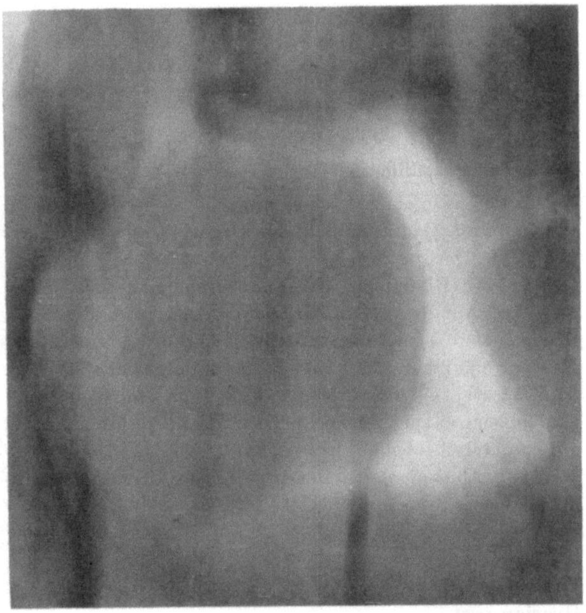

54

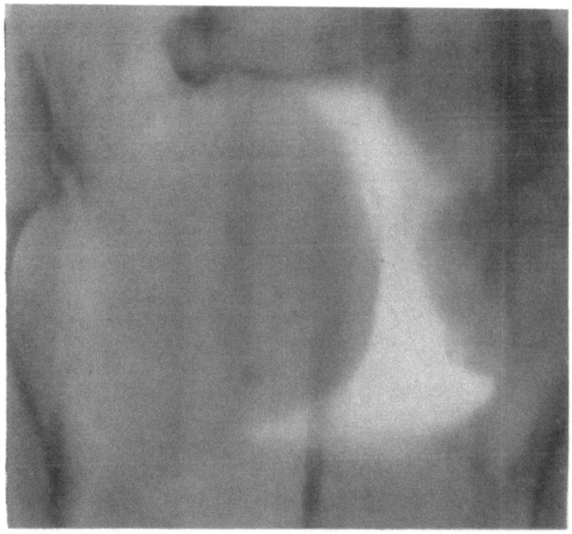

55

Abb. 52—56

Ovarialzysten beiderseits

Cystadenoma papilliferum, Status nach vaginaler Totalexstirpation des Uterus

55jähr. Patientin ohne Beschwerden. Die Entfernung der Gebärmutter erfolgte vor 7 Jahren wegen Uterus myomatosus

Tastbefund: In der Scheidennarbe hühnereigroßer höckriger Tumor

Indikation: Abgrenzung des Tumors

Abb. 52: Auf der *Übersichtsaufnahme* gut faustgroßer Ovarialtumor rechts und kleinerer Ovarialtumor links. Fehlen des Uterusschattens bei Zustand nach Totalexstirpation

Abb. 53—55: *Die Tomogramme* zeigen in 4 cm Tiefe Verwachsungsstränge des rechtsseitigen Tumors mit dem Harnblasenscheitel, in 7 cm und 9 cm Tiefe den Umfang der Geschwulst und mehrere Vorbuckelungen auch am linken Ovar

Verlauf: Salpingoophorektomie beiderseits

Abb. 56: Operationspräparat

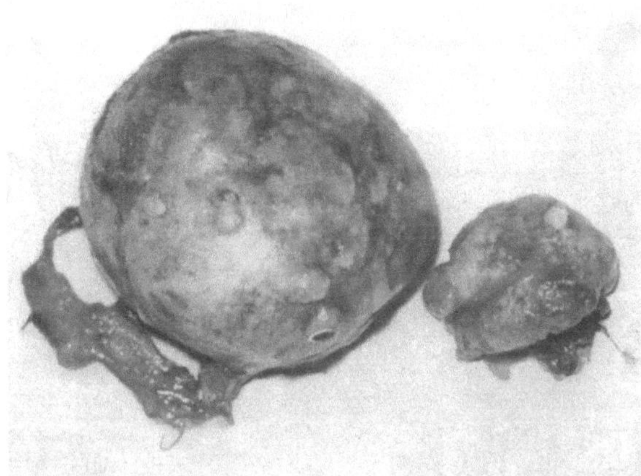

56

Figs. 52—56

Collateral ovarian cysts

Cystadenoma papilliferum, Condition after vaginal hysterectomy

Patient, 55, with no complaints, whose uterus had been removed seven years earlier for uterus myomatosus

Palpation finding: Presence of polycyclic tumor of hen-egg size in vaginal scar

Indication: Demarcation of tumor

Fig. 52 is a *standard radiograph* showing ovarian tumor of fist-size, on the right, and smaller ovarian tumor, on the left; no uterus shadow due to condition after hysterectomy

Figs. 53—55 are *tomograms*, 4 cm in depth, showing adhesive cords of right tumor with fundus of the bladder, or tomograms, 7 cm and 9 cm in depths, showing the outline of the tumor and, in addition, some bulgings at the left ovary

Course: Collateral salpingo-oophorectomy

Fig. 56: Surgical specimen

57
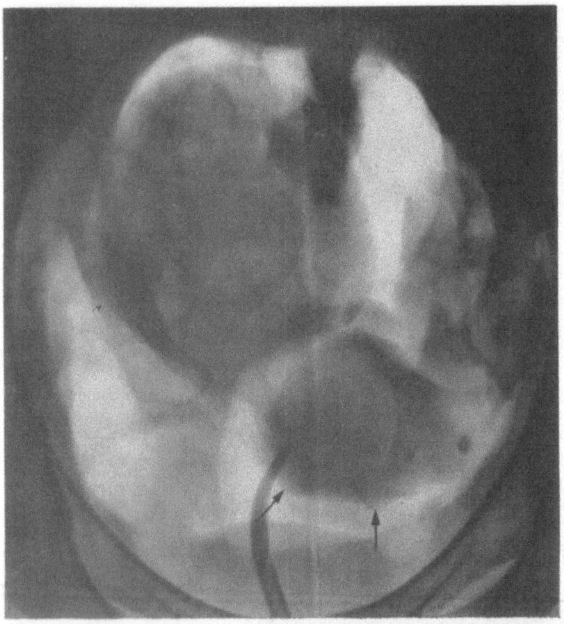

57a
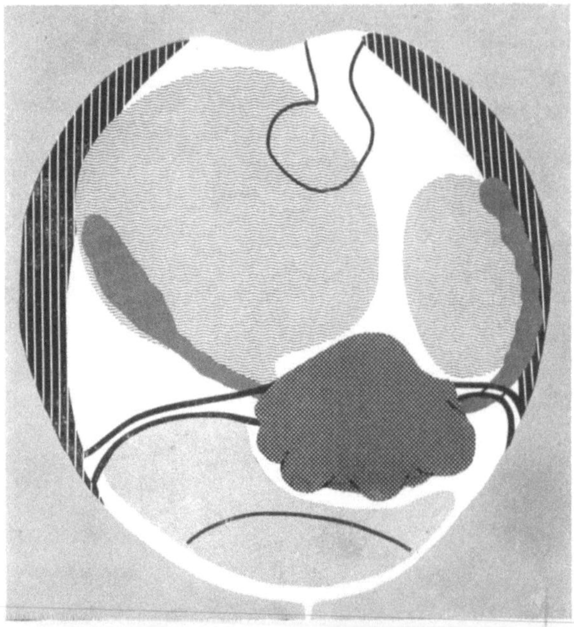

58
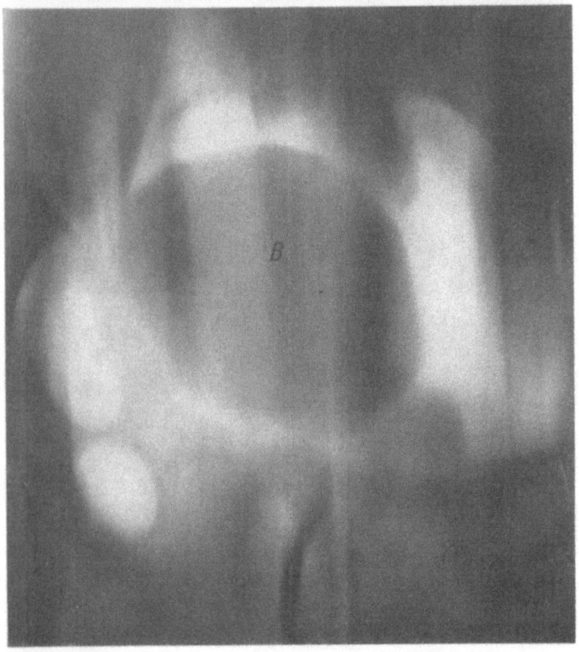

59
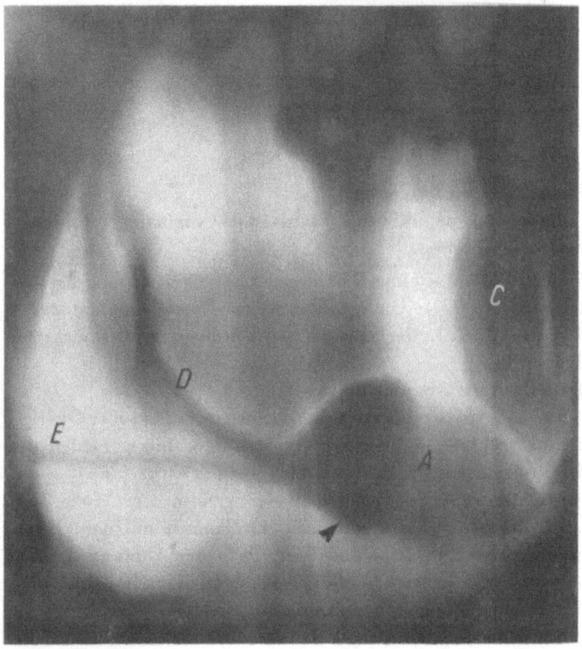

Abb. 57–59

Ovarialzyste

Cystadenoma serosum simplex mit Thekahaematom

23jähr. Frau mit Hirsutismus

Tastbefund: Gänseeigroßer zystischer Tumor rechts, Vergrößerung des linken Ovars

Indikation: Abgrenzung des Tumors, Darstellung der Ovarien

Abb. 57: Das *Übersichtsbild* zeigt einen gut faustgroßen rechtsseitigen Ovarialtumor, der den Uterus nach links abdrängt

→ = subseröse Myome

Abb. 58 und 59: Die *Tomogramme* ermöglichen zuverlässiger als die Summationsaufnahme eine Abgrenzung der rechten Tube, die über dem Tumor ausgespannt ist, und des nicht vergrößerten linken Ovars

A = Uterus; ▸ = Myom; B = Zyste des rechten Ovars; C = linkes Ovar; D = rechte Tube; E = Lig. teres uteri

Verlauf: Salpingoophorektomie rechts, Enukleation von zwei Myomknollen

Figs. 57–59

Ovarian cyst

Cystadenoma serosum simplex with thecahematoma

Patient, 23, afflicted with hirsutism

Palpation finding: Cystic tumor of goose-egg size on the right and enlargement of left ovary

Indication: Demarcation of tumor and visualisation of ovaries

Fig. 57 is a *standard radiograph* showing, on the right, ovarian tumor of fist-size displacing uterus to the left

→ = subserous myomas

Figs. 58 and 59 are *tomograms* that prove to be more reliable than standard radiography in delimitating the right tube, stretched above the tumor, and the unenlarged left ovary

A = uterus; ▸ = myoma; B = cyst of right ovary; C = left ovary; D = right tube; E = lig. teres uteri

Course: Salpingo-oophorectomy on the right, enucleation of two myoma bulbs

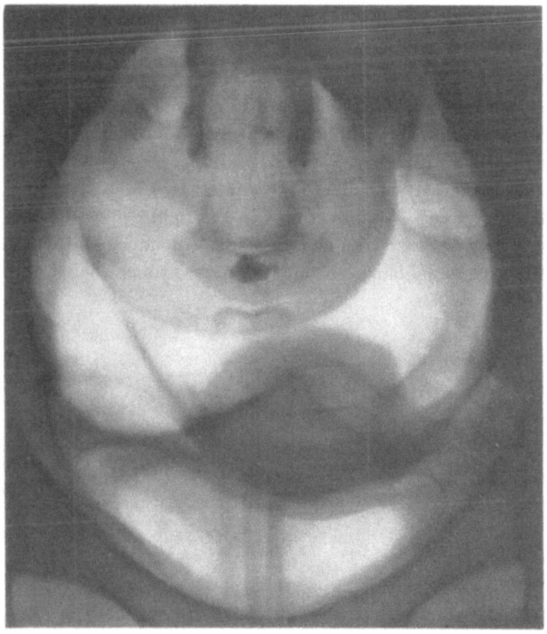

60

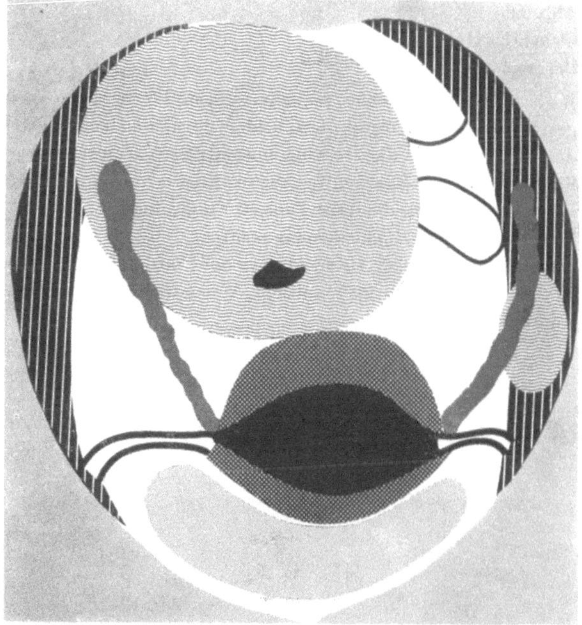

60 a

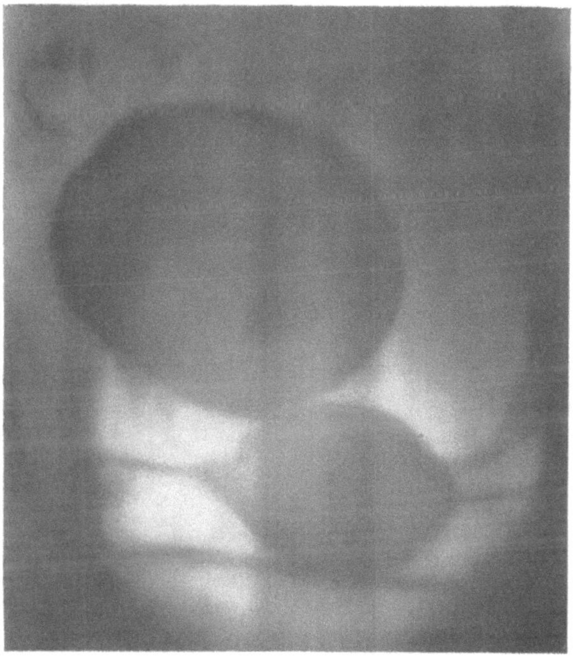

61

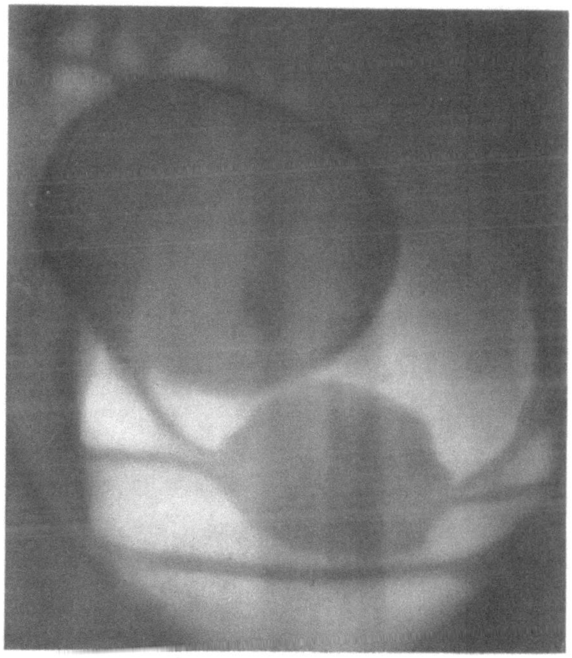

62

Abb. 60–62
Ovarialzyste
Dermoid

28jähr. Frau mit primärer Sterilität. Die Untersuchung erfolgt wegen dringenden Kinderwunsches

Tastbefund: Rechte Adnexe nach dorsal in den DOUGLASschen Raum verlagert, rechtes Ovar hühnereigroß tastbar, derb, nicht beweglich, linkes Ovar nicht palpabel

Indikation: Darstellung der Ovarien, Kombination mit Salpingographie zur Prüfung der Tubendurchgängigkeit

Abb. 60: *Übersichtsaufnahme.* Faustgroßer rundlicher Tumor des rechten Ovars, zwischen Rectum und Uterus eingeklemmt. Im Inneren wird eine Verkalkung mit der Form einer Zahnanlage dargestellt. Rechte Tube ausgezogen, linkes Ovar klein

Figs. 60–62
Ovarian cyst
Dermoid

Patient, 28, afflicted primarily with sterility; examination performed to meet urgent desire for children

Palpation finding: Right adnexum displaced dorsally into DOUGLAS' pouch, right ovary of hen-egg size palpable, hard, immovable, left ovary not palpable

Indication: Visualisation of ovaries, combination with salpingography to test tubal patency

Fig. 60 is a *standard radiograph* showing rounded fist-size tumor of right ovary impacted between rectum and uterus; demonstrated in the interior is a calcification of dental germ shape; right tube drawn out; left ovary small

Abb. 60–62
Ovarialzyste
Dermoid

Abb. 61 und 62: *Tomogramme* in 5 cm und 6 cm Tiefe. Dargestellt sind: Das Corpus uteri, beide Tuben, die Ovarialzyste, das Lig. teres und die Harnblasenwand. Bei der zusätzlichen Salpingographie zeigt sich der rechte Eileiter am ampullären Ende verschlossen, die linke Tube ist durchgängig

Verlauf: Salpingoophorektomie rechts

Histologischer Befund: Dermoidzyste mit Plattenepithel, Talgdrüsen, Haaren und Zahnanlagen, subepitheliale chronische Entzündung

Figs. 60–62
Ovarian cyst
Dermoid

Figs. 61 and 62: are *tomograms*, 5 cm and 6 cm in depths, showing corpus uteri, either tube, ovarian cyst, lig. teres, and wall of urinary bladder; additional *salpingography* shows right oviduct locked at ampullary end, while left tube ist patent

Course: Salpingo-oophorectomy on the right

Histological finding: Dermoid cyst with squamous epithelium, sebaceous glands, hairs, and dental germs; subepithelial chronic inflammation

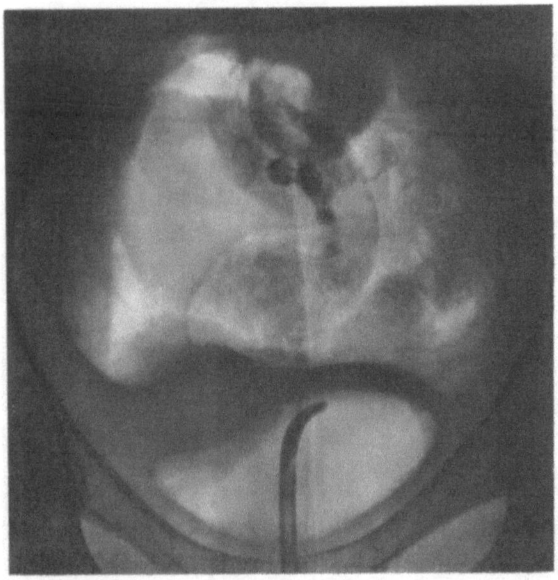

63

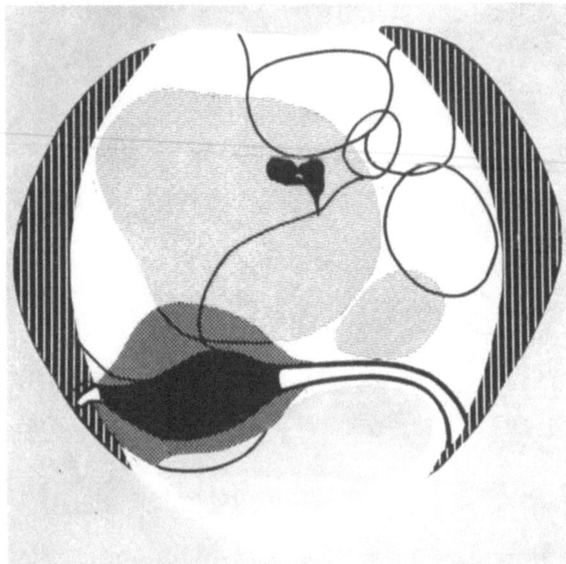

63 a

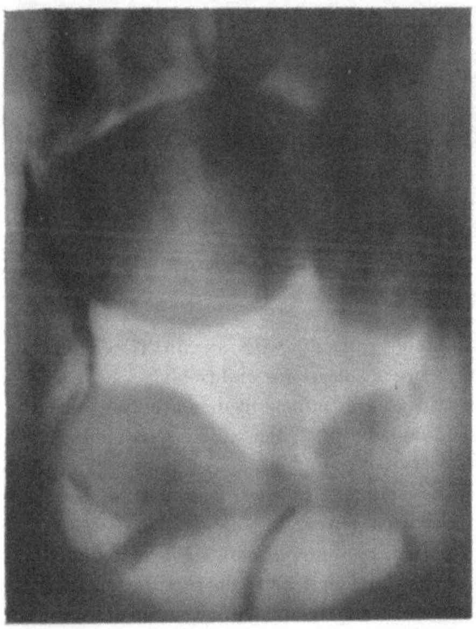

64

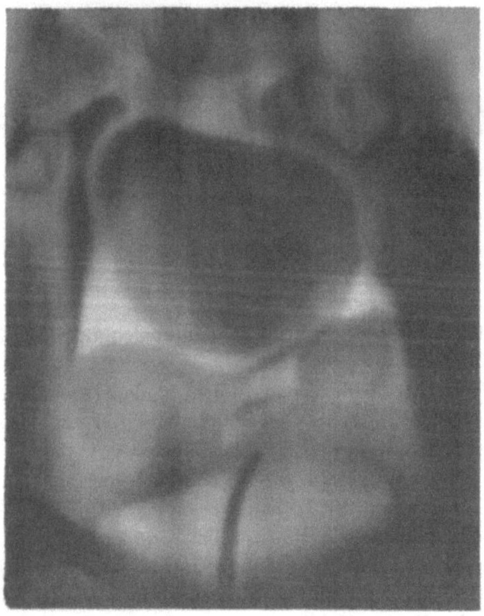

65

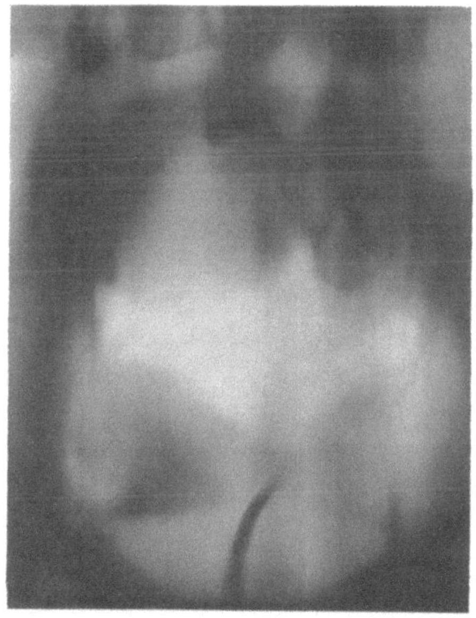

66

Abb. 63–66
Ovarialzyste
Dermoid

26jähr. Patientin mit Kreuzschmerzen, Druckgefühl im Unterbauch und Hirsutismus

Tastbefund: Hühnereigroßer derber Tumor in der Kreuzbeinhöhle rechts hinter dem Uterus gelegen, gut verschieblich

Indikation: Bestimmung der Organzugehörigkeit des Tumors, Darstellung der Ovarien

Abb. 63: Faustgroßer Ovarialtumor rechts mit Zahnanlagen, Verziehung des Uterus, normales linkes Ovar

Abb. 64–66: Nach den *Schichtaufnahmen* lassen sich die topographischen Verhältnisse im einzelnen beurteilen. Die linke Tube verläuft nach lateral und umgreift das Ovar. Die rechte Tube ist nach kranial gestreckt. Die Ligg. uteroovarica sind zwischen dem Seitenrand der Gebärmutter und beiden Ovarien erkennbar. Der Ovarialtumor hat sich vorwiegend extraligamentär entwickelt und enthält drei Zahnanlagen

Verlauf: Salpingoophorektomie rechts

Histologischer Befund: Dermoidzyste mit Plattenepithel, Talgdrüsen, Haaren und Zähnen

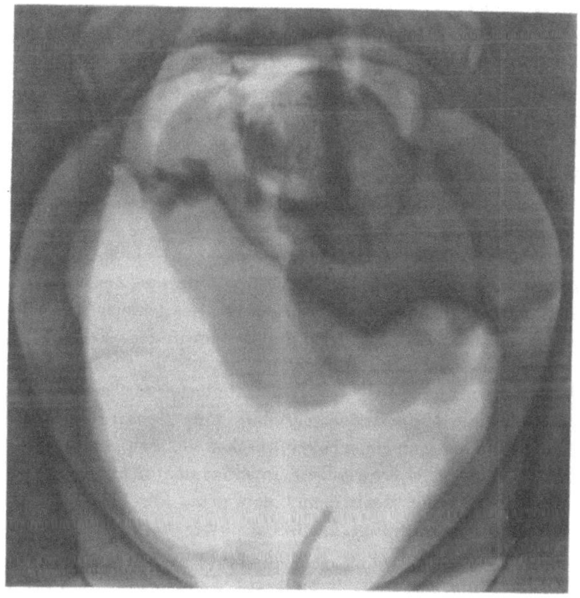

67

Figs. 63–66
Ovarian cyst
Dermoid

Patient, 26, complaining about lumbago, pressure feeling in lower abdomen, and hirsutism

Palpation finding: Hard tumor of hen-egg size located on the right behind the uterus in the hollow of the sacrum and readily displaceable

Indication: Identification of tumor-afflicted organ and visualisation of ovaries

Fig. 63 shows on the right fist-size ovarian tumor with dental germs, uterus distorted, but left ovary in normal condition

Figs. 64–66 are *tomograms* to enable more detailed assessment of topographic conditions; left tube extending laterally and encircling ovary; right tube stretched cranially; ligg. utero-ovarica are discernible between lateral margin of uterus and both ovaries; ovarian tumor has developed mainly in extraligamentous manner and contains three dental germs

Course: Salpingo-oophorectomy on the right

Histological finding: Dermoid cyst with squamous epithelium, sebaceous glands, hairs, and dental germs

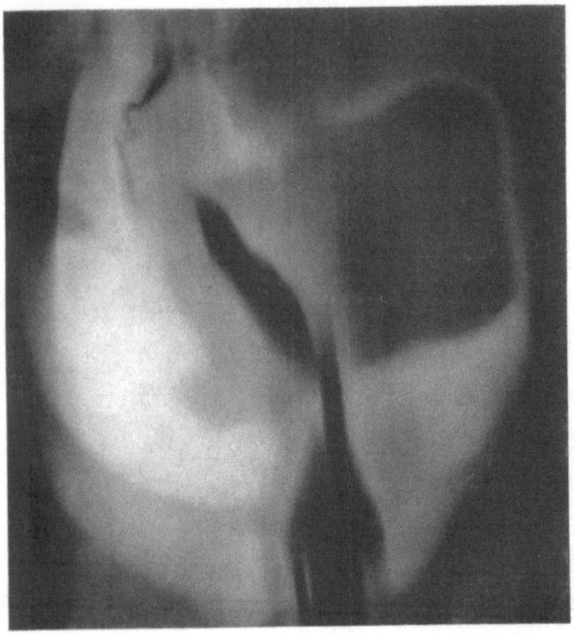

68

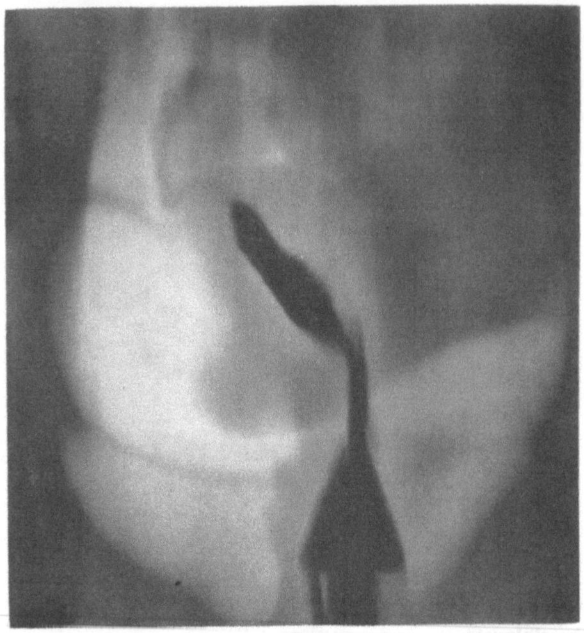

69

Abb. 67–69

Ovarialzyste, Uterus myomatosus

Teerzyste bei Endometriose des Ovars, subseröses Myom

36jähr. Patientin mit Schmerzen im linken Unterbauch, letzte Regelblutung abgeschwächt und verkürzt

Tastbefund: Linke Adnexe schmerzhaft, am Uterus nach links auslaufende derbe Vorbuckelungen

Indikation: Abgrenzung des Tumors und Feststellung der Organzugehörigkeit

Abb. 67: Auf der *Übersichtsaufnahme* wird ein großes, gebuckeltes Schattengebilde dargestellt, dessen Zentrum im kleinen Becken links dorsal gelegen ist. Bei genauer Betrachtung sind das rechte Lig. teres und der gewundene Verlauf des rechten Eileiters zu unterscheiden

Abb. 68 und 69: Zur weiteren Differenzierung erfolgt zusätzlich eine *Hysterosalpingographie* mit *Tomographie.* Die Schichtbilder zeigen einen polyzyklischen linksseitigen Ovarialtumor, der dem Uterus anliegt, intraligamentär lokalisiert ist und Verwachsungen mit dem Colon zeigt. Der Fundus uteri ist nach rechts verdrängt. Die Gebärmutterkontur wird auf der rechten Seite durch eine Myomknolle vorgebuckelt. Cavum uteri und rechter Eileiter sind mit Kontrastmittel gefüllt, linke Tube nicht gefüllt

Verlauf: Salpingoophorektomie links, Myomenukleation. Die Operation ergibt eine intraligamentär gelegene Teerzyste, die fast vollständig an den Uterus herangezogen und mit dem Darm und Netz verwachsen ist. Der linke Eileiter ist in den zystischen Tumor einbezogen. In der Vorderwand des Uterus subseröses Myom

Histologischer Befund: Im Ovar Endometrioseherde, chronische Entzündung der Zystenwand, chronische Salpingitis, Perisalpingitis

Figs. 67–69

Ovarian cyst, uterus myomatosus

Chocolade cyst with endometriosis of ovary, subserous myoma

Patient, 36, reporting pain in left lower abdomen as well as reduction and shortening of last menses

Palpation finding: Pain in left adnexum, hard bulgings at uterus extending to the left

Indication: Demarcation of tumor and identification of tumor-afflicted organ

Fig. 67 is a *standard radiograph* showing large, gibbous shadow, its centre being left-dorsal in the small pelvis; right lig. teres and curved shape of right oviduct differentiable on closer observation

Figs. 68 und 69 are *tomograms combined with hysterosalpingography* for more detailed differentiation, showing, on the left, polycyclic ovarian tumor situated close to the uterus, localised in intraligamentous position, and exhibiting adhesions with the colon; the fundus uteri is shown displaced to the right; the contour of the uterus is bulged to the right by a myoma bulb; cavum uteri and right oviduct are filled with contrast medium, but left tube is unfilled

Course: Salpingo-oophorectomy on the left, enucleation of myoma; surgery detecting an intraligamentous chocolate cyst, its length being almost entirely close to the uterus, with adhesion to both the intestine and omentum; the left oviduct is affected by the cystic tumor; a subserous myoma develops in the anterior uterine wall

Histological finding: Endometriosis foci in the ovary, chronic inflammation of cyst wall, chronic salpingitis, perisalpingitis

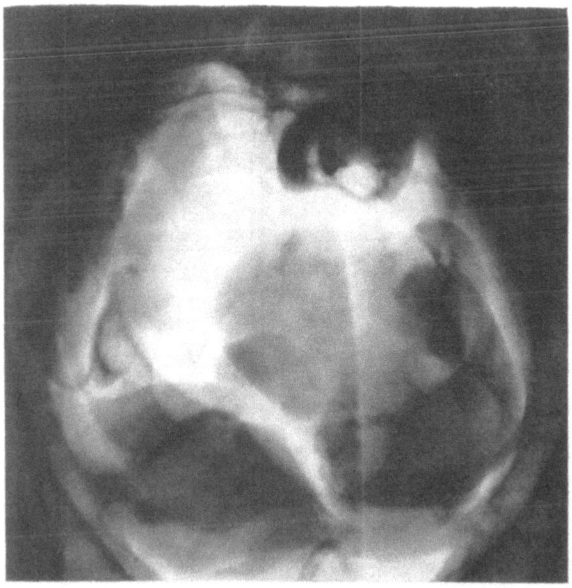

70

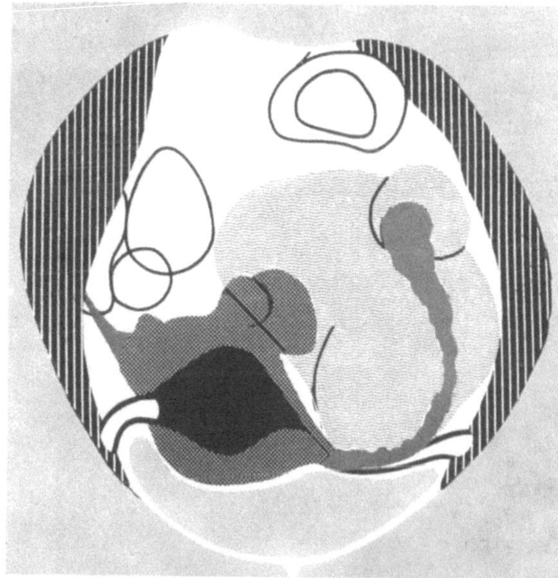

70 a

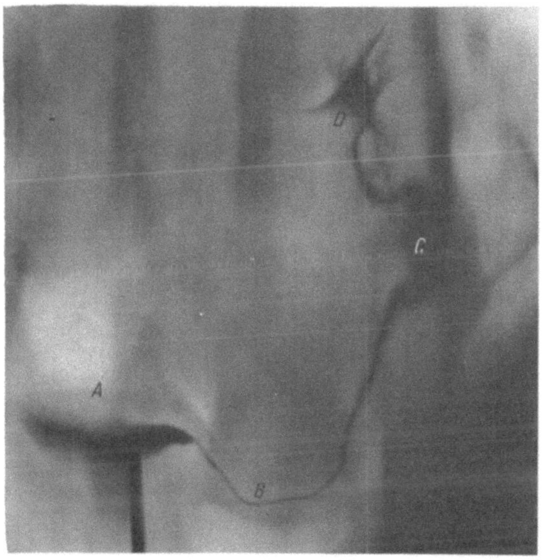

71

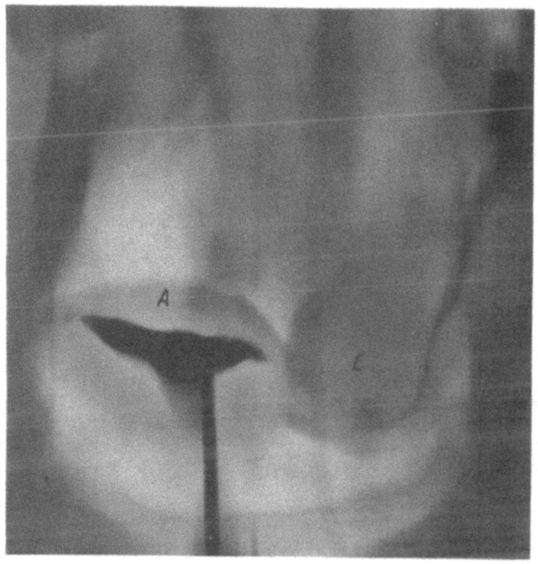

72

Abb. 70–76

Ovarialzyste, Uterus myomatosus

Corpus-luteum-Zyste, subseröses Myom, Status nach rechtsseitiger Salpingoophorektomie

31jähr Patientin mit dringendem Kinderwunsch. Primäre Sterilität, Schmerzen im Unterbauch, Kreuzschmerzen. Vor 5 Jahren wurden die rechten Adnexe wegen Hydrosalpinx und Ovarialzyste entfernt

Tastbefund: Nach rechts verzogener anteflektierter Uterus. Links dorsal langgestreckter, zystisch erscheinender Tumor, der sich nicht genau abgrenzen läßt

Indikation: Bestimmung der Organzugehörigkeit und Abgrenzung des Tumors, Salpingographie zur Klärung der Tubendurchgängigkeit

Abb. 70: Auf dem *Übersichtsbild* linksseitiger faustgroßer Ovarialtumor, dessen Oberfläche mehrere Vorbuckelungen aufweist. Der Tumor reicht intraligamentär an den Uterus heran und erstreckt sich nach dorsal bis zum Rectum. Die weitere Deutung der Schattenstrukturen erfolgte anhand der Tomogramme

Figs. 70–76

Ovarian cyst, uterus myomatosus

Corpus luteum cyst, subserous myoma, condition after salpingo-oophorectomy on the right

Patient, 31, reporting urgent desire for children; primary sterility, pain in lower abdomen, lumbago; adnexectomy on the right was performed five years ago for sactosalpinx and ovarian cyst

Palpation finding: Uterus anteflexed and distorted to the right, left-dorsal presence of elongated tumor of cystic appearance with no accurate demarcability

Indication: Identification of tumor-afflicted organ and demarcation of tumor, salpingography to test tubal patency

Fig. 70 is a *standard radiograph* showing, on the left, fist-size ovarian tumor with some bulging of its surface; the tumor is intraligamentous and extends to the uterus and, dorsally, to the rectum; detailed interpretation of shadow structures was based on tomograms

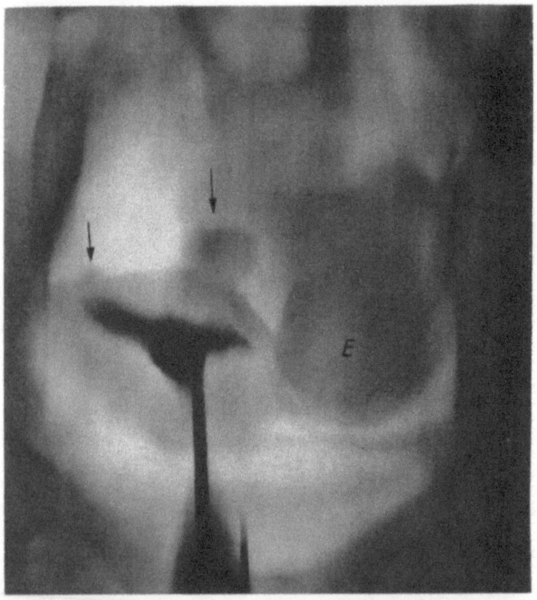

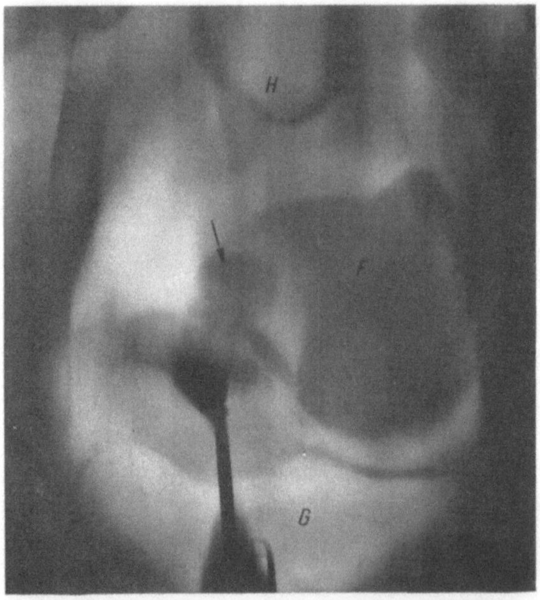

74

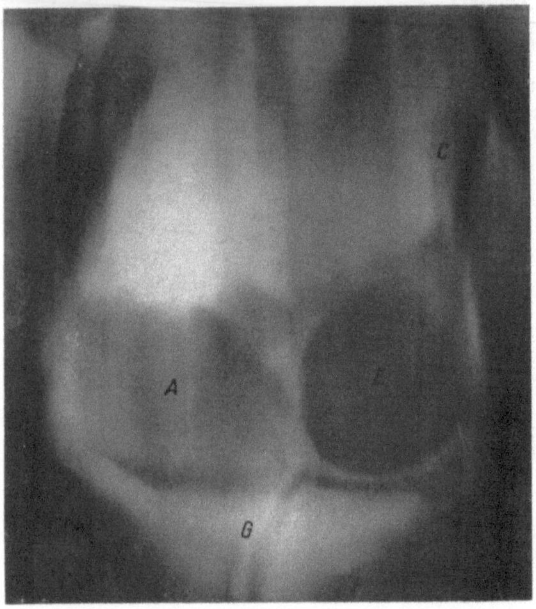

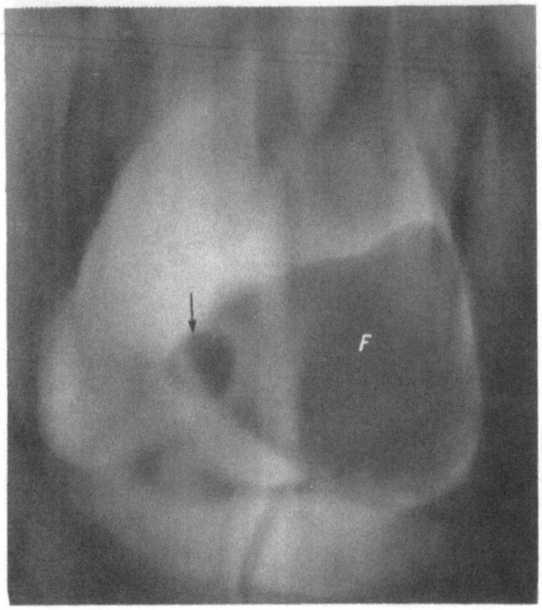

76

Abb. 71—76: Die *Tomogramme* zeigen in 4 cm bis 8 cm Tiefe drei subseröse Myome auf der dem Tumor zugekehrten Hinterwand des Uterus. Die *Salpingographie* ergibt einen durchgängigen linken Eileiter. Der Tubenverlauf vor dem Tumor ist in den ventralen Schichtebenen gut zu unterscheiden. Das Kontrastmittel fließt in die Bauchhöhle ein und verteilt sich zwischen Darmschlingen. Rechts im uterinen Tubenabschnitt Stop der Kontrastmittelfüllung bei Zustand nach Salpingoophorektomie

Abb. 75 und 76 zeigen Tomogramme ohne Hysterosalpingographie. Der Vergleich mit Abb. 70—74 ergibt, daß durch die Kombination von Pneumopelvigraphie, Hysterosalpingographie und Tomographie eine Erweiterung der diagnostischen Aussage gelingt, weil insbesondere der Ausschluß einer Saktosalpinx möglich wird

A = Corpus uteri; B = Isthmus tubae uterinae; C = Ampulla tubae uterinae; D = Kontrastmittel im Cavum peritonei; E = Ovarialzyste, intraligamentärer Teil; F = Ovarialzyste, extraligamentär dorsal gelegener Teil; G = Harnblase; H = Rectum; → = 3 subseröse Myomknollen, in verschiedenen Schichtebenen dargestellt

Figs. 71—76 are *tomograms*, 4 cm through 8 cm in depths, showing three subserous myomas on the tumor-oriented posterior uterine wall; *salpingography* reveals patency of left oviduct; tubes in front ot tumor are readily distinguishable in the ventral tomographic planes; contrast medium flows into peritoneal cavity and is distributed between intestinal loops; contrast medium flow is stopped in uterine tubal section, right, due to condition after salpingo-oophorectomy

Figs. 75 and 76 are tomograms without hysterosalpingography and suggest, by comparison with Figs. 70—74, that by combining pneumopelvigraphy, hysterosalpingography, and tomography more information will be available for diagnosis, mainly on account of the possibility to rule out sactosalpinx

A = corpus uteri; B = isthmus tubae uterinae; C = ampulla tubae uterinae; D = contrast medium in peritoneal cavity; E = ovarian cyst, intraligamentous part; F = ovarian cyst, extraligamentous part in dorsal position; G = urinary bladder; H = rectum; → = three subserous myoma bulbs represented in different tomographic planes

Verlauf: Bei der Laparotomie wird der Röntgenbefund bestätigt. Links besteht eine faustgroße Teerzyste des Ovars, die nach Punktion unter Erhaltung eines normal großen Restovars reseziert wird. Der Uterus zeigt eine erbsgroße und zwei weitere subseröse Myomknollen, die enukleiert werden
Histologischer Befund: Zystenwand mit Haematom in bindegewebiger Organisation, Corpus-luteum-Zyste, Fibromyome mit regressiven Veränderungen

Course: The radiological findings were confirmed by laparotomy which revealed, on the left, the presence of a fist-size ovarian chocolate cyst that was punctured and removed, with a residual ovary of normal size left; one pea-size and two subserous myoma bulbs were exhibited by the uterus and enucleated
Histological finding: Cyst wall with hematoma integrated in connective tissue, corpus luteum cyst, fibromyomas with regressive changes

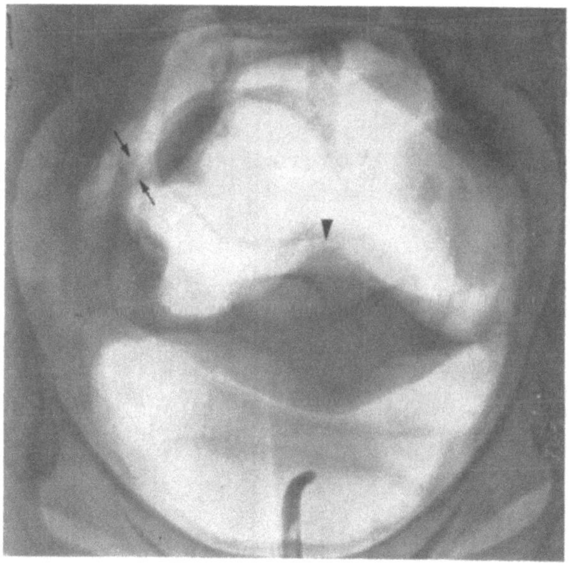

77

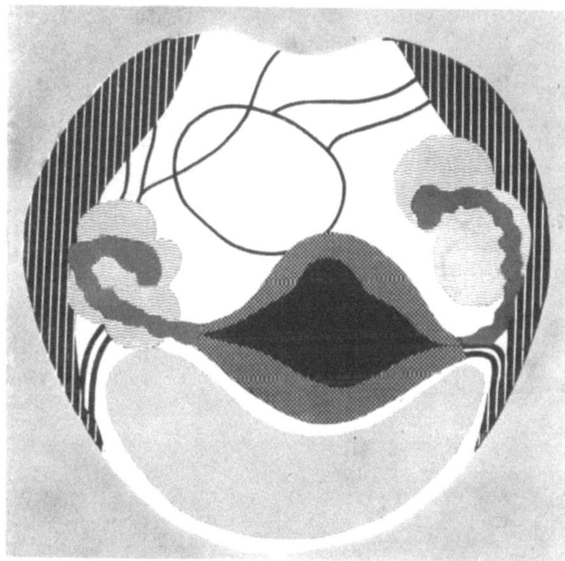

77a

Abb. 77—80
Kleinzystische Degeneration der Ovarien, Uterus myomatosus

32jähr. Patientin mit Zwischenblutungen
Tastbefund: Uterus normal groß, anteflektiert, mobil. Im Bereich der rechten Adnexe hühnereigroßer, der Beckenwand anliegender Tumor
Indikation: Bestimmung der Organzugehörigkeit und Abgrenzung des Tumors
Abb. 77: Auf der *Übersichtsaufnahme* polyzystische Ovarien ohne Vergrößerung, kein Tumor. Breiter Verwachsungsstrang zwischen rechtem Ovar und Rectum (→)
▸ = kleines Myom
Abb. 78—80: Die *Tomogramme* in 6 cm bis 8 cm Tiefe bestätigen den Befund. Der Verwachsungsstrang (→) hat bei der Palpation den Eindruck eines Tumors hervorgerufen
Verlauf: Keine Therapie

Figs. 77—80
Microcystic degeneration of ovaries, uterus myomatosus

Patient, 32, reporting menorrhagia
Palpation finding: Uterus of normal size, anteflexed, movable; hen-egg size tumor adjacent to pelvic wall, localised in right adnexal region
Indication: Identification of tumor-afflicted organ and demarcation of tumor
Fig. 77 is a *standard radiograph* showing polycystic ovaries without enlargement; no tumor discernible; visualisation of broad adhesive chord between right ovary and rectum (→);
▸ = small myoma
Figs. 78—80 are *tomograms*, 6 cm through 8 cm in depths, to confirm the above findings, with the adhesive chord (→) having produced the impression of a tumor, on palpation
Course: No therapy

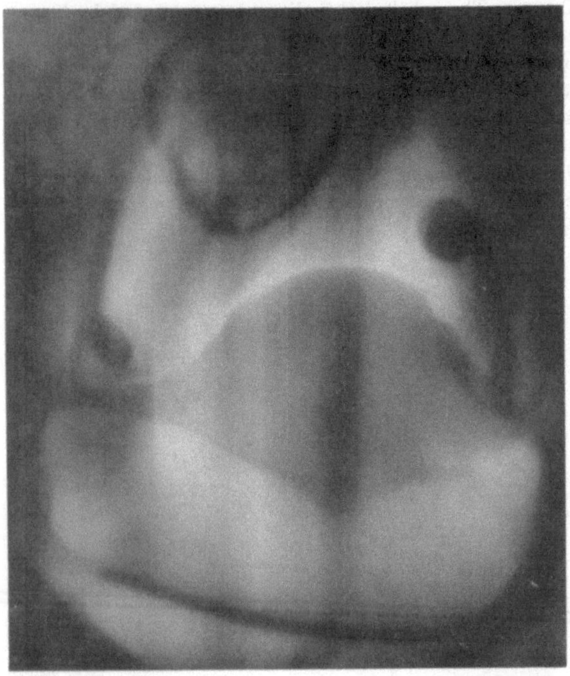

78

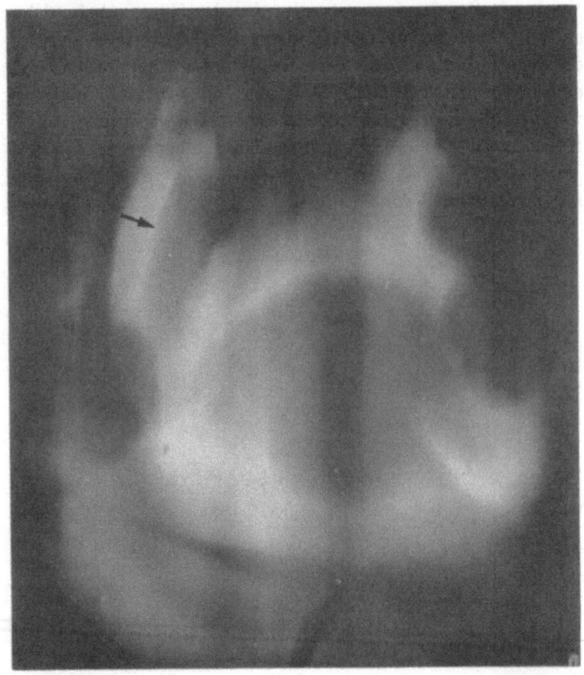

79

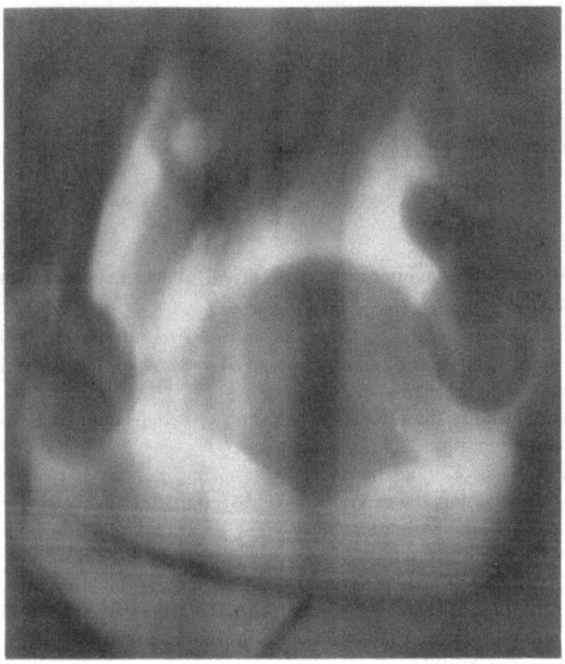

80

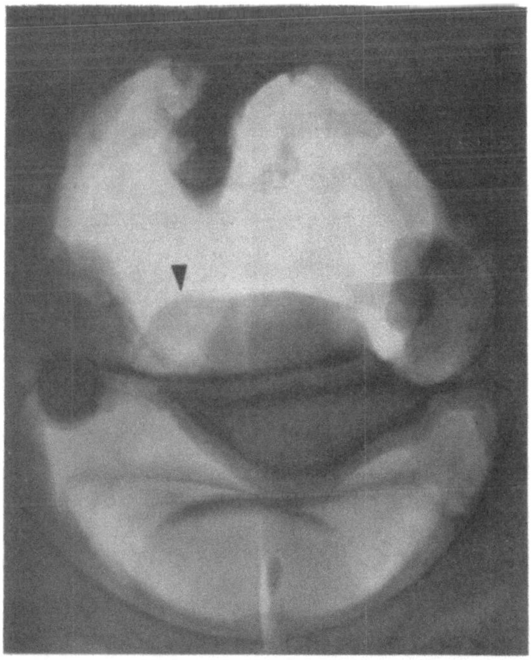

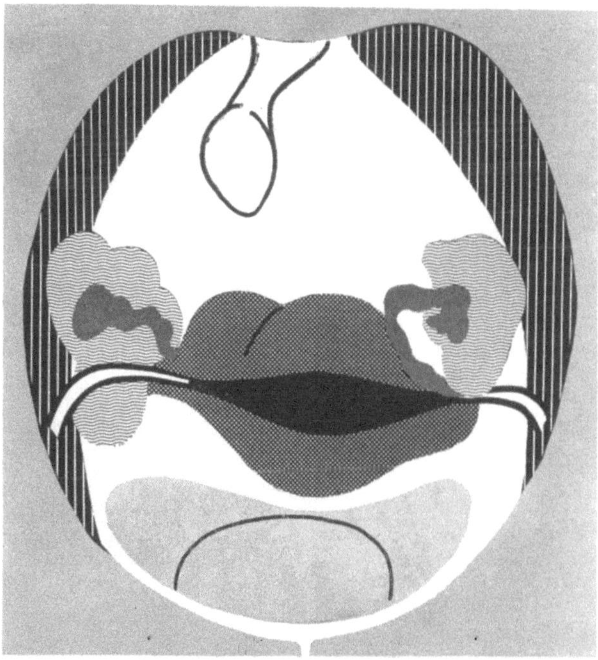

81 a

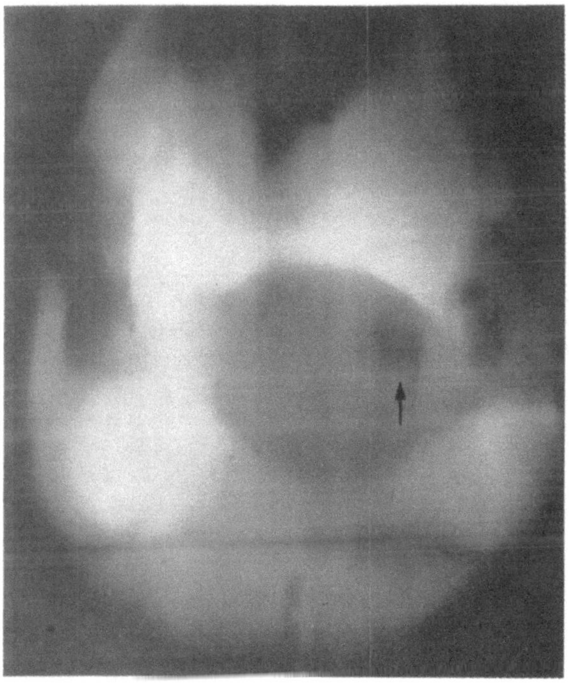

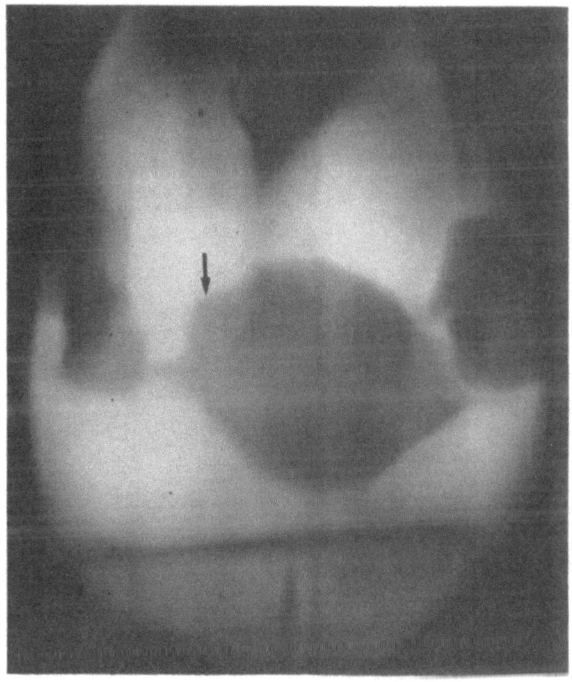

83

Abb. 81–83

Kleinzystische Degeneration der Ovarien, Uterus myomatosus

26jähr. Patientin mit Oligomenorrhoe

Tastbefund: Uterus normal groß, anteflektiert, mobil. Ovarialtumor rechts, dessen Ausdehnung nicht genau festzulegen ist

Indikation: Darstellung und Abgrenzung des Ovarialtumors

Abb. 81: Die *Übersichtsaufnahme* zeigt polyzystische, nicht vergrößerte Ovarien

▸ = Myom

Abb. 82 und 83: Auf den *Schichtbildern* sind zwischen den einzelnen erbsgroßen Zysten Einkerbungen zu sehen, die den Ovarien ein für das Krankheitsbild charakteristisches Aussehen verleihen. Im Corpus uteri eine subseröse Myomknolle rechts und ein weiteres intramurales Myom links (↓↑)

Figs. 81–83

Microcystic degeneration of ovaries, uterus myomatosus

Patient, 26, reporting oligomenorrhea

Palpation finding: Uterus of normal size, anteflexed, and movable; ovarian tumor on the right with no accurate assessment of expanse

Indication: Visualisation and demarcation of ovarian tumor

Fig. 81 is a *standard radiograph* showing polycystic, unenlarged ovaries

▸ = myoma

Figs. 82 and 83 are *tomograms* showing indentations between the pea-size cysts to give the ovaries an appearance characteristic of the disease; demonstrated in the corpus uteri are a subserous myoma bulb, right, and an additional intramural myoma, left (↑↓)

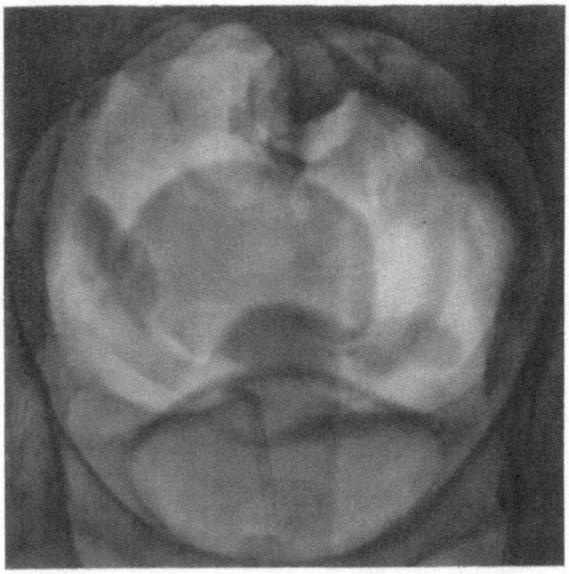

84

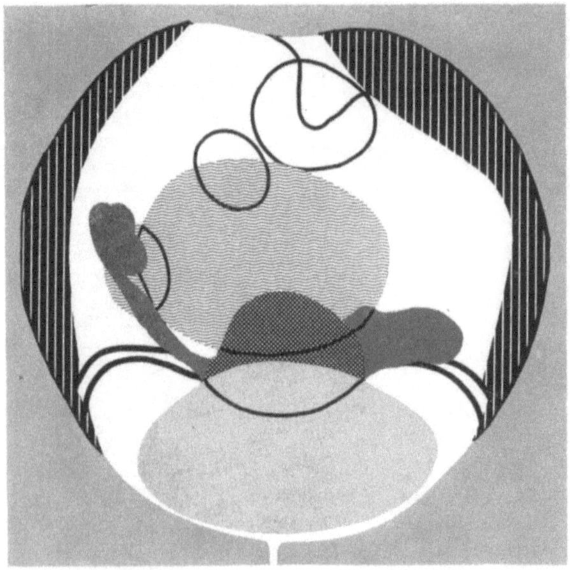

84 a

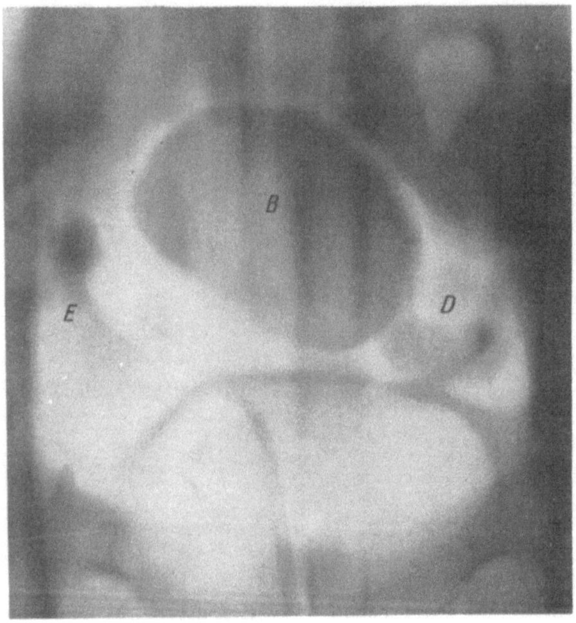

85

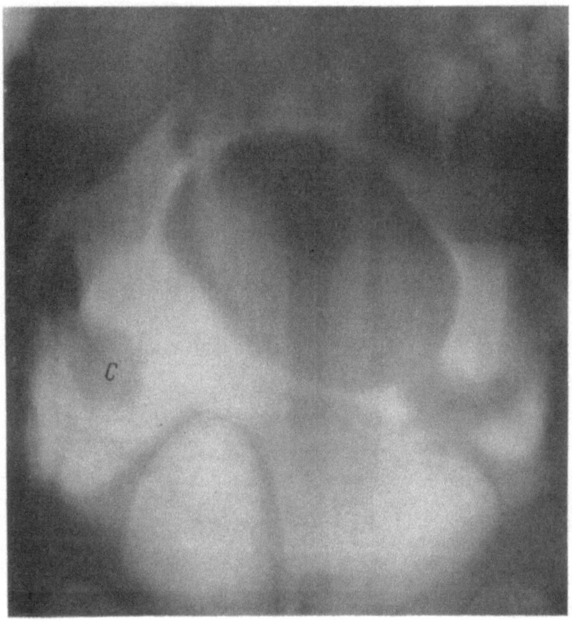

86

Abb. 84—88
Saktosalpinx, Ovarialtumor
Hydrosalpinx, Ovarialfibrom

57jähr. Patientin mit Gewichtsabnahme und Schmerzen im Unterbauch
Tastbefund: Links dorsal hühnereigroßer derber Tumor, Uterus atrophisch, rechte Adnexe frei.
Indikation: Bestimmung der Organzugehörigkeit des Tumors
Abb. 84: Auf der *Übersichtsaufnahme* projizieren sich Uterus und Tumorschatten aufeinander. Es läßt sich nicht entscheiden, ob die Geschwulst von den linken oder rechten Adnexen, oder vom Uterus ausgeht. Links und rechts sind je eine unregelmäßig geformte längliche Verschattung dargestellt, die man der Gestalt und Lage nach für atrophische Ovarien halten kann. Bei der Tomographie stellt sich jedoch heraus, daß diese Deutung nur für die rechte Seite zutrifft. Links liegt eine Saktosalpinx vor. Der palpierte Tumor gehört zum linken Ovar und erstreckt sich hinter dem Uterus nach rechts
Abb. 85—87: *Tomogramme* in 5 cm bis 7 cm Tiefe
A = Uterus; B = Tumor des linken Ovars (Fibrom); C = rechtes Ovar; D = Hydrosalpinx links; E = rechte Tube
Verlauf: Vaginale Totalexstirpation des Uterus mit beiden Adnexen
Abb. 88: Operationspräparat
A = Uterus; B = Tumor des linken Ovars (Fibrom); C = rechtes Ovar; D = Hydrosalpinx links; E = rechte Tube

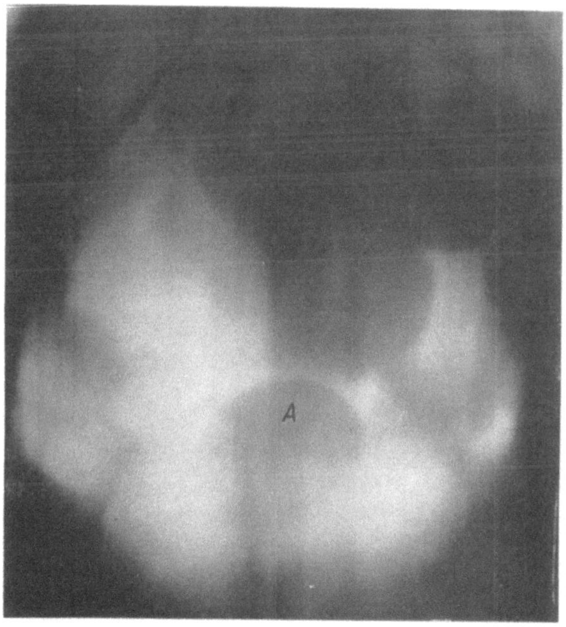

87

Figs. 84—88
Sactosalpinx, ovarian tumor
Hydrosalpinx, ovarian fibroma

Patient, 57, reporting loss of weight and pain in lower abdomen
Palpation finding: Left-dorsal presence of hen-egg size hard tumor, uterus atrophic, right adnexum unaffected
Indication: Identification of tumor-afflicted organ
Fig. 84 is a *standard radiograph* with a superimposed projection of the uterus and tumor shadow, no safe assessment is possible as to whether the tumor originates from the left or right adnexum or the uterus; one longish shadow of irregular shape is visualised on both the left and right, with their forms and positions offering themselves for interpretation as atrophic ovaries; tomography, however, revealed that such interpretation fell true only for the right side, whereas the left-side finding was a sactosalpinx; the palpated tumor was localised at the left ovary and extended dextrad behind the uterus
Figs. 85—87 are *tomograms*, 5 cm to 7 cm in depths, showing A = uterus; B = tumor of the left ovary (fibroma); C = right ovary; D = hydrosalpinx, left; E = right tube
Course: Vaginal hysterectomy, including removal of either adnexum
Fig. 88: Surgical specimen
A = uterus; B = tumor of the left ovary (fibroma); C = right ovary; D = hydrosalpinx, left; E = right tube

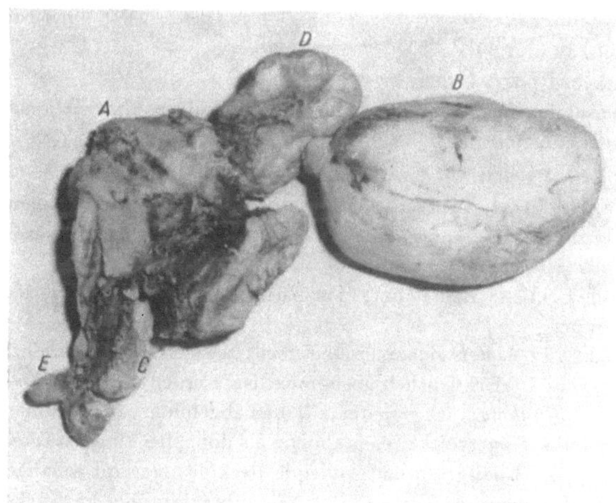

88

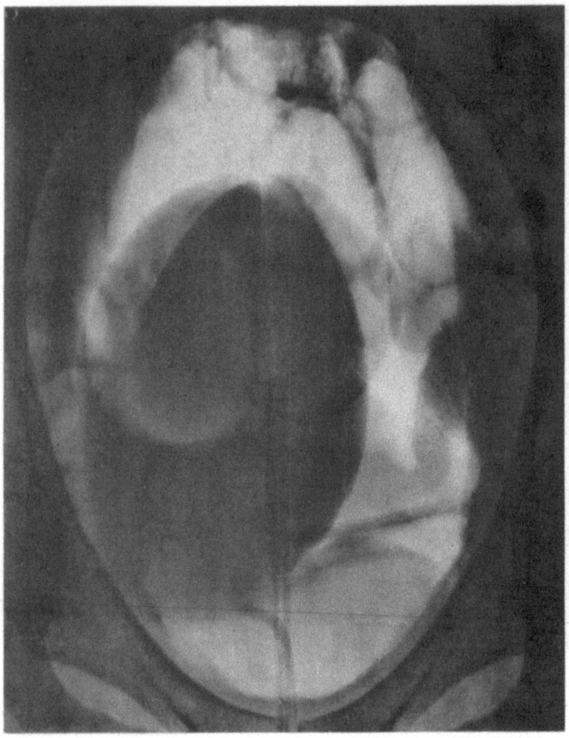

89

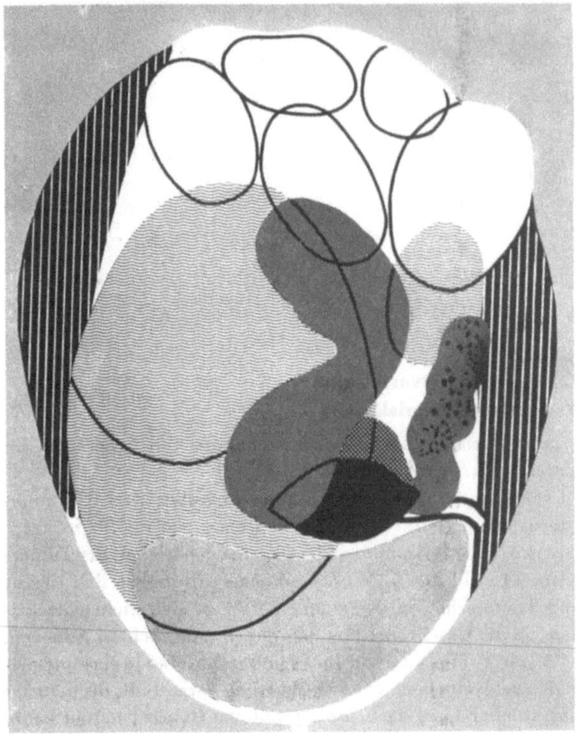

89 a

Abb. 89 und 90

Saktosalpinx, Ovarialzyste

Pyosalpinx bei Tubentuberkulose, multilokuläres Cystadenoma pseudomucinosum

22jähr. Patientin mit primärer Amenorrhoe

Tastbefund: Zystischer Tumor, dicht neben und hinter dem Uterus gelegen, stark dolent. Linke Adnexe narbig verdickt, nicht schmerzhaft

Indikation: Beurteilung der Adnexe und Darstellung des Tumors

Abb. 89: Außer einem großen rechtsseitigen Ovarialtumor, der vom Uterus deutlich abgegrenzt ist, werden auf der *Übersichtsaufnahme* stark erweiterte Tuben abgebildet. Ihr Kaliber hat links Fingerstärke, rechts mehr als doppelte Fingerstärke. Der linke Eileiter enthält multiple fleckförmige und schalige Verkalkungen. Außerdem bestehen strangförmige Verwachsungen des Tumors mit der Beckenwand und beider Tuben mit dem Darm

Verlauf: Oophorektomie rechts und ampulläre Tubenresektion bds. unter Streptomycinschutz. Aus beiden Tuben entleeren sich käsige Massen

Abb. 90: Operationspräparat

1 = Zyste des rechten Ovars

2 = Pyosalpinx links

3 = Pyosalpinx rechts

Histologischer Befund: In den Eileitern zahlreiche verkäsende, links verkalkte Nekrosen mit randständigen Epitheloidzellen, Tuberkulom in der linken Tube

Figs. 89 and 90

Sactosalpinx, ovarian cyst

Pyosalpinx concomitant with tubal tuberculosis, multilocular pseudomucinous cystadenoma

Patient, 22, afflicted primarily with amenorrhea

Palpation finding: Cystic tumor localised closely adjacent to and behind uterus, highly dolent; left adnexum scarred and thickened, but no pains

Indication: Assessment of adnexa, visualisation of tumor

Fig. 89 is a *standard radiograph* showing, on the right, large ovarian tumor, demarcated sharply from uterus, and strongly dilated tubes, their diameters being finger thickness, on the left, and more than double finger thickness, on the right; multiple speckled and shell-like calcifications are present in the left oviduct; funicular adhesions are recorded for the tumor with the pelvic wall and for either tube with the intestine

Course: Oophorectomy on the right and ampullary salpingectomy with streptomycin shield on either side; caseous matter discharged from either tube

Fig. 90: Surgical specimen

1 = cyst of the right ovary

2 = pyosalpinx, left

3 = pyosalpinx, right

Histological finding: Presence of numerous caseating necroses in the oviducts, on the left calcification with marginal epitheloid cells; tuberculoma in the left tube

Organdifferenzierung gelingt mit Hilfe der Tomographie (Abb. 84—88). Auch von der simultan durchgeführten Hysterosalpingographie kann man in manchen Fällen eine Befunderweiterung erwarten. Der Kombination von Pneumopelvigraphie, Hysterosalpingographie und Tomographie sollte deshalb nach Möglichkeit der Vorzug gegeben werden.
Kalkeinlagerungen in den Tuben sind ein wichtiger Hinweis auf eine Adnextuberkulose. Die Kalkschatten werden zwar auch auf gewöhnlichen Übersichtsaufnahmen des Beckens abgebildet, ihre genaue Lokalisation im Adnexbereich gelingt aber nur mit Hilfe des Pneumopelvigramms (Abb. 89 und 90).

5.1.4. *Postoperative Verwachsungen*

Tumorverdächtige Tastbefunde nach Operationen werden mitunter durch massive Verwachsungen der Genitalien mit dem Darm verursacht. Ein rascher Befundwechsel kann dabei die Deutung besonders schwierig gestalten. Die Pneumopelvigraphie gibt in solchen Fällen zuverlässig darüber Auskunft, ob der palpierte Tumor durch adhärente Darmschlingen nur vorgetäuscht wird oder einem morphologischen Substrat der Genitalien entspricht.
Bei *Verwachsungen des Uterus und der Adnexe mit dem Intestinum* bleiben Darmschlingen trotz vorschriftsmäßiger Lagerung der Patientin im kleinen Becken fixiert. Liegen ausgedehnte Adhäsionen vor, so werden die inneren Genitalien von den verwachsenen Darmschlingen oft vollständig umhüllt. Auf Übersichtsaufnahmen ist in solchen Fällen eine Differenzierung kaum möglich. Mit Hilfe der Tomographie gelingt dagegen fast regelmäßig eine Klärung (Abb. 91—94).

pyosalpinx, *hematosalpinx* or *tubal hydrops*. Additional problems will be added to the analysis of a radiograph as a result of distortion caused by perisalpingitis. A more successful differentiation of the affected organ will be possible by means of tomography (Figs. 84—88). Under certain circumstances, improved findings can be expected also from simultaneous hysterosalpingography. Whenever possible, preference should, therefore, be given to the combination of pneumopelvigraphy with hysterosalpingography and tomography.
Calcareous infiltration of the tubes is an important indication to the presence of adnexal tuberculosis. While calcareous patches are represented also by ordinary radiographs of the pelvis, their accurate localisation within the adnexal region requires the use of a pneumopelvigram (Figs. 89 and 90).

5.1.4. *Postoperative adhesions*

Postsurgical palpation findings that give rise to tumor suspicion are sometimes caused by massive adhesions of the genitals with the intestine. Such findings are subject to considerable change, which adds to the difficulty of interpretation. In such cases, safe information will be obtained from pneumopelvigraphy as to wether the palpated tumor is merely simulated by adherent intestinal loops or based on a morphological substrate of the genitals. In the event of *adhesion of both the uterus and adnexa with the intestines*, some intestinal loops will remain fixed to the minor pelvis even though the patient is positioned properly. In cases of larger adhesions, the internal genitals will often be encased entirely by the adherent intestinal loops. In such cases, differentitation will hardly be possible on the basis of standard radiographs, while elucidation will be achieved in almost all cases by means of tomography (Figs. 91—94).

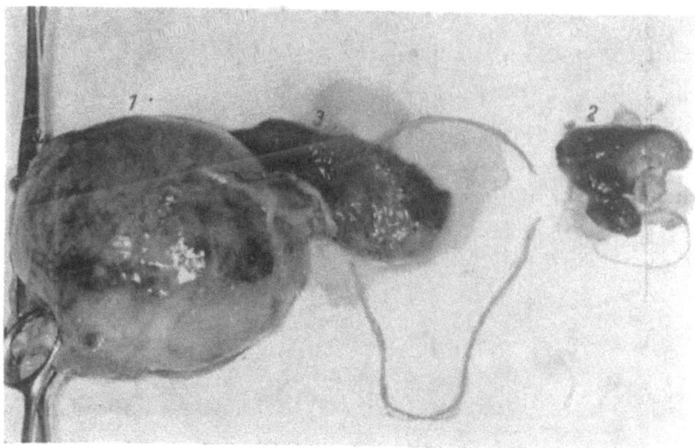

90

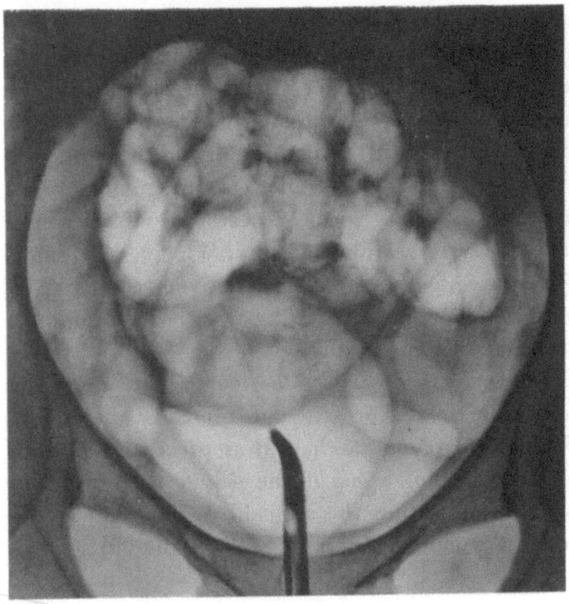

91

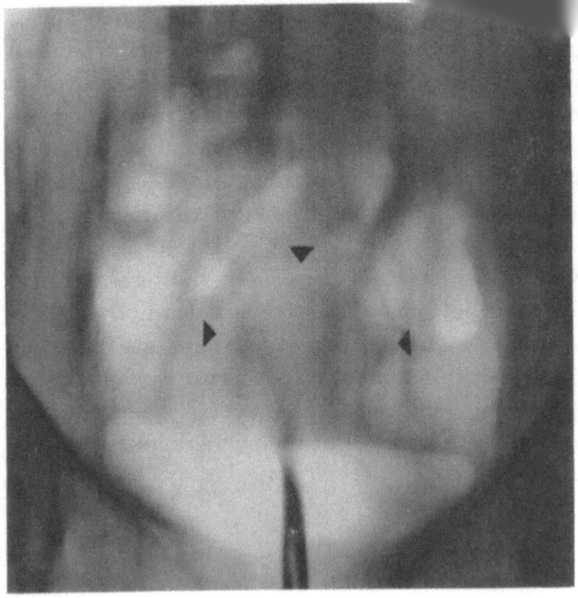

92

Abb. 91 und 92
Postoperative Darmverwachsungen
Zustand nach 3maliger Laparotomie

38jähr. adipöse Patientin mit Schmerzen im Unterbauch
Tastbefund: Der Uterus imponiert vergrößert, die Adnexe sind nicht sicher palpabel
Indikation: Nachweis oder Ausschluß eines Uterus myomatosus und Differenzierung von Verwachsungen
Abb. 91: Das kleine Becken ist von Darmschlingen ausgefüllt, die auch nach Beckenhochlagerung fixiert bleiben. Auf der *Übersichtsaufnahme* ist eine Differenzierung der Genitalorgane nicht möglich
Abb. 92: Das *Tomogramm* in 8 cm Tiefe zeigt, daß der Uterus (◂) von Darmschlingen eingehüllt und mit diesen im Bereich seines gesamten Serosaüberzuges verwachsen ist. Kein Uterus myomatosus. Beide Adnexe sind in die massiven Verwachsungen einbezogen

Figs. 91 and 92
Postoperative intestinal adhesions
Condition after three laparotomies

Patient, 38, afflicted with adiposity and reporting pain in lower abdomen
Palpation finding: The uterus appears to be enlarged, with the adnexa not being safely palpable
Indication: Confirmation or ruling out of uterus myomatosus and differentiation of adhesions
Fig. 91 is a *standard radiograph* showing the small pelvis to be filled up with intestinal loops which remain fixed even after elevation of pelvis; differentiation of genital organs impossible
Fig. 92 is a *tomogram*, 8 cm in depth, showing the uterus to be encased (◂) by intestinal loops and adherent to them over the entire region of its serous coat; no uterus myomatosus; both adnexa being involved in massive adhesions

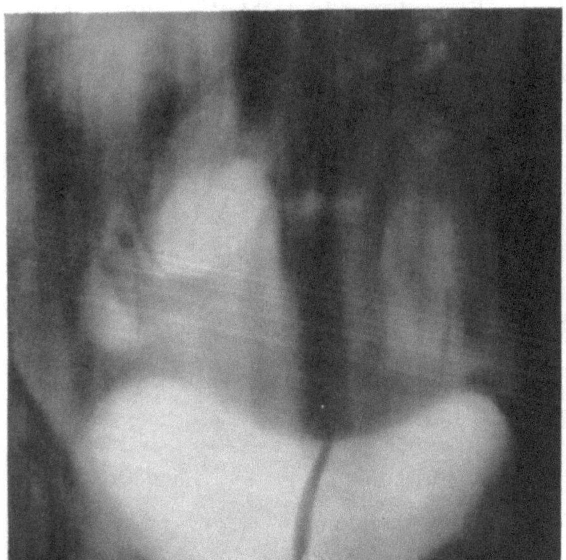

93

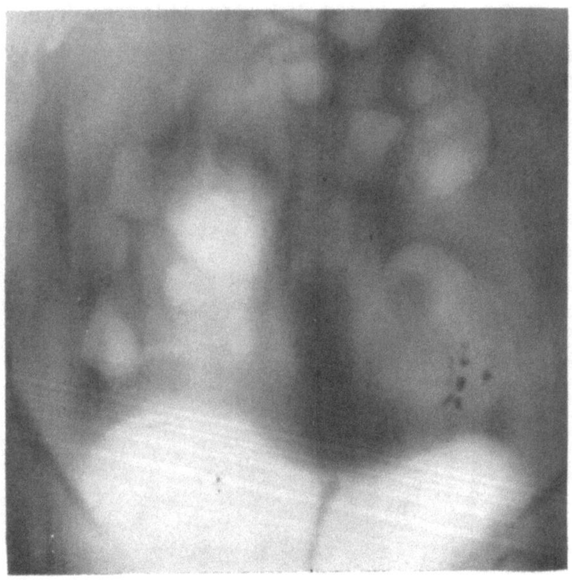

94

...moren

...n der Diagnostik maligner Tumoren des Beckens spielt die Pneumopelvigraphie bei einigen Fragen eine wichtige Rolle. In Verbindung mit der Lymphographie ist sie zur Erkennung von Rezidiven und Metastasen maligner Genitaltumoren und zur Beurteilung des Stadiums maligner Harnblasengeschwülste hervorragend geeignet. Der Wert der Methode liegt in der Darstellung von Tumorpartien, die sich sonst dem Nachweis entziehen. Demgegenüber betrachten wir das unbehandelte Uteruskarzinom und das Rektumkarzinom nicht als Indikationsgebiete, da sich bei diesen Krankheitsbildern mit der Pneumopelvigraphie in der Regel keine wesentliche Befunderweiterung erzielen läßt.

5.2.1. *Rezidive und Metastasen maligner Genitaltumoren*

Die rechtzeitige Erkennung von Tumorrezidiven[1]) nach Radikaloperationen und Bestrahlungen bereitet dem Gynäkologen häufig Schwierigkeiten. Ischialgien, Lymph- oder Blutstauungen an den unteren Extremitäten geben meistens ersten Anlaß zur Verdachtsdiagnose. Diese Symptome sind jedoch für ein Tumorrezidiv oder für retroperitoneale Lymphknotenmetastasen nicht beweisend. Der Palpationsbefund bleibt in vielen Fällen negativ oder zweifelhaft. Nicht nur lokale sondern auch aus-

[1]) Die Bezeichnung „Rezidiv" bezieht sich auf das klinische Geschehen. Pathologisch-anatomisch handelt es sich überwiegend um fortschreitendes Tumorwachstum oder regionale Lymphknotenmetastasen.

Abb. 93 und 94
Postoperative Darmverwachsungen
Zustand nach Oophoro-Salpingektomie links wegen Ovarialcystoms

34jähr. Patientin mit Schmerzen im rechten Unterbauch
Tastbefund: Uterus normal groß, anteflektiert, rechts hühnereigroßer weicher Tumor palpabel. Bei Kontrolluntersuchungen werden unterschiedliche und wechselnde Befunde erhoben. Teils tastet man einen zystischen Tumor, anderenteils derbe strangförmige Adnexe
Indikation: Darstellung des Uterus und der Adnexe zur Klärung des Tastbefundes
Abb. 93 und 94: Die *Tomogramme* in 6 cm und 7 cm Tiefe zeigen ein kleines rechtes Ovar mit erbsgroßer Verkalkung am oberen Pol. Die rechten Adnexe und der Uterus sind auf breiter Fläche mit Darmschlingen verwachsen. Links im Bereich der ektomierten Adnexe fleckförmige Verkalkungen und massive Verwachsungen mit dem Intestinum

5.2. Malignant tumors

Pneumopelvigraphy has proved to play an important role in connection with certain problems related to the diagnosis of malignant tumors of the pelvis. Combined with lymphography, it is a highly efficient method to detect recurrences and metastases of malignant genital tumors and to assess the phases of malignant tumors of the urinary bladder, its suitability being implied mainly in its capacity to represent those tumor sections that would otherwise escape detection. Untreated hysterocarcinoma and untreated carcinoma of the rectum, however, are not considered to be indications, since, as a rule, no essential enlargement of findings may be achieved in such cases by means of pneumopelvigraphy.

5.2.1. *Recurrences and metastases of malignant tumors of the genitals*

Gynecologists often have to face problems regarding the early detection of recurrent tumors[1]) following both radical surgery and irradiation. Ischialgia, lymphostasis or vascular congestion in the lower extremities are frequent findings to give rise to a tentative diagnosis. Such symptoms, however, cannot substantiate the presence of a recurrent tumor or the development of retroperitoneal lymphatic node metastasation. The palpation findings will often remain negative or dubious. Not only localised but

[1]) The term of recurrence is defined with reference to the clinical course. Pathologico-anatomically, it primarily describes progressing tumor growth or localised lymph node metastases.

Figs. 93 and 94
Postoperative intestinal adhesions
Condition after left-side oophoro-salpingectomy for ovarian cystoma

Patient, 34, reporting pain in lower abdomen, right
Palpation finding: Uterus of normal size and anteflexed; soft hen-egg size tumor palpable on the right; differing and changing findings obtained from control checks, with alternating palpation of cystic tumor or hard funicular adnexa
Indication: Visualisation of uterus and adnexa to elucidate palpation findings
Figs. 93 and 94 are *tomograms*, 6 cm and 7 cm in depths, showing on the right small ovary with pea-size calcification at upper pole; right adnexum and uterus with massive adhesions to intestinal loops; speckled calcifications and massive adhesions with intestines on the left, in the region of the removed adnexum

95 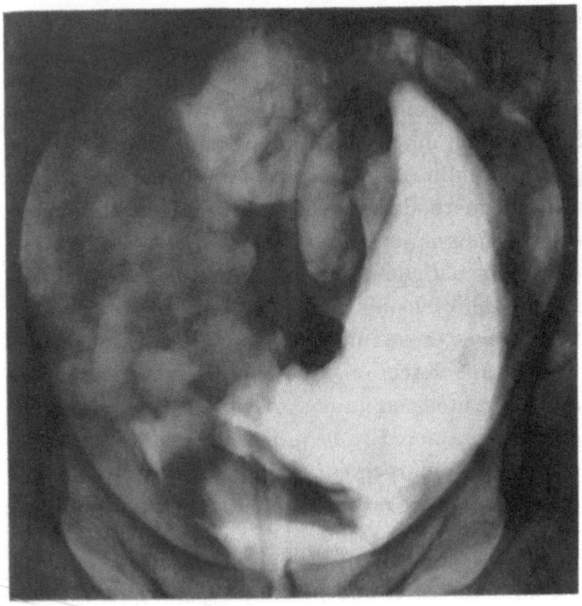

95 a 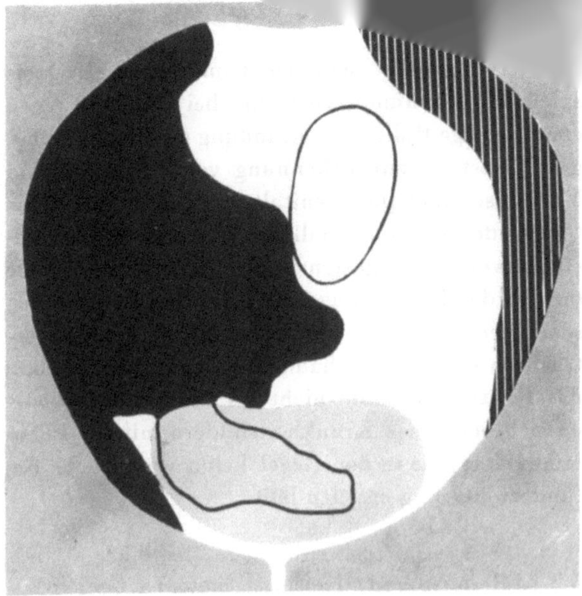

Abb. 95
Rezidiv eines Zervixkarzinoms III

2 Jahre nach Radiumvorbestrahlung, vaginaler Radikaloperation mit Entfernung beider Adnexe und Röntgennachbestrahlung
51jähr. Patientin mit Schwellung des rechten Beines
Tastbefund: Keine tumorverdächtige Resistenz
Indikation: Suche nach hochgelegenem Beckenwandrezidiv
Abb. 95: Großes Tumorrezidiv, das sich mit höckriger Oberfläche weit in das Cavum peritonei vorwölbt, die rechte Bekkenseite verschattet und mit der Harnblasenwand verwachsen ist. Das Rectum ist am Tumor adhaerent
Verlauf: Trotz zytostatischer Behandlung fortschreitendes Tumorwachstum mit Einbruch in die Harnblase, Urämie, Exitus

Fig. 95
Recurrent carcinoma of the cervix, III

Two years after pre-surgical radium treatment, vaginal radical hysterectomy and radical adnexectomy, and postoperative X-ray irradiation
Patient, 51, with swelling of right leg
Palpation finding: No tumor-suspicious resistance
Indication: Search for elevated recurrence at pelvic wall
Fig. 95 shows large recurrent tumor, with its polycyclic surface bulging far into peritoneal cavity, casting shadow on the right side of the pelvis, and adhering to the wall of the urinary bladder; the rectum is found adherent to the tumor
Course: Cytostatic treatment fails to prevent progressive tumor growth; infiltration of urinary bladder; uremia, exitus

gedehnte Tumorrezidive können dem Nachweis entgehen, wenn sie wegen hoher Lage im Becken für den tastenden Finger nicht erreichbar sind. Andererseits lassen sich palpable Rezidive von postoperativen Vernarbungen und radiogenen Fibrosen des Beckenraumes nicht immer unterscheiden. Parametrane Schwielen, ausgedehnte Verwachsungen zwischen Darmschlingen, Netz, Harnblase und Beckenwand führen zu pathologischen Resistenzen, geben Anlaß zu Täuschungen und machen es oft unmöglich, eine sichere Entscheidung zu treffen. In der Bestrahlungsplanung wirken sich diese diagnostischen Unsicherheiten besonders nachteilig aus.

Wie unsere Untersuchungen an Patientinnen mit klinischem Verdacht auf ein Tumorrezidiv ergaben, können mit der Pneumopelvigraphie Rezidive maligner Genitaltumoren viel sicherer erkannt, wesentlich besser lokalisiert und eindeutiger abgegrenzt werden, als es auf Grund manueller Untersuchungen möglich ist. Das untersuchte Krankengut umfaßt überwiegend *Situationen nach vaginalen oder abdominalen Radikaloperationen mit Röntgennachbestrah-*

also extended tumor recurrences may escape detection, if they are not palpable for their elevated position within the pelvis. On the other hand, palpable recurrences cannot always be differentiated from postoperative cicatrisations or radiogenic fibroses of the pelvic cavity. Parametric callosities, extended adhesions located between intestinal loops, omentum, urinary bladder, and pelvic wall often are causes of pathological resistance and simulated phenomena, so that no safe judgement will be possible. Such uncertainties in diagnosis have unfavourable effects mainly when it comes to irradiation planning.

Our own examinations of patients clinically suspicious of recurrent tumors have shown that by pneumopelvigraphy detection, localisation, and delimination of recurrent malignant genital tumors is much safer, more efficient, and consistent than it would be by manual examination. The patients examined include mainly *cases to reflect situations following vaginal or obdominal radical surgery with postoperative irradiation, with recurrent processes of the pelvic wall* following *surgery of carcinomas of the*

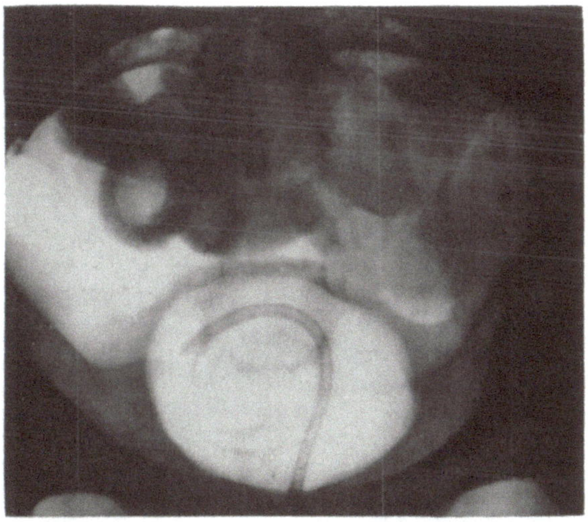

96

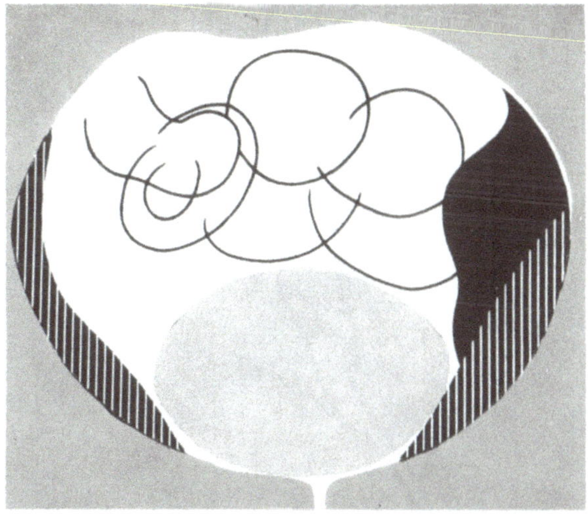

96a

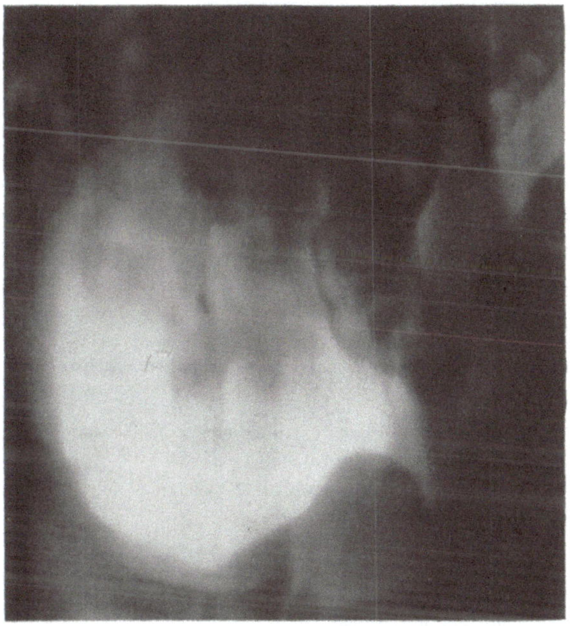

97

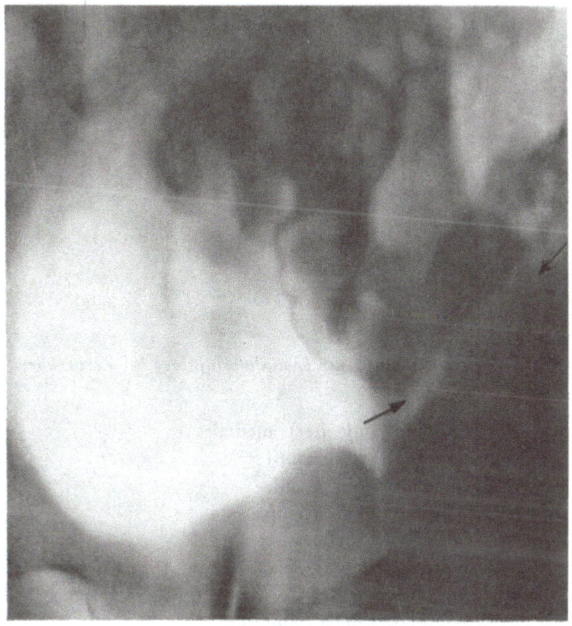

98

Abb. 96—98

Rezidiv eines Zervixkarzinoms II

$1^1/_2$ Jahre nach vaginaler Radikaloperation und Röntgennachbestrahlung

61jähr. Patientin mit Schmerzen im linken Bein.

Tastbefund: Derbe Resistenz im linken Parametrium

Indikation: Feststellung der Tumorausdehnung vor Telekobalttherapie

Abb. 96: Die *Übersichtsaufnahme* läßt eine vom Darm nicht genau abgrenzbare Verschattung an der linken Beckenwand erkennen, die dem Tumorrezidiv entspricht

Abb. 97 und 98: Die *Schichtbilder* zeigen an der linken Beckenwand in großer Ausdehnung vom Os sacrum bis zur Symphyse zahlreiche knollige Verschattungen. Abb. 97 zeigt eine ventrale, Abb. 98 eine mittlere Schichtebene mit Tumorknoten. Das Colon sigmoideum haftet an mehreren Stellen an der Tumoroberfläche, zeigt jedoch keine breitflächigen Verwachsungen. Zwischen Tumor und Darmwand ist ein schmaler Gasspalt nachweisbar (→)

Verlauf: Telekobalttherapie

Figs. 96—98

Recurrent carcinoma of the cervix, II

Condition 18 months after vaginal radical hysterectomy and postoperative X-ray irradiation

Patient, 61, reporting pain in left leg

Palpation finding: Hard resistance in left parametrium

Indication: Identification of tumor extent for decision of tele-cobalt therapy

Fig. 96 is a *standard radiograph* showing at the left pelvic wall a shadow cast apparently by the recurrent tumor and being not safely demarcable from the intestine

Figs. 97 and 98 are *tomograms* showing numerous bulbiform shadows to extend widely at the left pelvic wall from the os sacrum to the symphysis; Fig. 97 shows a ventral and Fig. 98 a central tomographic plane with tumor bulbs; while several parts of the colon sigmoideum are adherent to the tumor surface, no massive adhesions are discernible; a narrow gas gap is detectable between the tumor and intestinal wall (→)

Course: Tele-cobalt therapy

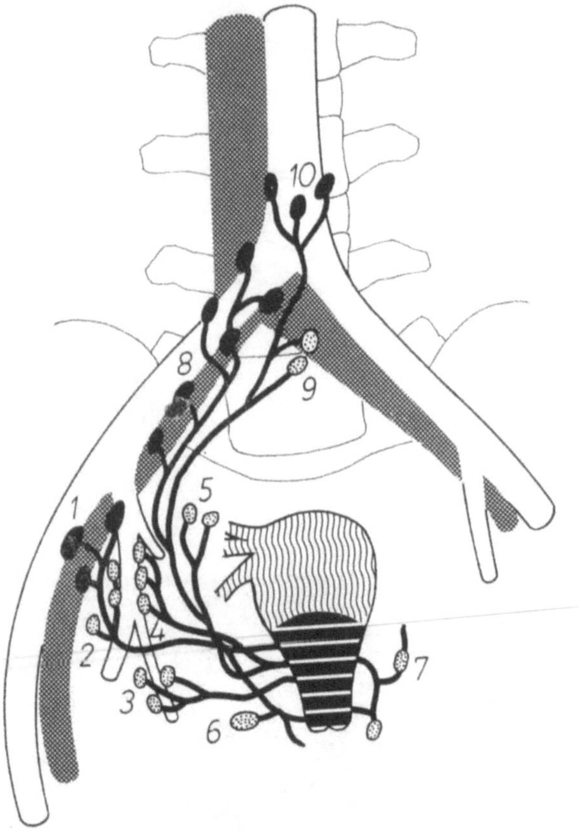

99a

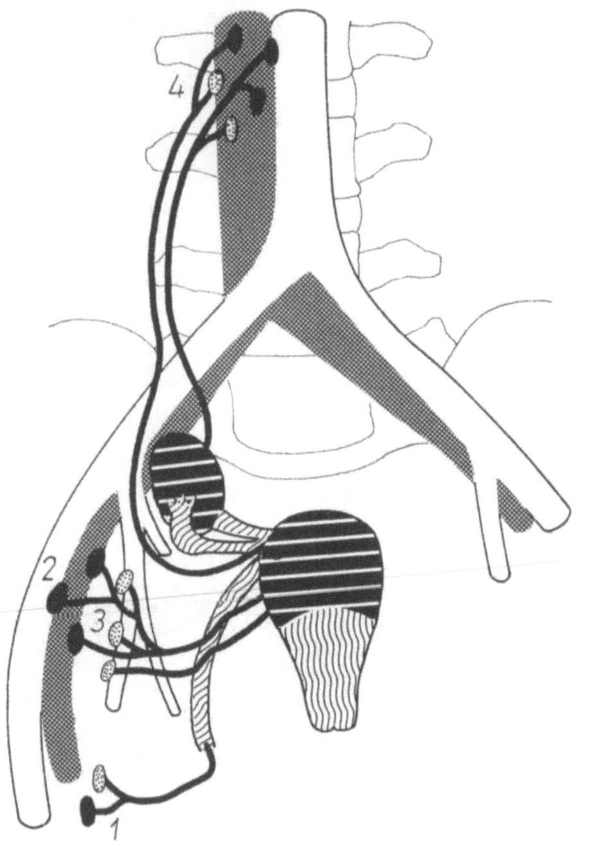

99b

Abb. 99a
Schematische Darstellung der Lymphabflußwege bei Zervixkarzinom

1 = Nodi lymphatici iliaci ext. mediales
2 = Nodi lymphatici obturatorii
3 = Nodi lymphatici glutaei inf.
4 = Nodi lymphatici glutaei sup.
5 = Nodi lymphatici sacrales
6 = Nodi lymphatici paravesicales
7 = Nodi lymphatici rectales
8 = Nodi lymphatici iliaci communes
9 = Nodi lymphatici subaortici
10 = Nodi lymphatici aortici

Schwarz = lymphographisch darstellbare Lymphknoten
Punktiert = lymphographisch nicht darstellbare Lymphknoten

Fig. 99a
Diagram of lymphatic discharge tracts in patients afflicted with carcinoma of the cervix

1 = nodi lymphatici iliaci ext. mediales
2 = nodi lymphatici obturatorii
3 = nodi lymphatici glutaei inf.
4 = nodi lymphatici glutaei sup.
5 = nodi lymphatici sacrales
6 = nodi lymphatici paravesicales
7 = nodi lymphatici rectales
8 = nodi lymphatici iliaci communes
9 = nodi lymphatici subaortici
10 = nodi lymphatici aortici

Black = lymphatic nodes demonstrable by lymphography
Dotted = lymphatic nodes not demonstrable by lymphography

Abb. 99b
Schematische Darstellung der Lymphabflußwege bei Korpus- und Ovarialkarzinom

1 = Nodi lymphatici inguinales superficiales
2 = Nodi lymphatici iliaci externi mediales
3 = Nodi lymphatici obturatorii
4 = Nodi lymphatici aortici

Schwarz = lymphographisch darstellbare Lymphknoten
Punktiert = lymphographisch nicht darstellbare Lymphknoten

Fig. 99b
Diagram of lymphatic discharge tracts in patients afflicted with corpus and ovarian carcinomas

1 = nodi lymphatici inguinales superficiales
2 = nodi lymphatici iliaci externi mediales
3 = nodi lymphatici obturatorii
4 = nodi lymphatici aortici

Black = lymphatic nodes demonstrable by lymphography
Dotted = lymphatic nodes not demonstrable by lymphography

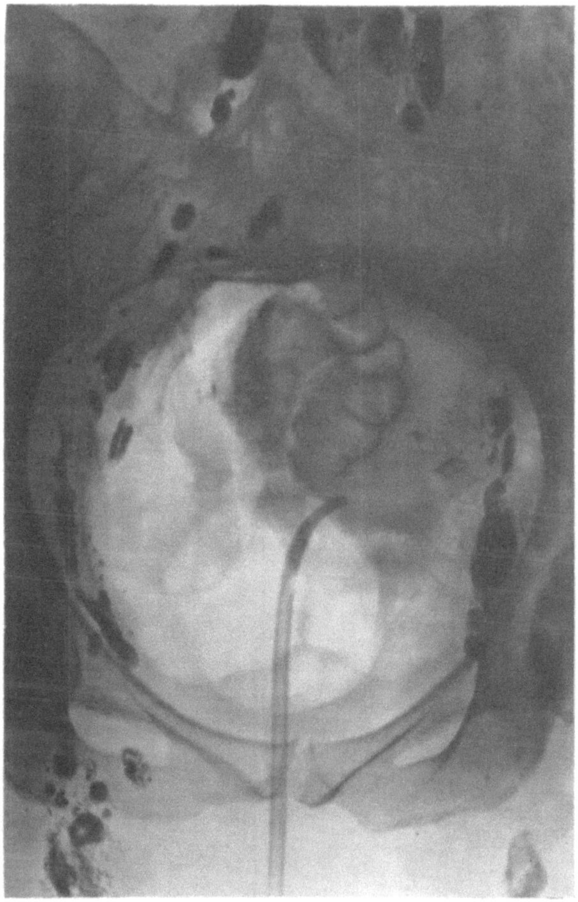

100

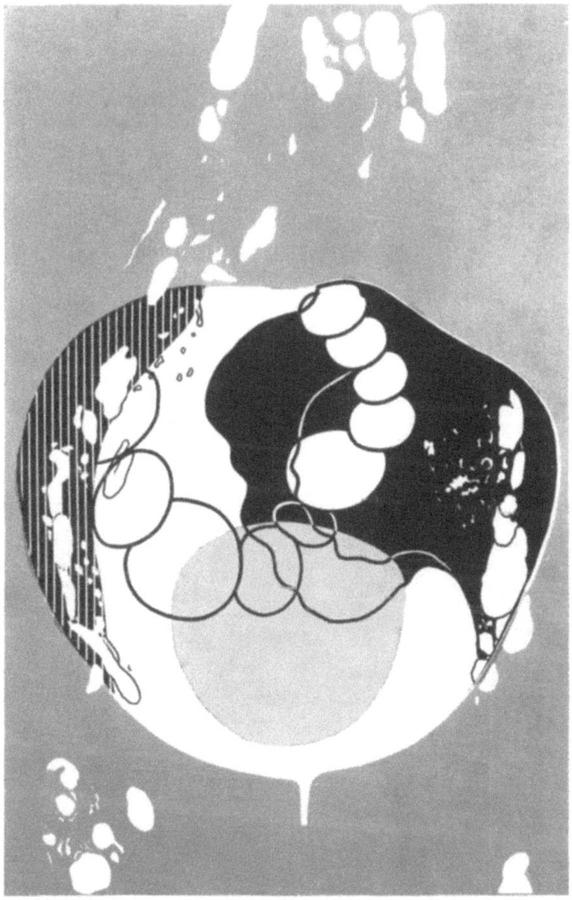

100a

Abb. 100–102

Rezidiv eines Zervixkarzinoms II

1 Jahr nach Radiumvorbestrahlung, vaginaler Radikaloperation ohne Adnexe und Röntgennachbestrahlung

38jähr. Patientin mit Ischialgie, Miktionsbeschwerden und röntgenologisch „stummer Niere" links

Tastbefund: Parametrium beiderseits derb infiltriert, links knotig mit Einengung des Rectum

Indikation: Suche nach weiteren Metastasen, *Kombination mit Lymphographie*

Abb. 100: *Übersichtsaufnahme.* Tumorrediziv links, das sich weit in den Beckenraum vorwölbt. Massive Lymphknoteninfiltration in der Basis des Beckenwandrezidivs, Füllungsausfall, Vergrößerung und Konglomeratbildung der Nodi lymph. iliac. comm.

Abb. 101 und 102: *Schichtaufnahmen* in 5 cm und 7 cm Tiefe. Große polyzyklisch begrenzte Verschattung im kleinen Becken links durch Tumorknoten. Das Colon sigmoideum wird durch die Geschwulst verdrängt und ist an deren Oberfläche abhärent

Verlauf: Telekobalttherapie, 6 Monate später nach fortschreitender Tumorausbreitung Exitus

Figs. 100–102

Recurrent carcinoma of the cervix, II

Condition one year after presurgical radium treatment, vaginal radical hysterectomy, without removal of adnexa, and postsurgical X-ray irradiation

Patient, 38, with ischialgia, micturition difficulties, and left kidney not responsive to urography

Palpation finding: Hard bilateral infiltration of parametrium, bulbiform phenomena on the left accompanied by narrowing of rectum

Indication: Search for additional metastases, combination with lymphography

Fig. 100 is a *standard radiograph* showing, on the left recurrent tumor bulging widely into pelvic cavity; massive infiltration of lymphatic nodes in the base area of the pelvic wall recurrence; stop of filling; enlargement and conglomeration of nodi lymphatici iliaci communes

Figs. 101 and 102 are *tomograms*, 5 cm and 6 cm in depths, showing in the small pelvis large (left) shadow of polycyclic bordering and caused by tumor bulb; the colon sigmoideum is found to be displaced by the tumor and adherent to its surface

Course: Tele-cobalt therapy, exitus after six months following to progressive tumor proliferation

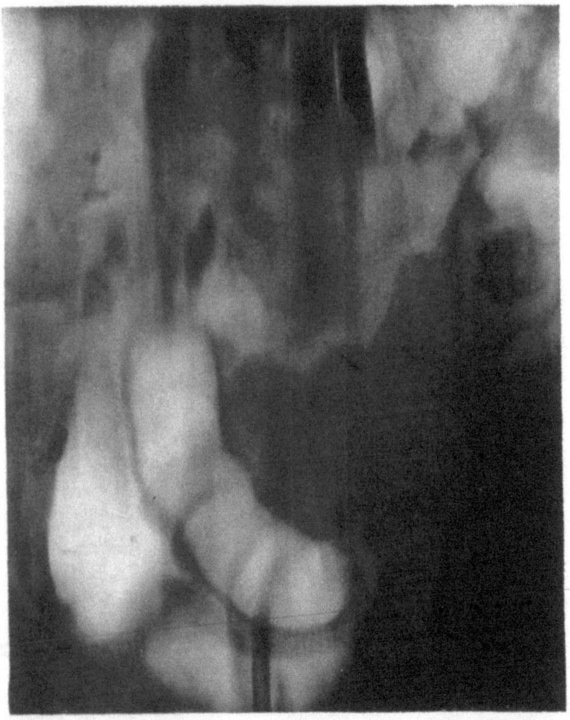

101

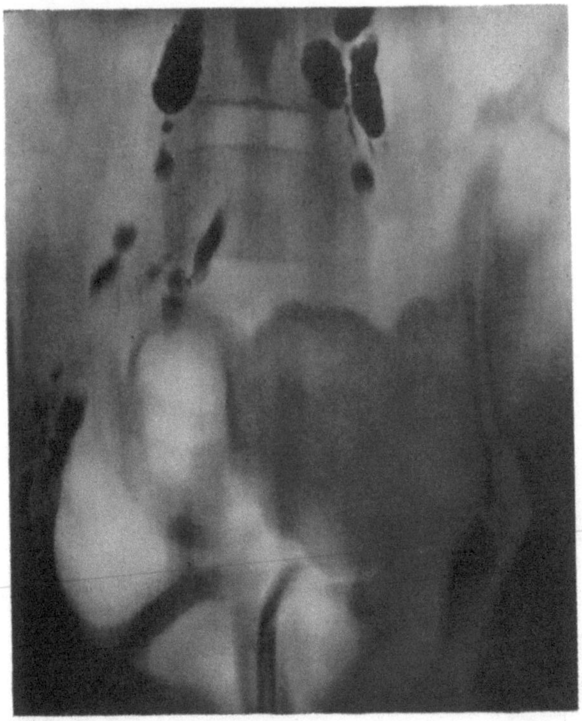

102

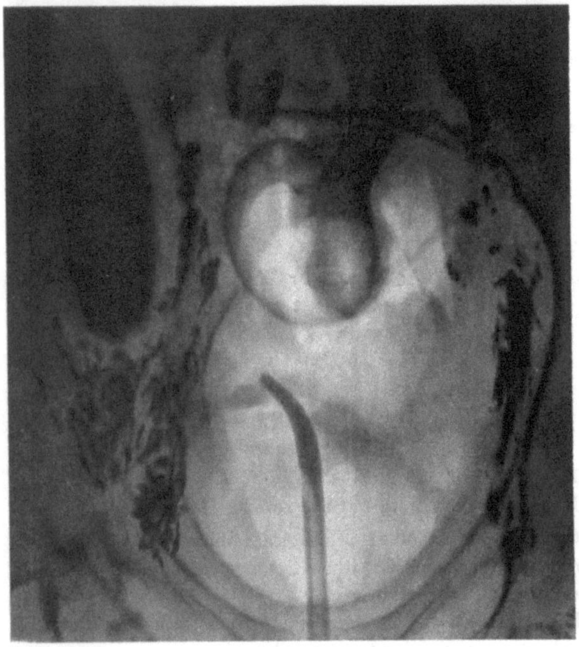

103

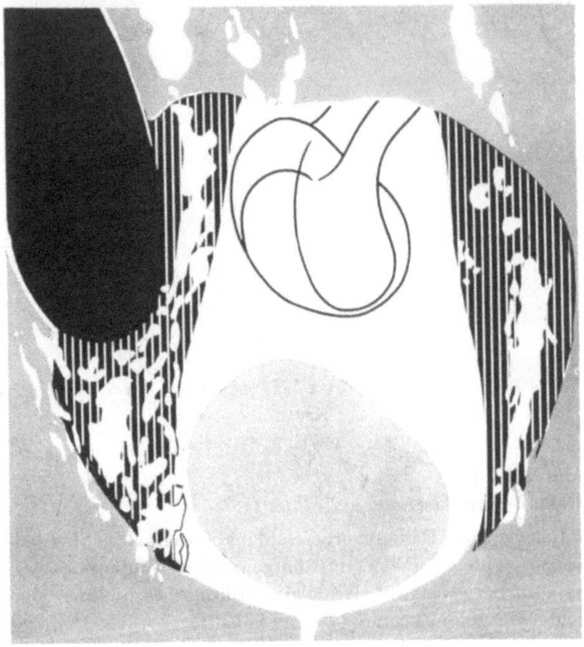

103 a

Abb. 103

Rezidiv eines Zervixkarzinoms II

7 Monate nach vaginaler Radikaloperation ohne Adnexe
41jähr. Patientin mit rechtsseitiger Ischialgie
Tastbefund: Derbe Resistenz auf der rechten Seite
Indikation: Tumornachweis und Suche nach weiteren Metastasen, *Kombination mit Lymphographie*
Abb. 103: Vorwölbung eines ausgedehnten Tumorschattens an der rechten Beckenwand. Füllungsabbrüche von Lymphgefäßen und Extravasate an der Tumorbegrenzung, Darstellung von Kollateralgefäßen in der Tumorumgebung
Verlauf: Telekobalttherapie

Fig. 103

Recurrent carcinoma of the cervix, II

Seven months after vaginal radical hysterectomy, without removal of adnexa
Patient, 41, with ischialgia on the right
Palpation finding: Hard resistance on the right
Indication: Confirmation of tumor and search for additional metastases; *combination with lymphography*
Fig. 103 shows bulging of extended tumor shadow on right pelvic wall; filling stopped at lymphatic vessels, points of extravasation along tumor bordering; visualisation of collateral vessels in region surrounding the tumor
Course: Tele-cobalt therapy

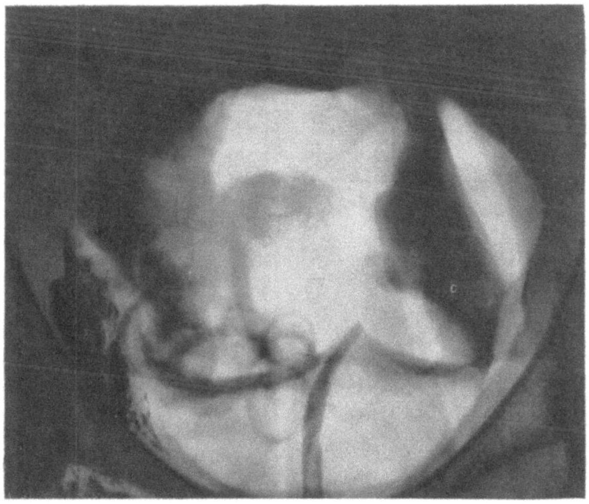

104

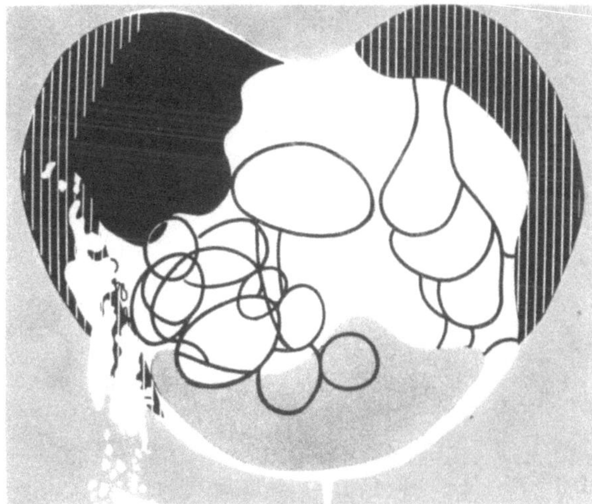

104 a

Abb. 104
Rezidiv eines Zervixkarzinoms II

5 Jahre nach vaginaler Radikaloperation und Röntgennachbestrahlung
56jähr. Patientin mit Schwellung des rechten Beines
Tastbefund: Flache, derbe Resistenz an der rechten Beckenwand
Indikation: Differenzierung zwischen Tumorrezidiv und Fibrose. *Kombination mit Lymphographie*
Abb. 104: Polyzyklische Verschattung im kleinen Becken rechts durch Tumorknoten eines Beckenwandrezidivs. Füllungsabbruch der Lymphgefäße mit Kontrastmittelstop und Kontrastmittelextravasaten, Füllungsausfall der Nodi lymph. iliac. ext. und comm. in der Tumorbasis. Ausgedehnte Verwachsungen zwischen Darm, Harnblase und Beckenwand
Verlauf: Telekobalttherapie

Fig. 104
Recurrent carcinoma of the cervix, II

Condition five years after vaginal radical hysterectomy followed by postsurgical X-ray irradiation
Patient, 56, with swelling of right leg
Palpation finding: Flat, hard resistance on the right pelvic wall
Indication: Differentiation between recurrent tumor and fibrosis; *combination with lymphography*
Fig. 104 shows polycyclic shadow in minor pelvis, right, cast by bulb of recurrent tumor of the pelvis; filling interrupted at lymphatic vessels with stop and extravasation of contrast medium as well as filling stop at nodi lymphatici iliaci ext. and communes in the tumor base; expanded adhesions between intestine, urinary bladder, and pelvic wall
Course: Tele-cobalt therapy

lung. Den größten Anteil bilden *Beckenwandrezidive operierter Zervixkarzinome.* Bei einer Reihe von Patientinnen war eine alleinige Strahlentherapie vorausgegangen.
Methodisch ist zu berücksichtigen, daß die Übersichtsaufnahme nur relativ selten eine sichere Beurteilung zuläßt. Operationen und Bestrahlungen führen regelmäßig zu Verwachsungen des Rectum, Colon sigmoideum, Cecum und Ileum. Diese Darmschlingen bleiben nach Beckenhochlagerung im kleinen Becken fixiert und machen eine exakte Analyse der Summationsaufnahmen of unmöglich, so daß der anatomische Situs unübersichtlich bleibt. Diese Erfahrung veranlaßte andere Untersucher, vorausgegangene gynäkologische Operationen zu den Kontraindikationen der Pneumopelvigraphie zu zählen. Schichtuntersuchungen erweisen sich als aufschlußreicher und sollten für die Deutung stets herangezogen werden. Um Darmschlingen und Verwachsungsstränge von Tumorschatten besser unterscheiden zu können, füllen wir Rectum und Colon über ein Darmrohr zusätzlich mit Luft. *Tumorknoten werden als unregelmäßige, höckerig begrenzte*

cervix. Some of the patients had undergone solely radiotherapy.
Regarding the methodical approach, it should be borne in mind that a safe diagnosis is possible but rarely on the basis of standard radiography. Both surgery and irradiation will cause regularly adhesions of the rectum, colon sigmoideum, cecum, and ileum. When the pelvis has been elevated, these intestinal loops tend to remain fixed in the minor pelvis and often render impossible an accurate analysis of the given standard radiograph, so that the anatomic site will remain obscured. Such experience caused other examiners to consider previous gynecological operations as contraindications to pneumopelvigraphy. Diagnostic tomography has been found to yield more information and, therefore, should always be used for interpretation. Additional air is insufflated into the rectum and colon through an intestinal tube for better differentiation of intestinal loops and adhesive chords from tumor shadows. *Tumorous nodes are projected as shadows with irregular and humpy limitations,* which will either protrude from the pelvic wall or be accommo-

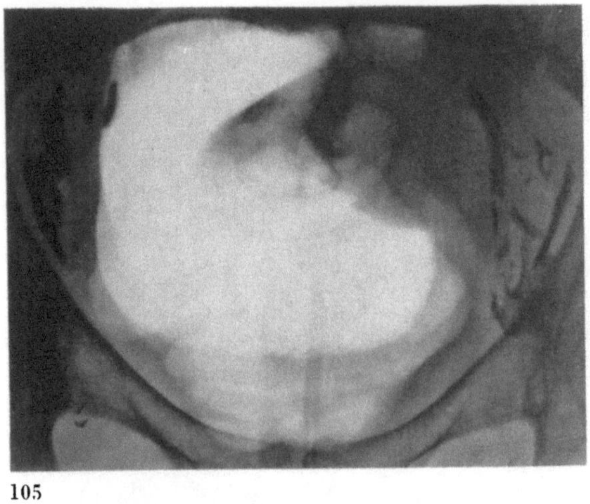

105

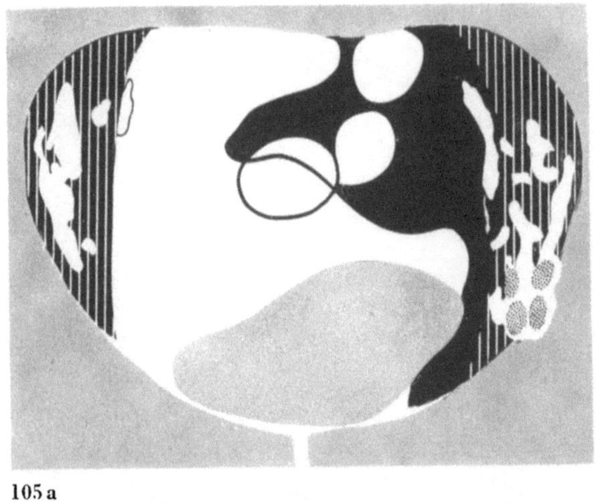

105a

Abb. 105 und 106

Rezidiv eines Zervixkarzinoms III

1 Jahr nach vaginaler Radikaloperation mit Entfernung beider Adnexe, Teilresektion der Harnblase und Röntgennachbestrahlung

46jähr. Patientin mit röntgenologisch „stummer Niere“ links und Schwellung des linken Beines

Tastbefund: Derber Tumor an der linken Beckenwand

Indikation: Tumorlokalisation und Suche nach weiteren Metastasen vor Telekobalttherapie, *Kombination mit Lymphographie*

Abb. 105: Die *Übersichtsaufnahme* zeigt einen knolligen Tumor an der linken Beckenwand. Marginale Füllungsdefekte in den externen iliakalen Lymphknoten im Bereich des Tumorrezidivs

Der Befund läßt sich ohne Kenntnis des Pneumopelvigramms von Bestrahlungsfolgen oder anderen degenerativen Lymphknotenveränderungen nicht unterscheiden

Abb. 106: *Tomogramm* in 9 cm Tiefe. Der Tumorschatten (→) sitzt der Beckenwand breitbasig auf

Figs. 105 and 106

Recurrent carcinoma of the cervix, III

Condition one year after vaginal radical hysterectomy, including radical adnexectomy and partial resection of the urinary bladder, followed by postsurgical X-ray irradiation

Patient, 46, with left kidney not responsive to urography and swelling of left leg

Palpation finding: Hard tumor on left pelvic wall

Indication: Localisation of tumor and search for additional metastases for decision of tele-cobalt therapy; *combination with lymphography*

Fig. 105 is a *standard radiograph* showing a bulbiform tumor on the left pelvic wall and marginal filling defects in the external iliac lymphatic nodes within the region of the recurrent tumor; the finding would not be differentiable from damage by irradiation or other degenerative changes of the lymphatic nodes, had it not been for the pneumopelvigram

Fig. 106 is a *tomogram*, 9 cm in depth, showing the tumor shadow (→) rest with wide base on the pelvic wall

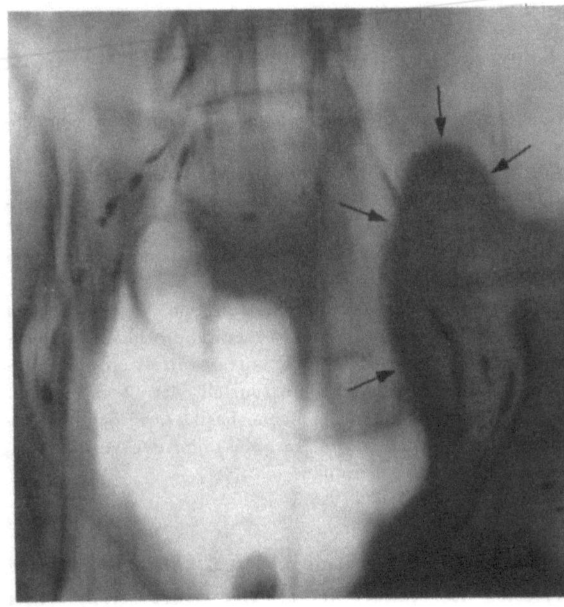

106

Abb. 107–109

Rezidiv eines Zervixkarzinoms I

10 Monate nach vaginaler Radikaloperation mit Entfernung beider Adnexe und Röntgennachbestrahlung

49jähr. Patientin ohne Beschwerden

Tastbefund: Beide Parametrien imponieren gleichmäßig derb infiltriert

Indikation: Differenzierung zwischen Tumorrezidiv und Fibrose, Suche nach Metastasen, *Kombination mit Lymphographie*

Figs. 107–109

Recurrent carcinoma of the cervix, I

Condition ten months after vaginal radical hysterectomy, including radical adnexectomy, and postsurgical X-ray irradation

Patient, 49, with no complaints

Palpation finding: Both parametria appear to be infiltrated with equal hardness

Indication: Differentiation between recurrent tumor and fibrosis; search for metastases; *combination with lymphography*

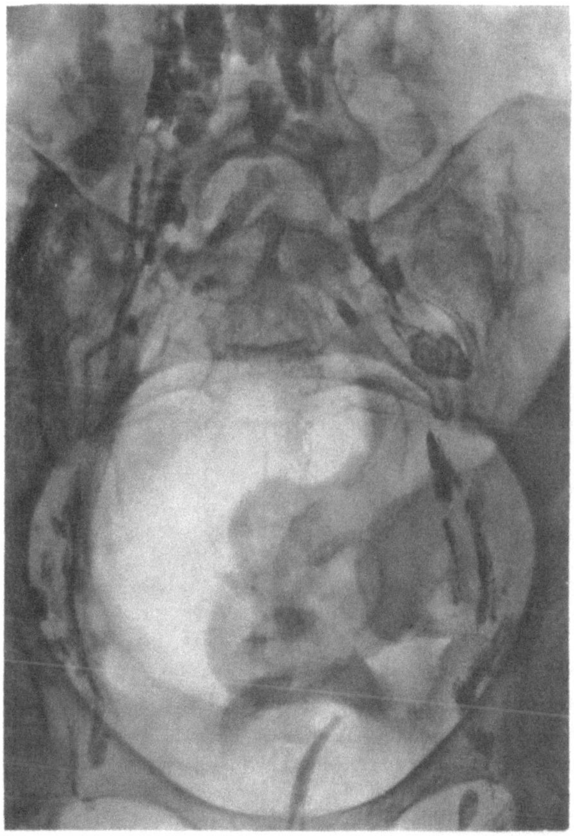

107

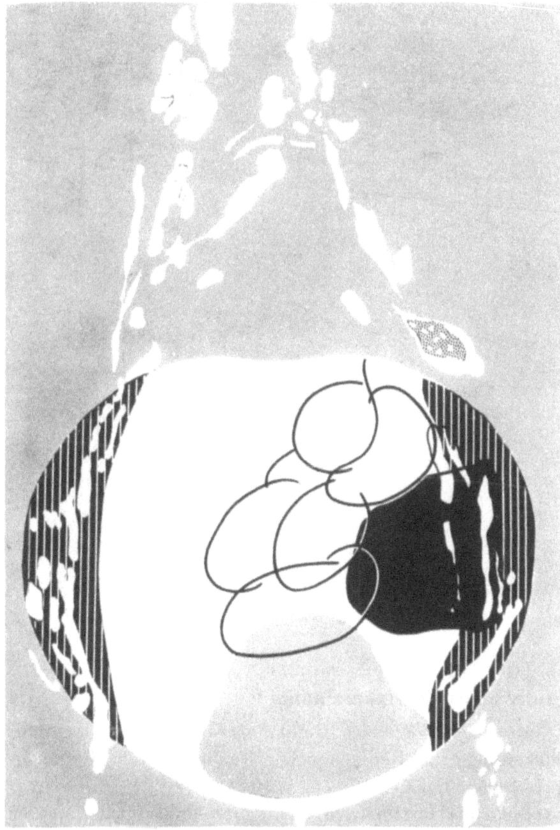

107a

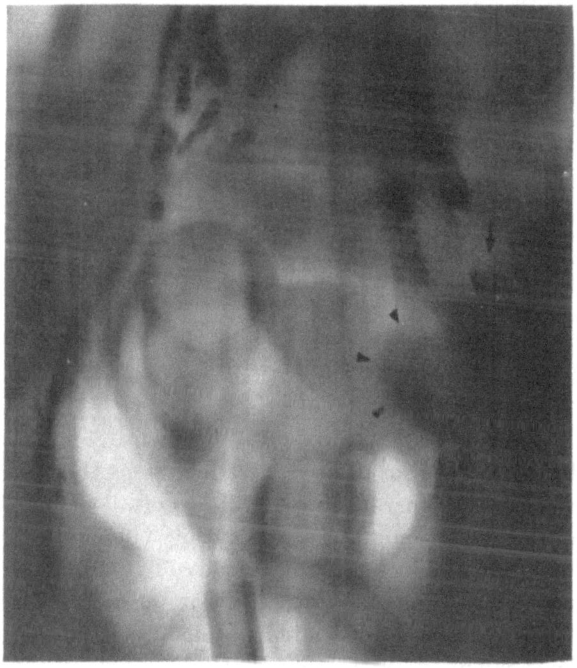

108

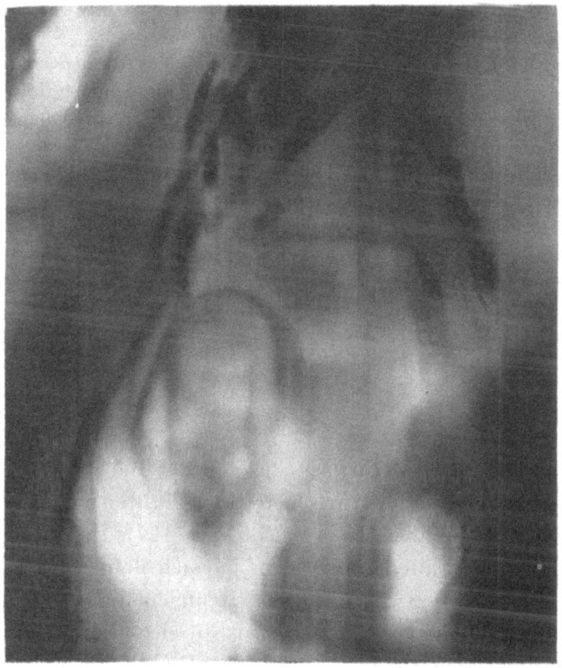

109

Abb. 107: Auf der *Übersichtsaufnahme* pathologische Verschattungen durch ein Tumorrezidiv im Becken links, teilweise vom Colon sigmoideum überlagert, Lymphknotenmetastase

Abb. 108 und 109: Die *Schichtbilder* ermöglichen eine sichere Differenzierung von Tumorknoten (▸), an denen das abgedrängte Colon sigmoideum adhärent ist. Metastase in einem iliakalen Lymphknoten (→)

Verlauf: Telekobalttherapie

Fig. 107 is a *standard radiograph* showing, on left side of pelvis, pathological shadows caused by recurrent tumor and to some extent overshadowed by the colon sigmoideum; metastasation of lymphatic nodes

Figs. 108 and 109 are *tomograms* which facilitate safe differentiation of tumor bulbs (▸) to which the displaced colon sigmoideum is adherent; metastasation of one iliac lymphatic node (→)

Course: Tele-cobalt therapy

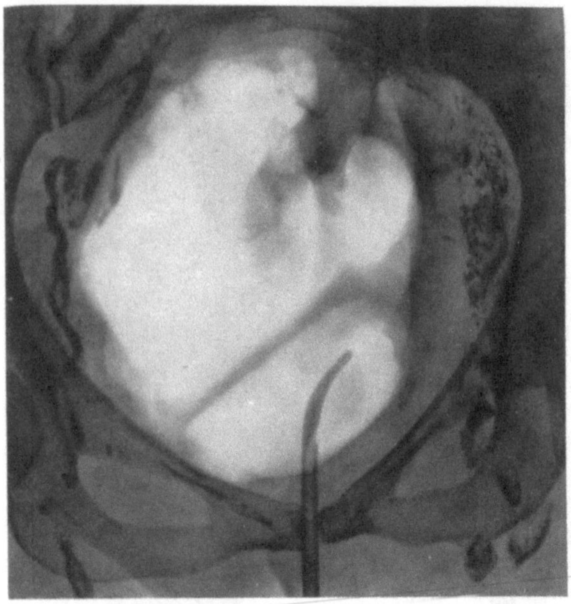

110

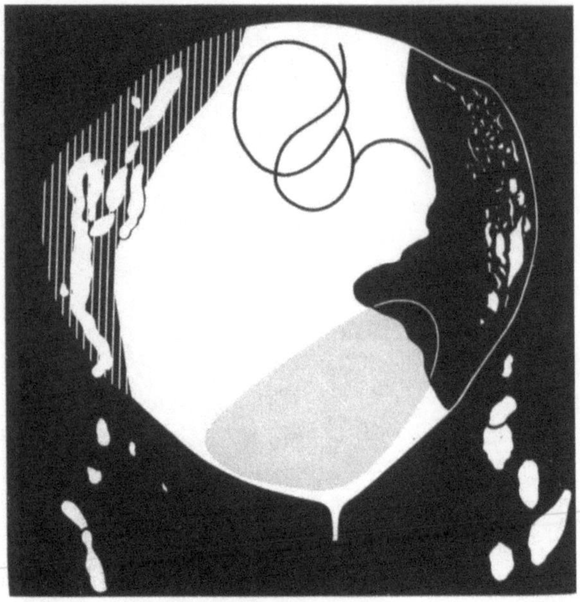

110 a

Abb. 110–112

Rezidiv eines Zervixkarzinoms I

$4^1/_2$ Jahre nach vaginaler Radikaloperation mit Entfernung beider Adnexe und Röntgennachbestrahlung. 51jähr. Patientin mit Ischialgie links

Tastbefund: Parametrien rechts frei, links flacher derber Tumor an der Beckenwand

Indikation: Tumorabgrenzung und Suche nach weiteren Metastasen, *Kombination mit Lymphographie*

Abb. 110: *Übersichtsaufnahme.* Von der linken Beckenwand vorspringende knollige Verschattung durch ein Tumorrezidiv mit breitem Kontakt zur Harnblasenwand, die an den Tumor herangezogen ist. Massive Tumorinfiltration mit Vergrößerung, Konglomeratbildung und Füllungsdefekten der Nodi lymph. iliac. ext. in der seitlichen Tumorbasis

Abb. 111 und 112: Die *Tomogramme* in 7 cm und 8 cm Tiefe zeigen in die Harnblasenwand einwachsende Tumorknollen

Verlauf: Telekobalttherapie. 10 Monate später fortschreitendes Tumorwachstum, nach 14 Monaten Exitus

Figs. 110–112

Recurrent carcinoma of the cervix, I

Condition four-a-half years after vaginal radical hysterectomy, including radical adnexectomy, and postsurgical X-ray irradiation

Patient, 51, with ischialgia on the left

Palpation finding: Parametria on the right unaffected; flat, hard tumor on the pelvic wall, left

Indication: Demarcation of the tumor and search for additional metastases; *combination with lymphography*

Fig. 110 is a *standard radiograph* showing bulbiform shadow, caused by recurrent tumor, protruding from left pelvic wall and being in wide-base contact with the urinary bladder wall which is drawn close to the tumor; massive tumor infiltration with enlargement, conglomeration, and filling defects of the nodi lymph. iliac. ext. in lateral tumor base

Figs. 111 and 112 are *tomograms*, 7 cm and 8 cm in depths, showing tumor bulbs growing into the wall of the urinary bladder

Course: Tele-cobalt therapy, followed, after ten months, by progressive tumor growth, exitus after 14 months

Verschattungen abgebildet, die von der Beckenwand vorspringen oder zwischen luftgefüllten Darmschlingen lokalisiert sind (Abb. 95–127). Bei nicht operierten Fällen findet man je nach dem Tumorstadium polyzyklische Verschattungen des Lig. latum und seiner seitlichen Basis durch parametrane Infiltrationen (Abb. 121 und 122). Da sich die Wand der luftgefüllten Harnblase gut erkennen läßt, kann die Lage des Tumors zur Blasenwand leicht beurteilt werden (Abb. 110–112). Nach Luftfüllung des Rectum und Colon läßt sich außerdem die Beziehung des Tumors zur Darmwand klären (Abb. 125–127). Die negative Kontrastgebung durch Gasfüllung der Harnblase, des Cavum peritonei pelvis und des Darmlumens bringt den anatomischen Situs auf

dated between insufflated intestinal loops (Figs. 95 to 127). Non-operated cases will exhibit, depending on the given tumor stage, polycyclic shadows of the lig. latum and its lateral base, caused by parametric infiltration (Figs. 121 and 122). The position of the tumor relative to the wall of the bladder may be defined safely, since the wall is clearly visible due to air insufflation of the bladder (Figs. 110–112). The local relationship between the tumor and the intestinal wall may be elucidated, too, as soon as air has been insufflated into the rectum and colon (Figs. 125–127). In the tomogram a detailed projection of the given anatomic site is achieved due to the negative opacification effectuated by filling gas into the urinary bladder, cavum peritonei pel-

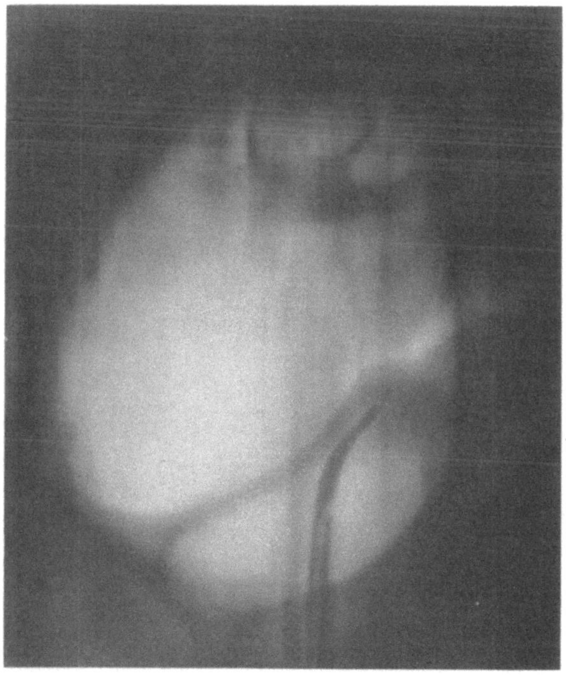

111

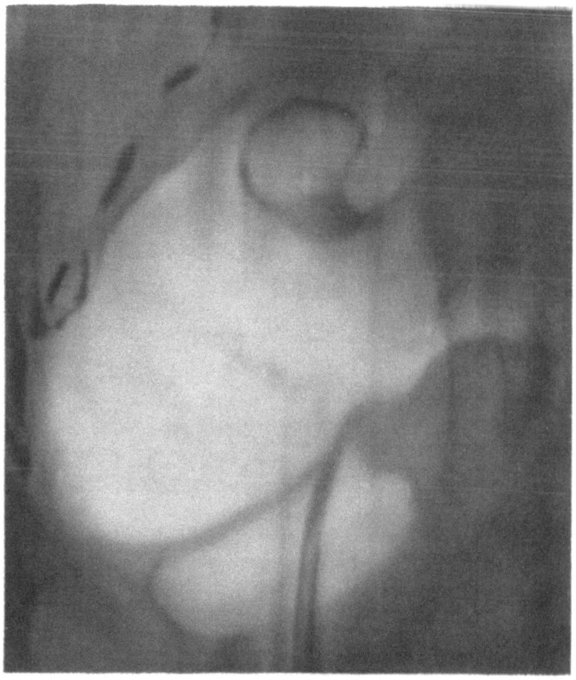

112

Schichtbildern detailliert zur Darstellung. Dadurch gelingt es auch, tumorverdächtige Tastbefunde in manchen Fällen als postoperative oder radiogene Verschwielungen zu klären und makroskopische Tumorrezidive mit ausreichender Sicherheit auszuschließen (Abb. 128).

Eine Erweiterung der diagnostischen Möglichkeiten ergibt die *Kombination von Pneumopelvigraphie und Lymphographie* (Abb. 99—122). Die Anlage des Pneumoperitoneum erfolgt einen oder wenige Tage nach Durchführung der Lymphographie (s. Seite 21). Lymphographische Befunde (Füllungsdefekte in Lymphknoten, Füllungsabbrüche mit Kontrastmittelrückstauung in den Lymphgefäßen, Kollateralbahnen) und Befunde des Pneumoperitoneum (Tumorvorwölbungen in den gasgefüllten intraperitonealen Beckenraum) ergänzen sich zu einer guten morphologischen Übersicht. Dadurch wächst der Informationsgehalt der Röntgenbilder. Die vorangegangene Lymphographie erweitert das Urteil bezüglich der regionären Lymphknotenstationen. Andererseits gewinnt auch die Interpretation mehrdeutiger Lymphogramme durch die Pneumopelvigraphie wesentlich an Sicherheit. Degenerative Veränderungen und Reaktionen der Lymphknoten und Lymphgefäße durch vorangegangene Radikaloperationen (Lymphknotenausräumung), Bestrahlungen (Fibrosierung) und begleitende pathologische Prozesse an den Venen (Thrombosen, Obstruktionen) erschweren bekanntlich die Deutung mancher Lymphogramme, denn Strahlenreaktionen und postoperative Prozesse können zu ähnlichen lympho-

vis, and the intestinal lumen. Such approach also helps to elucidate palpation findings suspicious of tumor, which in some cases may be merely postoperative or radiogenic callosities, and to rule out safely macroscopic tumor recurrences (Fig. 128).

An even wider range of diagnostic possibilities is offered by a *combination of pneumopelvigraphy with lymphography* (Figs. 99—122). The pneumoperitoneum is to be applied, in such cases, one or a few days after lymphography (see p. 21). A fairly complete morphological picture may then be achieved on the basis of the lymphographic findings (filling defects in the lymphatic nodes, discontinuation of filling with reflux of contrast medium into the lymphatic vessels, collateral pathways) together with the findings obtained from the pneumoperitoneum (bulging of the tumor into the gas-filled intraperitoneal pelvic cavity). It goes without saying that such approach will add considerably to the amount of information provided by the radiographs. Lymphography, when preceding pneumopelvigraphy, will help to improve assessment of the regional lymph node sites, while ambiguous lymphograms, on the other hand, may be interpreted much more safely by adding pneumopelvigraphy. It is well known that problems are faced in the interpretation of certain lymphograms due to the presence of degenerative changes and reactions of both the lymphatic nodes and vessels, with such phenomena being caused by earlier radical surgery (removal of lymphatic nodes), irradiation (fibrotisation), and concomitant pathological venous processes (thrombosis, obstruc-

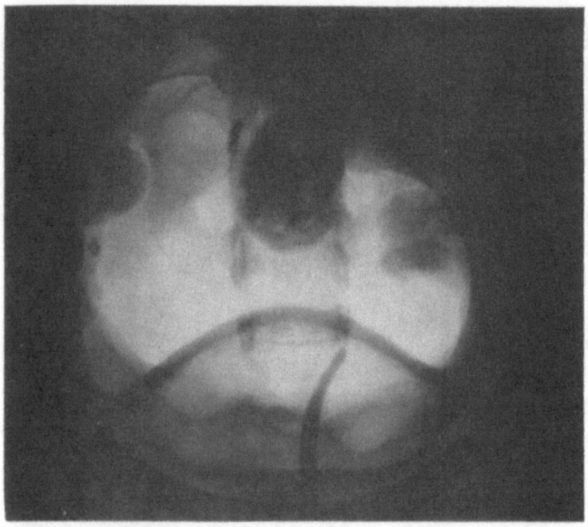

113

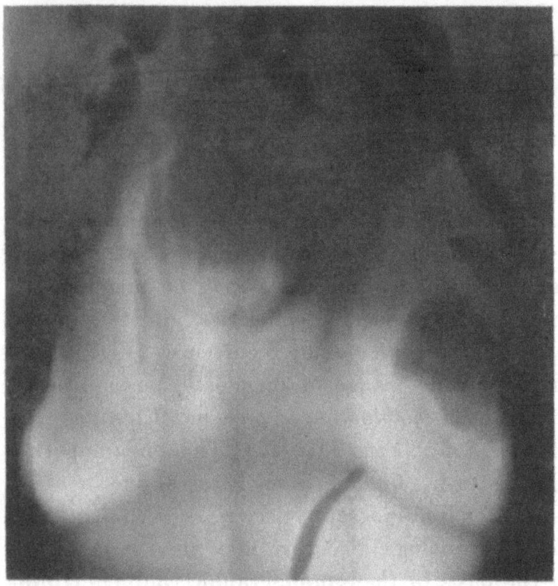

114

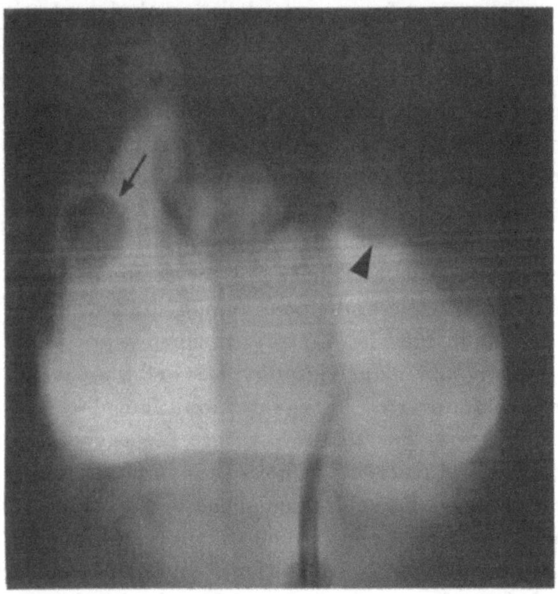

115

Abb. 113–117

Rezidiv eines Zervixkarzinoms III

3 Jahre nach vaginaler Radikaloperation ohne Adnexe. 41jähr. Patientin mit Ischialgie und Schwellung des linken Beines

Tastbefund: unauffällig

Indikation: Metastasensuche, *Kombination mit Lymphographie*

Abb. 113: Die *Übersichtsaufnahme* zeigt die bei der Operation zurückgelassenen Adnexe. Links neben dem Rectum glatt begrenzte glatte Vorwölbung, die einem Tumorrezidiv entspricht, irrtümlich jedoch als fibrotische Schwiele gedeutet wurde

Abb. 114 und 115: Auf den *Tomogrammen* imponieren die Adnexe links größer als rechts. Das linke Ovar läßt sich von der Tumorbegrenzung (▸) deutlich unterscheiden

Abb. 116: Lymphadenogramm

Abb. 117: Kontrollaufnahmen nach 5 Monaten. Wachstum einer Metastase (→) im Bereich der Nodi lymph. iliac. comm.

Verlauf: Bei einer erneuten Pneumopelvigraphie 5 Monate später ist die linke Beckenseite von Tumorknoten ausgefüllt. Telekobalttherapie

Figs. 113–117

Recurrent carcinoma of the cervix, III

Condition three years after vaginal radical hysterectomy, without removal of adnexa

Patient, 41, with ischialgia and swelling of left leg

Palpation finding: Unpathological

Indication: Search for metastases; *combination with lymphography*

Fig. 113 is a *standard radiograph* showing the adnexa, left in place when uterus was removed; left to the rectum is visualised a smoothly demarcated smooth bulging which while caused by a recurrent tumor, was misinterpreted as a fibrotic callosity

Figs. 114 and 115 are *tomograms* in which the left adnexum appears to be larger than the right one and where the left ovary can be differentiated clearly from the tumor bordering (▸)

Fig. 116: Lymphadenogram

Fig. 117: Check-up radiographs taken after five months showing growth of a metastasis (→) in the area of the nodi lymph. iliac. comm.

Course: Repetition of pneumopelvigraphy after five months shows left side of the pelvis filled up with tumor bulbs; telecobalt therapy

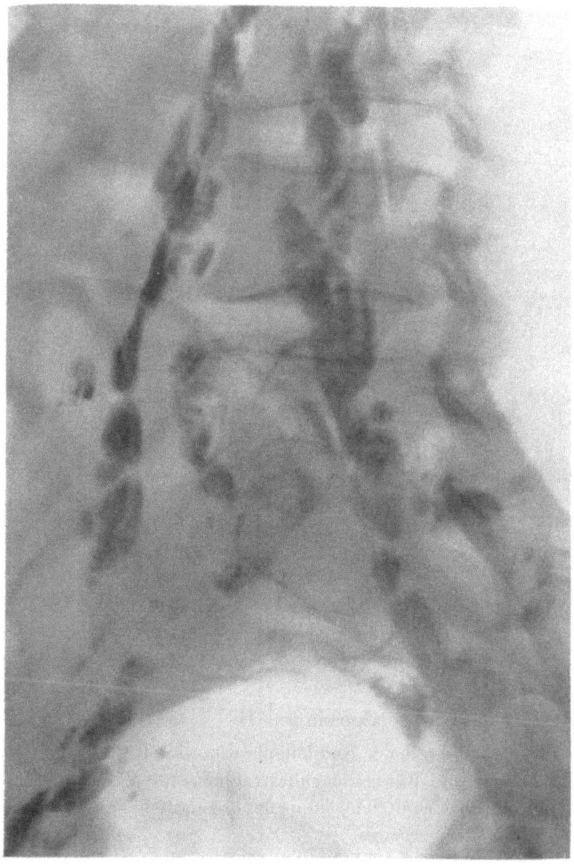

116

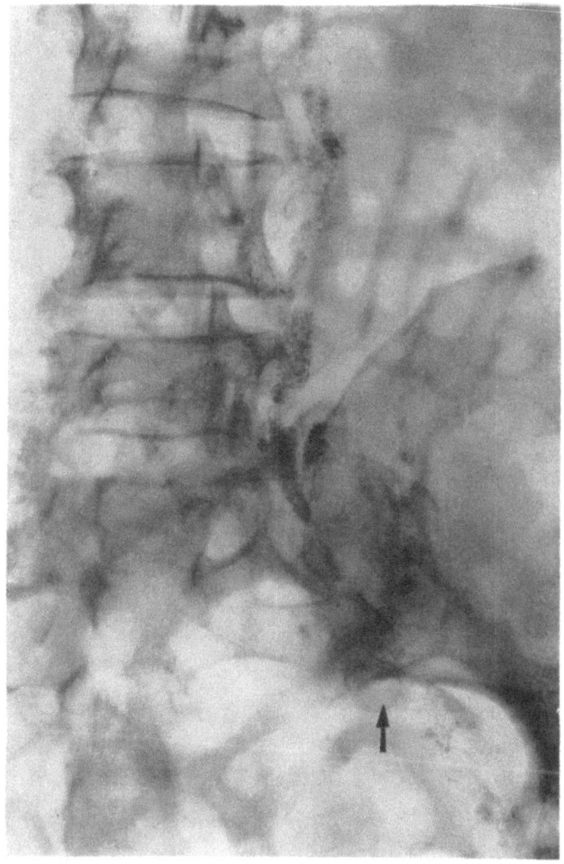

117

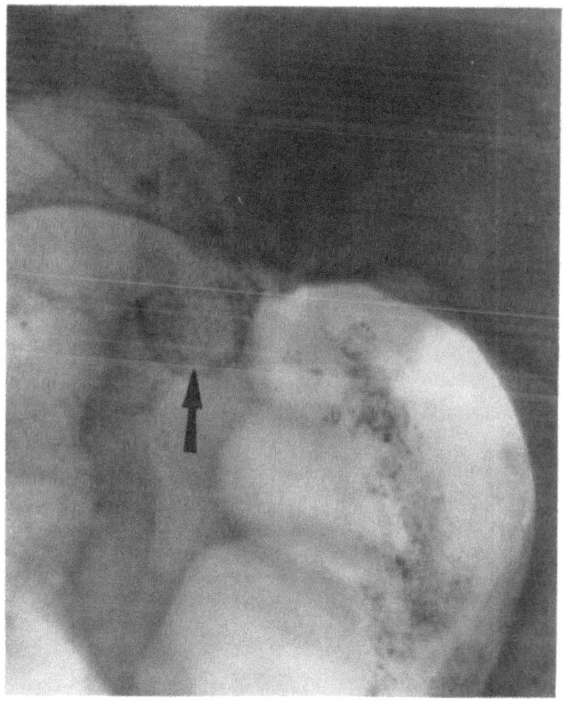

117a

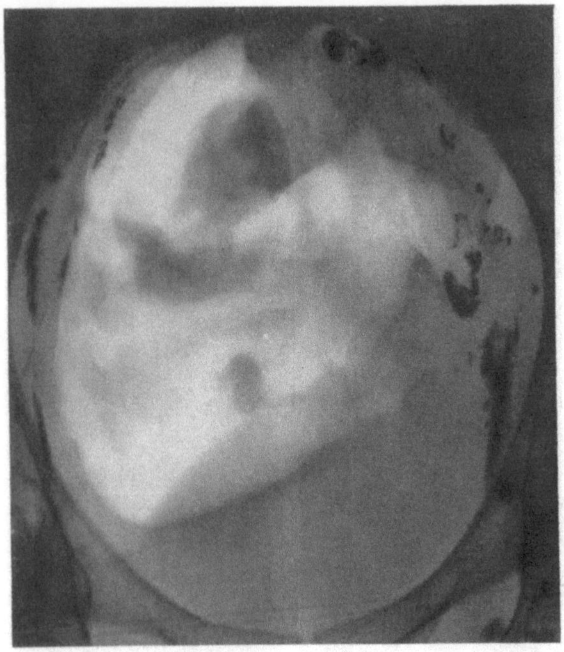

118

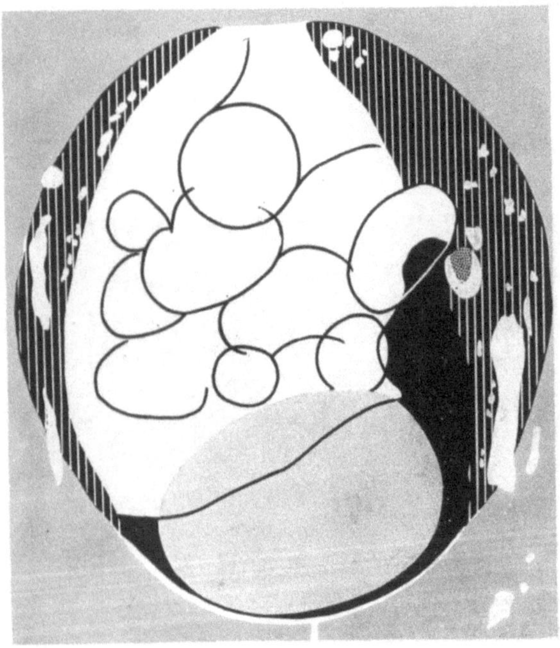

118a

Abb. 118—120

Rezidiv eines Zervixkarzinoms II

6 Jahre nach vaginaler Radikaloperation mit Entfernung beider Adnexe und Röntgennachbestrahlung

44jähr. Patientin mit Schwellung des linken Beines und Schmerzen in der Leistenbeuge

Tastbefund: Kein sicherer Anhalt für ein Tumorrezidiv

Indikation: Nachweis bzw. Ausschluß eines Tumorrezidivs, *Kombination mit Lymphographie*

Abb. 118: Auf der *Übersichtsaufnahme* höckrig begrenzter Tumorschatten auf der linken Beckenseite, der sich ventral bis hinter die Symphyse erstreckt. Metastase in einem externen iliakalen Lymphknoten (Füllungsdefekt)

Abb. 119 und 120: Nach Lufteinblasung in das Rectum wird der Befund durch *Zonographie* (kreisförmige Verwischung, Pendelwinkel 3°, Abb. 119) und *Tomographie* (Linearverwischung, Pendelwinkel 20°, Abb. 120) dargestellt. Es zeigen sich Verwachsungen des Colon sigmoideum (→) mit der Tumoroberfläche (▸)

Verlauf: Telekobalttherapie

Figs. 118—120

Recurrent carcinoma of the cervix, II

Condition six years after vaginal radical hysterectomy, including radical adnexectomy, and postsurgical X-ray irradiation

Patient, 44, with swelling of left leg and pain in the groin

Palpation finding: No safe suggestion to presence of recurrent tumor

Indication: Confirmation or ruling out of recurrent tumor; *combination with lymphography*

Fig. 118 is a *standard radiograph* showing, on the left side of the pelvis, tumor shadow with polycyclic bodering which extends ventrally to an area behind the symphysis; metastasis present in an external iliac lymphatic node (filling defect)

Figs. 119 and 120: Rectal insufflation is used to represent the finding by *zonography* (circular blurring, angle of pendulum 3 deg., Fig. 119) and *tomography* (linear blurring, angle of pendulum 20 deg., Fig. 120); parts of the colon sigmoideum (→) are shown to be adherent to the surface of the tumor (▸)

Course: Tele-cobalt therapy

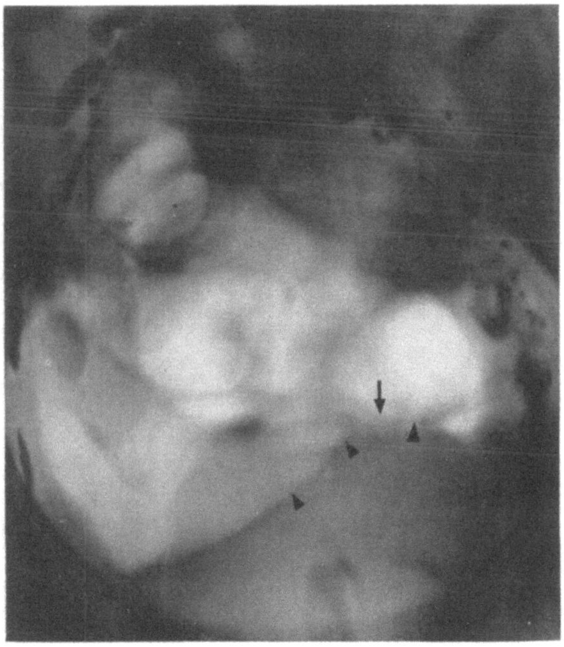

119

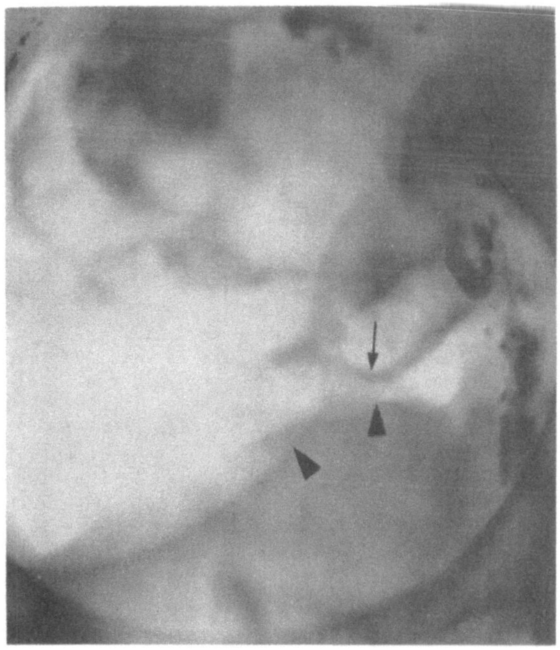

120

graphischen Mustern führen wie Metastasen. Der pneumopelvigraphische Nachweis von Tumorknoten ist deshalb wertvoll, wenn im Lymphogramm mehrdeutige, auf einen Karzinombefall verdächtige, aber nicht hinreichend sichere Befunde erfaßt werden. Außerdem muß man berücksichtigen, daß eine Reihe von Lymphknotengruppen des Beckenraumes bei der Lymphographie nicht dargestellt, andere nur inkonstant gefüllt werden. Wie aus Abb. 99 hervorgeht, können in den Lymphknotenstationen der Genitalorgane Tumorinfiltrationen lymphographisch erkannt werden, wenn die Nodi lymphatici iliaci externi, iliaci communes, aortici und die entsprechenden Lymphgefäße befallen sind. Demgegenüber sind Metastasen in den Nodi lymphatici interni, die bei Zervixkarzinom in der Regel als die primäre Filterstation wirken, nur selten nachweisbar. Eine Kontrastmittelfüllung der Iliaka-interna-Gruppe erfolgt nur in einem Teil der Fälle über inkonstante Lymphbahnen aus den Nodi lymphatici iliaci externi. Da sich die Exkavationen des Bauchfells nach caudal erstrecken, können mit Hilfe der Pneumopelvigraphie häufig auch in dieser Region Tumorpartien entdeckt werden, wenn das Lymphogramm negativ ist. Nach unserer Erfahrung an 250 gynäkologischen Tumorrezidiven gewinnt die Diagnostik durch die Kombination von *Pneumopelvigraphie und Lymphographie* beträchtlich an Sicherheit und ist in dieser Form als die zur Zeit *aufschlußreichste Methode* zu bezeichnen.

tion), because radioreactions and postoperative processes may lead to lymphographic patterns similar to those caused by metastases. Pneumopelvigraphic confirmation of tumor nodes will be of interest, if ambiguous findings are provided by the lymphogram, such as phenomena indicating but not confirming the presence of carcinoma. In addition, it should be borne in mind that by lymphography certain groups of lymphatic nodes of the pelvic cavity are not represented, while others are filled inconstantly. As may be seen from Fig. 99, tumor infiltration of the lymphatic node sites of the genital organs may be detected by lymphography, provided that the nodi lymphatici iliaci externi, iliaci communes, aortici, and the pertinent lymphatic vessels are affected. On the other hand, metastasation of the internal lymphatic nodes, usually the primary filtering site in cases of cervical carcinoma, is detectable but rarely. Only in some cases, contrast medium is filled from the external iliac lymphatic nodes via inconstant lymphatic channels into the internal iliac group. Since the excavations of the peritoneum extend caudally, tumorous foci can be detected by means of pneumopelvigraphy also in this region, even in cases where the lymphogram had been negative. The authors' experience, obtained from the investigation of 250 cases of recurrent gynecological tumors, seems to suggest quite strongly that a *combination of pneumopelvigraphy with lymphography* does not merely improve essentially the reliability of diagnosis, but that it even may be considered *the most informative method* available to this purpose for the time being.

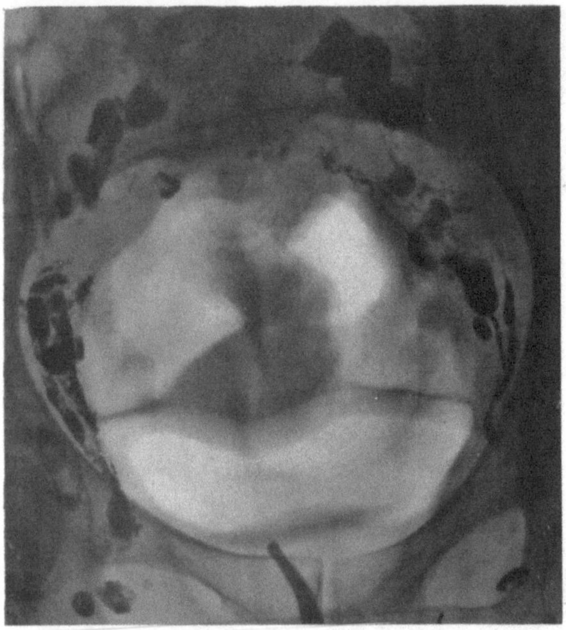

121

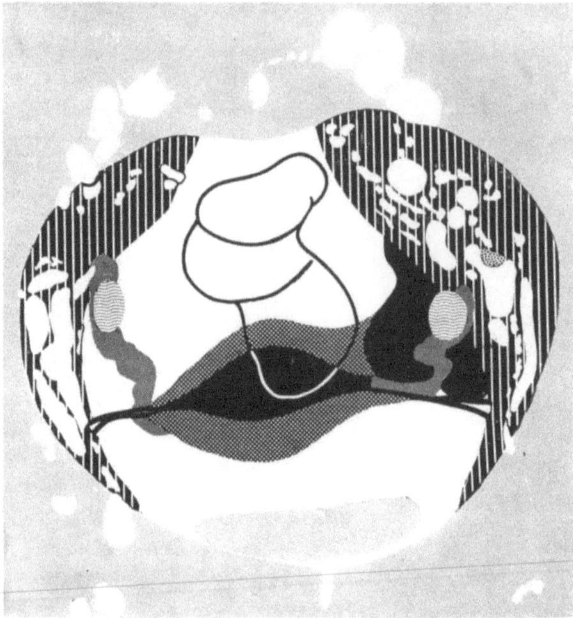

121 a

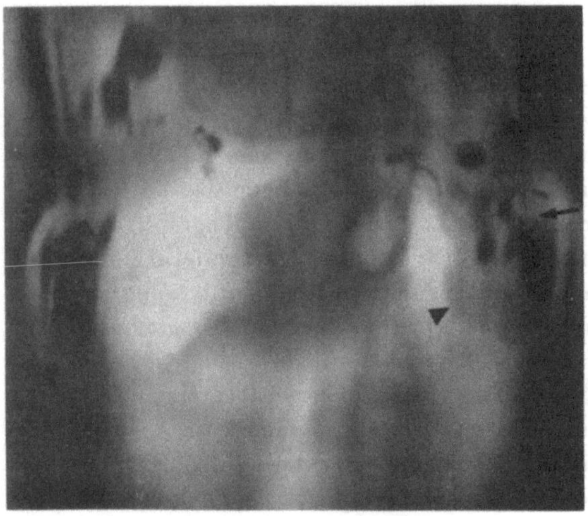

122

Abb. 121 und 122

Rezidiv eines Zervixkarzinoms III

6 Monate nach Radium- und Röntgentherapie
50jähr. Patientin mit Ischialgie links
Tastbefund: Beide Parametrien derb
Indikation: Metastasensuche, *Kombination mit Lymphographie*
Abb. 121: Die *Übersichtsaufnahme* zeigt eine Verdickung des Lig. latum links mit starker Verbreiterung ihrer seitlichen Basis durch parametrane Tumorinfiltration, Lymphknotenmetastase
Abb. 122: Auf dem *Schichtbild* werden im linken Parametrium knollige Verschattungen durch Tumorknoten abgebildet (▸). In gleicher Höhe findet sich in einem externen iliakalen Lymphknoten ein Füllungsdefekt infolge Tumorinfiltration (→)
Verlauf: Trotz zytostatischer Therapie rasche Tumorausbreitung. 4 Monate später Exitus

Figs. 121 and 122

Recurrent carcinoma of the cervix, III

Condition six months after radium and X-ray treatment
Patient, 50, with ischialgia on the left
Palpation finding: Both parametria hardened
Indication: Search for metastases; *combination with lymphography*
Fig. 121 is a *standard radiograph* showing the lig. latum, left, thickened, with its base strongly broadened due to tumor infiltration of the parametrium; metastasis of lymphatic node
Fig. 122 is a *tomogram* showing in the left parametrium bulbiform shadows cast by tumor bulbs (▸); filling defect due to tumor infiltration is found on the same level in a external iliac lymphatic node (→)
Course: Cytostatic therapy fails to prevent rapid proliferation of tumor; exitus after four months

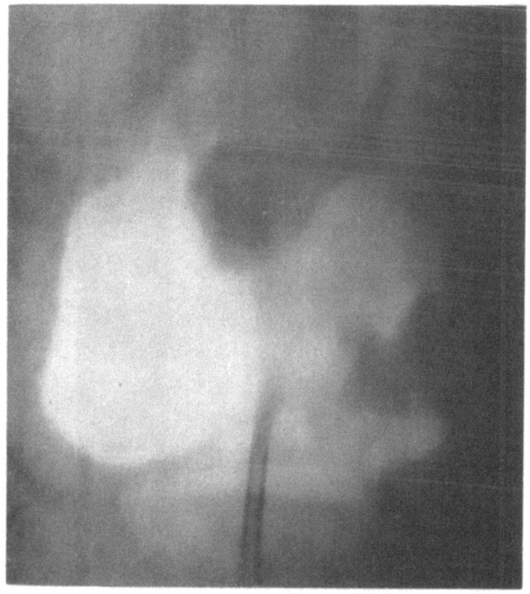

123

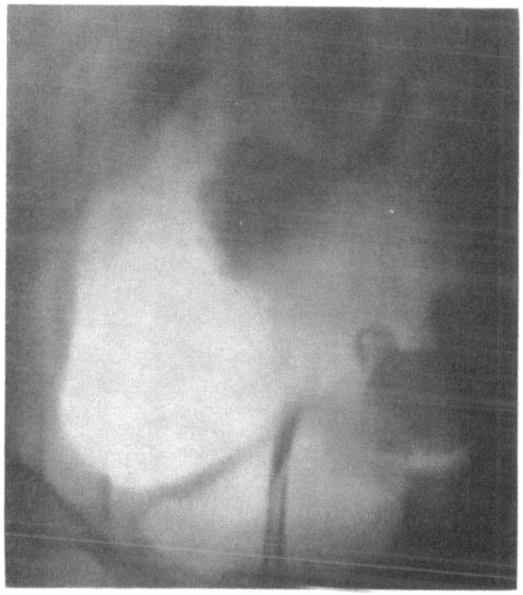

124

Abb. 123 und 124

Rezidiv eines Granulosazelltumors

4 Jahre nach abdominaler Totalexstirpation des Uterus mit Entfernung beider Adnexe

53jähr. Patientin ohne Beschwerden

Tastbefund: Weiche Resistenz in Höhe des linken Adnexstumpfes, Befund nicht eindeutig

Indikation: Nachweis oder Ausschluß eines Tumorrezidivs

Abb. 123 und 124: Die *Schichtaufnahmen* zeigen einen Tumorschatten, welcher der linken Beckenwand anliegt und von einem Konglomerat rundlicher Verschattungen gebildet wird. Dorsal ist das Rectum, ventral die Harnblase zu erkennen, deren Wand von der Katheterspitze angehoben wird

Verlauf: Die Relaparotomie bestätigt die Diagnose eines Tumorrezidivs. Ein Konglomerat blau-roter Tumorknoten ist in größerer Ausdehnung mit der Beckenwand und dem Serosaüberzug des Colon sigmoideum verbacken. Exstirpation der Geschwulstknoten und anschließende intraperitoneale Radiogoldinstillation

Figs. 123 and 124

Recurrent granulosa cell tumor

Condition four years after abdominal radical hysterectomy, including radical adnexectomy

Patient, 52, with no complaints

Palpation finding: Soft resistance on the level of the left adnexal stump; ambiguous finding

Indication: Confirmation or ruling out of recurrent tumor

Figs. 123 and 124 are *tomograms* showing tumor shadow attached to the left pelvic wall and formed by a conglomerate of rounded shadows; visualised dorsally is the rectum and ventrally the urinary bladder, with the latter's wall being elevated by the catheter tip

Course: Diagnosis of recurrent tumor confirmed by relaparotomy; a conglomerate of bluish-red tumor bulbs is found to adhere massively to the pelvic wall and the serous coat of the colon sigmoideum; extirpation of the tumor bulbs followed by intraperitoneal application of radioactive gold implants

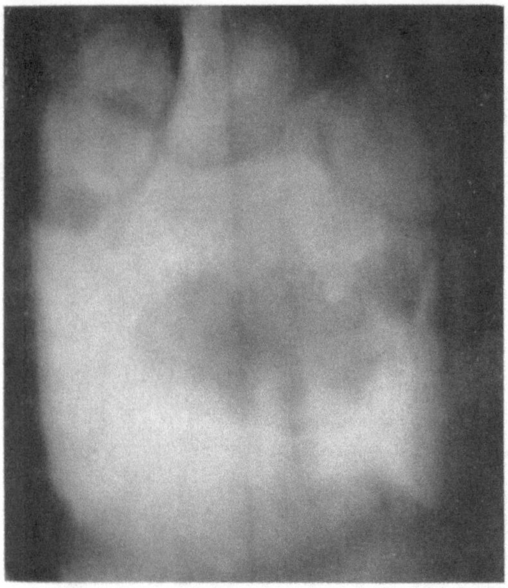

125

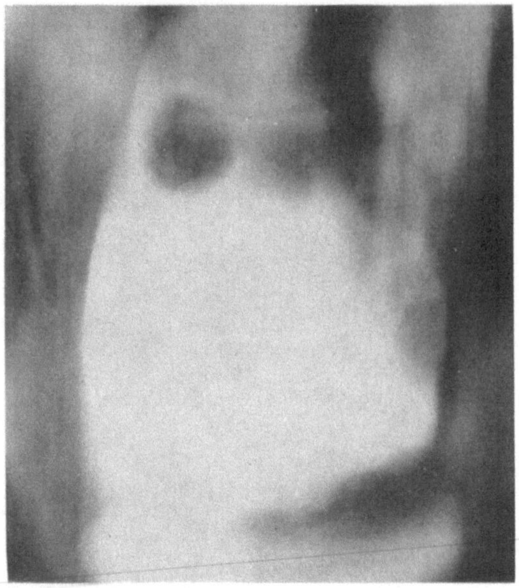

127

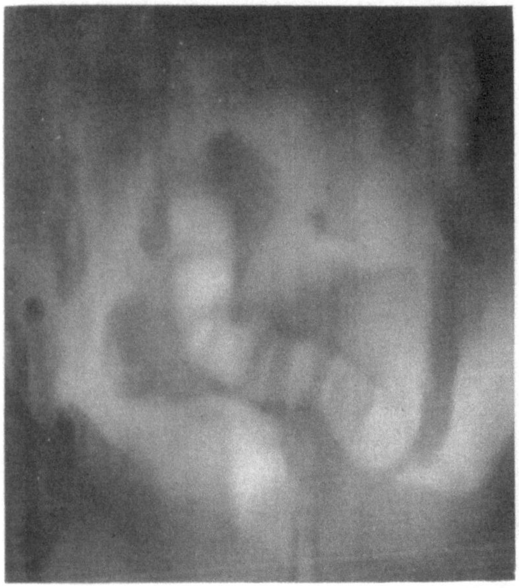

126

Abb. 125—127

Metastasen eines Granulosazelltumors

4 Monate nach abdominaler Totalexstirpation des Uterus und beider Adnexe

42jähr. Patientin mit Aszites

Tastbefund: Im Douglasschen Raum beweglicher derber Tumor, der mit dem Vaginalstumpf verbunden ist

Indikation: Suche nach weiteren Metastasen

Abb. 125: Das *Tomogramm* in 6 cm Tiefe zeigt eine pathologische Verschattung in Beckenmitte, die sich aus einem Konglomerat von Knotenbildungen zusammensetzt

Abb. 126: Multiple Tumorschatten werden in 9 cm zwischen Darmschlingen dargestellt. Sie zeigen breiten Kontakt zur Darmwand

Abb. 127: In 12 cm Tiefe wird eine weitere Metastase in einem Mesenteriallymphknoten in Höhe des Promontorium abgebildet

Verlauf: Relaparotomie, Resectio omenti und Exstirpation von peritonealen Metastasen

Figs. 125—127

Metastases of a grunulosa cell tumor

Condition four months after abdominal radical hysterectomy, including radical adnexectomy

Patient, 42, afflicted with ascites

Palpation finding: Movable hard tumor connected with vaginal stump is palpated in Douglas' pouch

Indication: Search for additional metastases

Fig. 125 is a *tomogram*, 6 cm in depth, showing in centre of pelvis pathological shadow composed of a conglomerate of nodes

Fig. 126 is a *tomogram*, 9 cm in depth, showing multiple tumor shadows between intestinal loops; wide-base contact with intestinal wall

Fig. 127 is a *tomogram*, 12 cm in depth, showing another metastasis in a mesenterial lymphatic node on promontory level

Course: Relaparotomy, resectio omenti, and extirpation of peritoneal metastases

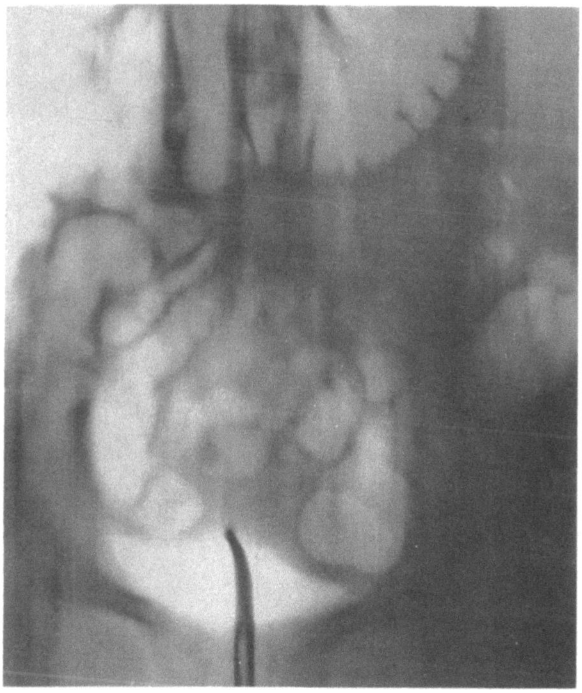

128

Abb. 128

Darmverwachsungen im Becken

2 Jahre nach abdominaler Radikaloperation mit Entfernung beider Adnexe wegen Ovarialkarzinoms. 42jähr. Patientin ohne Beschwerden

Tastbefund: Tumorverdächtige Resistenz im linken mittleren Beckenraum

Indikation: Darstellung und Abgrenzung des fraglichen Tumors

Abb. 128: Die *Schichtuntersuchung* klärt den Befund als ein Konvolut miteinander verwachsener und an der Beckenwand adhärenter Darmschlingen, die das gesamte kleine Becken ausfüllen. Ein Tumorschatten ist in keiner Ebene sichtbar

Verlauf: Während fünf Jahren weiterer Beobachtung kein Tumorrezidiv

Fig. 128

Intrapelvic intestinal adhesions

Condition two years after abdominal radical surgery, including radical adnexectomy, for ovarian carcinoma

Patient, 42, with no complaints

Palpation finding: Tumor-suspicious resistance left in the central pelvic cavity

Indication: Visualisation and demarcation of eventual tumor

Fig. 128 is a *tomogram* to elucidate the finding as a convolution of intestinal loops filling up the entire minor pelvis and being adherent to each other and to the pelvic wall; no tumor shadow is detectable on any plane

Course: No recurrence of tumor during five years of follow-up

5.2.2. *Maligne Harnblasentumoren*[1])

Bei malignen Tumoren der Harnblase kann mit der Pneumopelvigraphie die *perivesikale Infiltration und Tumorausbreitung* beurteilt werden (Abb. 129 bis 131). Auch für eine *Infiltration der Tunica muscularis* sind Anhaltspunkte zu gewinnen, da die Dicke der Harnblasenwand sichtbar wird. Die Frage der Infiltrationstiefe läßt sich besonders bei Tumoren der Blasenhinterwand durch die Darstellung im Pneumopelvigramm oftmals klären.

Das perivesikale Wachstum maligner Harnblasengeschwülste kann in fortgeschrittenen Stadien die in der Blase selbst gelegenen Tumorpartien an Masse und Ausdehnung übertreffen (Abb. 130 u. 131). Für die Bestrahlungsplanung ist der pneumopelvigraphische Befund in solchen Fällen von besonderem Interesse. Gleichzeitig werden Verwachsungen mit dem Darm und den inneren Genitalien erfaßt. Ebenso wie bei malignen Genitaltumoren ist die *Kombination mit der Lymphographie* zur gleichzeitigen Darstellung der regionären Lymphknoten zu empfehlen.

[1]) Die Pneumopelvigraphie ist auch bei männlichen Patienten zur Darstellung von Harnblasentumoren gut geeignet.

5.2.2. *Malignant tumors of the urinary bladder*[1])

Pneumopelvigraphy is a method to assess in malignant tumors of the urinary bladder both *perivesical infiltration and propagation* (Figs. 129—131). Since the thickness of the urinary bladder wall is rendered visible, information may be obtained also regarding an *infiltration of the tunica muscularis*. The depth of infiltration, mainly of tumors located at the posterior wall of the bladder, is another problem which may often be elucidated by pneumopelvigraphic representation.

In advanced stages of malignant tumors of the urinary bladder, both the amount and extension of the perivesical growth may be much more serious than that of the tumor parts within the bladder (Figs. 130 and 131). In such cases, irradiation planning may benefit considerably from pneumopelvigraphic findings. Adhesions with the intestines and the internal genital organs may be recorded, as well. A *combination of pneumopelvigraphy with lymphography* is recommended not only to detect genital tumors, but to represent, at the same time, the regional lymphatic nodes.

[1]) Pneumopelvigraphy is suitable to demonstrate tumors of the urinary bladder also in male patients

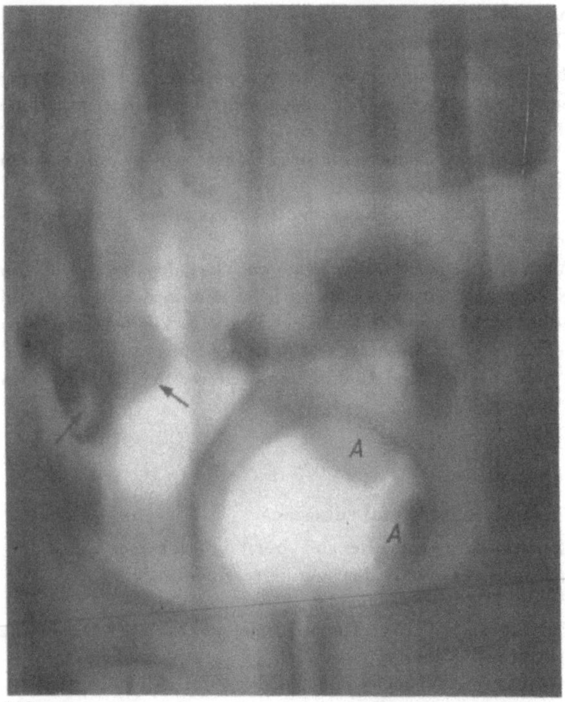

129

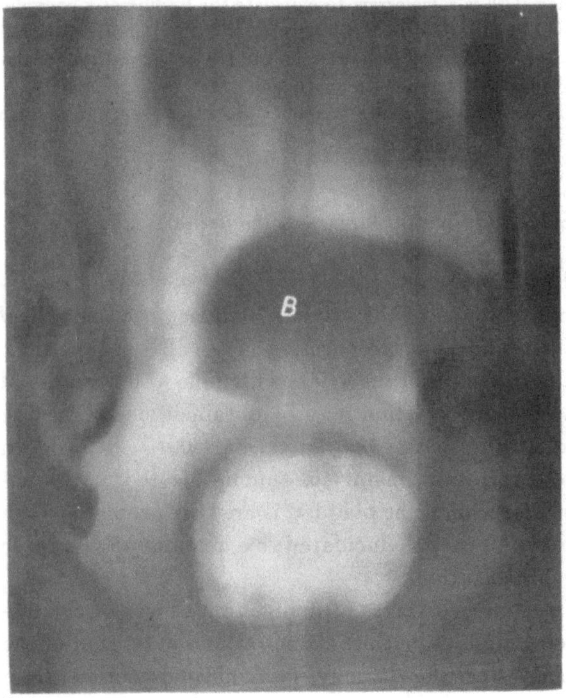

130

Abb. 129–131
Harnblasenkarzinom

62jähr. Patientin mit Haematurie und Schmerzen im Unterbauch. Zustand nach abdominaler Totalexstirpation des Uterus und beider Adnexe wegen Uterus myomatosus

Tastbefund: Vom vorderen Scheidengewölbe aus weicher Tumor im Harnblasenbereich palpabel. Die *Zystoskopie* ergibt einen ausgedehnten, vorwiegend papillären Tumor

Histologischer Befund: Übergangsepithelkarzinom

Indikation: Feststellung der perivesikalen Infiltrationstiefe, Tumorausdehnung und Metastasensuche, *Kombination mit Lymphographie*

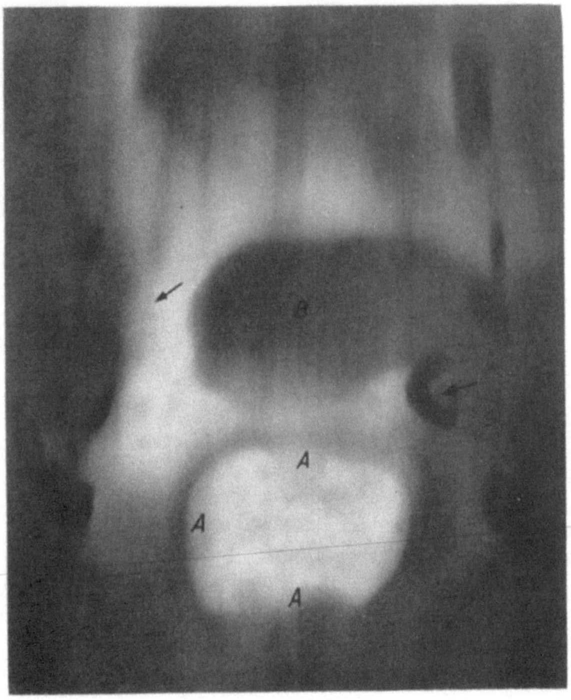

131

Abb. 129–131: Die *Tomogramme* in 5 cm, 7 cm und 9 cm Tiefe zeigen eine Verdickung der gesamten Harnblasenwand, multiple, ins Blasenlumen vorspringende knollige und papilläre Tumorpartien (A) auf allen Schnittflächen und einen kinderfaustgroßen perivesikalen Tumoranteil (B), der von der Blasenhinterwand ausgeht und die Mitte des kleinen Beckens einnimmt. Füllungsdefekt und gleichzeitige Vorwölbung vergrößerter iliakaler Lymphknoten auf beiden Seiten durch Metastasen (←).

Verlauf: Telekobalttherapie

Figs. 129–131
Carcinoma of the urinary bladder

Patient, 62, afflicted with hematuria and reporting pain in the lower abdomen

Condition after abdominal radical hysterectomy; including radical adnexectomy, for uterus myomatosus

Palpation finding: Soft tumor extending from the anterior fornix palpable in the region of the urinary bladder

Expanded and predominantly papillary tumor revealed by cystoscopy

Histological finding: Transitional epithelial carcinoma

Indication: Determination of depth of perivesical infiltration, expanse of tumor, and metastases; *combination with lymphography*

Figs. 129–131 are *tomograms*, 5 cm, 7 cm and 9 cm in depths, showing thickening of the entire urinary bladder wall and multiple bulbiform and papillary tumor parts (A) that are found to protrude on all planes into the vesicular lumen as well as a perivesical tumor part (B) of child's fist size, the latter originating from the posterior wall of the bladder and covering the centre of the minor pelvis; metastases have caused filling defect together with bulging of enlarged iliac lymphatic nodes on either side (←)

Course: Tele-cobalt therapy

Pneumopelvigraphie und perivesikale Gasinsufflation werden mit prinzipiell gleichartiger Indikation eingesetzt. Die Wahl zwischen beiden Verfahren richtet sich vor allem nach der Tumorlokalisation, da die Dicke der Harnblasenwand mit Hilfe des Pneumoperitoneum nicht in allen Abschnitten sichtbar gemacht werden kann.

Basically, there is one and the same indication ruling the use of pneumopelvigraphy and perivesical gas insufflation. The choice of methods will have to depend mainly on the localisation of the tumor, since only some sections of the urinary bladder wall and its thickness can be visualised by means of the pneumoperitoneum.

5.3. Funktionsstörungen der Ovarien und Mißbildungen der Genitalien

Für die Diagnostik der Ovarialsuffizienz und die Klärung verschiedener Syndrome, die mit makroskopischen Veränderungen der Keimdrüsen einhergehen, ergeben sich aus der Kenntnis der Gonadengröße entscheidende Anhaltspunkte. Das gilt besonders für den Nachweis des großen polyzystischen Ovars bei STEIN-LEVENTHAL-Syndrom und für die Klärung der Gonadendysgenesie. Ferner kann die Darstellung der inneren Genitalstrukturen bei Intersexformen und uterovaginalen Mißbildungen von Wert sein, besonders wenn operative Korrekturen geplant werden. Dabei ist die röntgenmorphologische Übersicht der digitalen Beurteilung immer überlegen.

5.3. Ovarian dysfunction and malformation of the genitals

Knowledge of gonodal size is found to be of decisive importance to the diagnosis of ovarian insufficiency and the elucidation of certain syndromes which are accompanied by macroscopic changes of the gonads. This applies mainly to the detection of the enlarged polycystic ovary in cases of STEIN-LEVENTHAL's syndrome and to the elucidation of gonodal dysgenesis. The demonstration of the internal genital structures may be of interest also in cases of hermaphroditism and uterovaginal malformation, particularly when surgical correction is intended. In this context it has become commonplace that a radiographical demonstration of the morphological picture will always be superior to any digital assessment.

5.3.1. STEIN-LEVENTHAL-*Syndrom*

Die *Größenbestimmung der Ovarien* trägt zur diagnostischen Klärung des Krankheitsbildes wesentlich bei. Vom Nachweis vergrößerter Ovarien ist die Indikation zur operativen Therapie (Resectio ovarii) abhängig. Palpatorisch gelingt die Feststellung jedoch nur bei einem Teil der Fälle. Für eine exakte Beurteilung der Ovariengröße ist die Pneumopelvigraphie daher kaum zu entbehren und als Untersuchungsmethode der Wahl zu bezeichnen. Die Volumenzunahme betrifft beide Ovarien und geht meistens ohne Veränderung ihrer Form einher. Die dem Operateur als große graue Ovarien bekannten Befunde rufen charakteristische Röntgenbilder hervor (Abb. 132–140). Das wesentliche Kriterium sind bilateral gleichmäßig vergrößerte Keimdrüsen bei sonst regelrechten Strukturen des inneren Genitales.

Die genauesten Maße erhält man mit Hilfe der Tomographie. Bei der Bewertung der Abmessungen im Tomogramm ist der vom Schichtgerätetyp abhängige Vergrößerungsfaktor zu berücksichtigen. Nach Abzug der Vergrößerung legen wir als obere Grenzwerte der Norm bei jungen Frauen eine Länge von 5 cm und eine Breite von 3 cm zugrunde (STIEVE). Auch auf dem Summationsbild läßt sich aus dem Größenvergleich zwischen Uterus und

5.3.1. STEIN-LEVENTHAL'S *syndrome*

Diagnostic elucidation of a given clinical picture is supported essentially by a *determination of ovarian size.* The indication for therapeutic surgery (resectio ovarii) depends on whether or not the presence of enlarged ovaries can be confirmed. Palpation, however, will yield such confirmation only in some of the cases. Therefore, pneumopelvigraphy is rather indispensable for an accurate assessment of ovarian size, and it may be considered as the method of choice for examination. Expansion usually takes place in either ovary and is, generally, not accompanied by deformation. Very characteristic radiographs are obtainable from the findings known to the surgeon as large grey ovaries (Figs. 132–140). The major criterion includes the presence of bilaterally and equally enlarged gonads, with the remaining structures of the internal genital organ being normal.

Most accurate measurement will be possible by means of tomography. The dimensions visualised by the tomogram should be interpreted and assessed with due consideration of the magnifying factor which depends on the type of tomograph used. The upper limits adopted as normal for young women are 5 cm in length and 3 cm in width after substracting the magnification (STIEVE). Quite a fair picture of the situation may be obtained also from a standard ra-

132 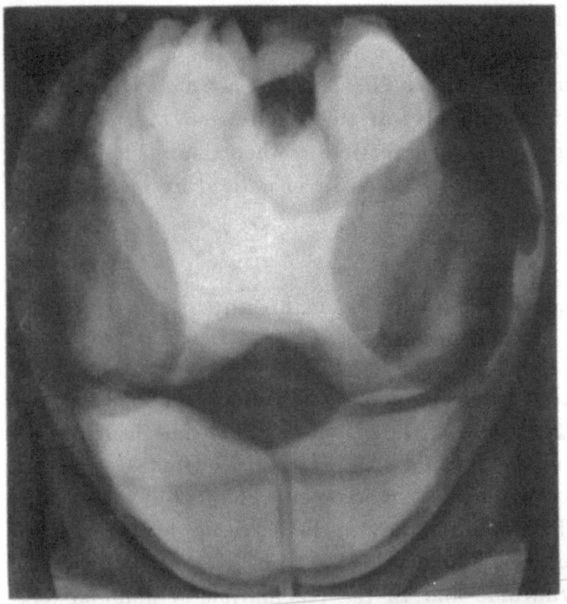 132a 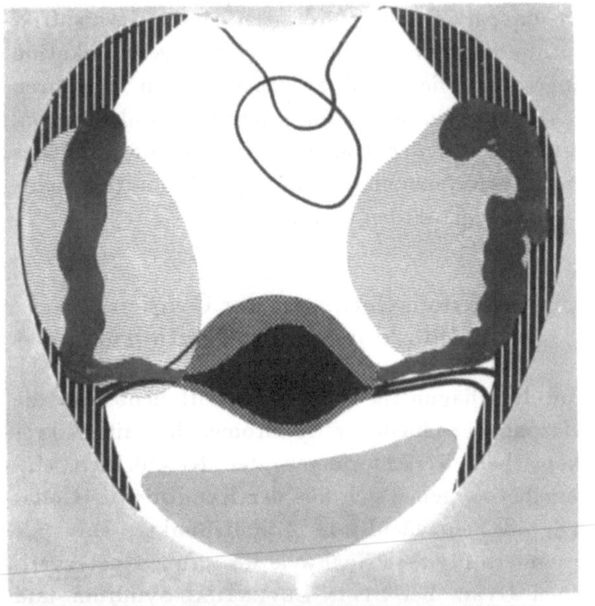

133 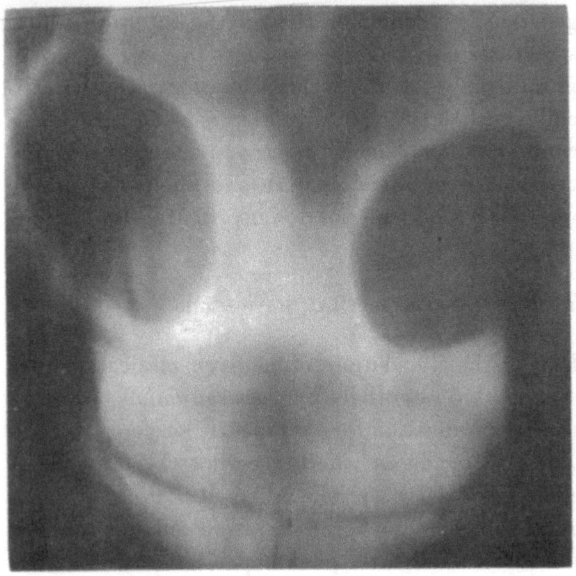 134 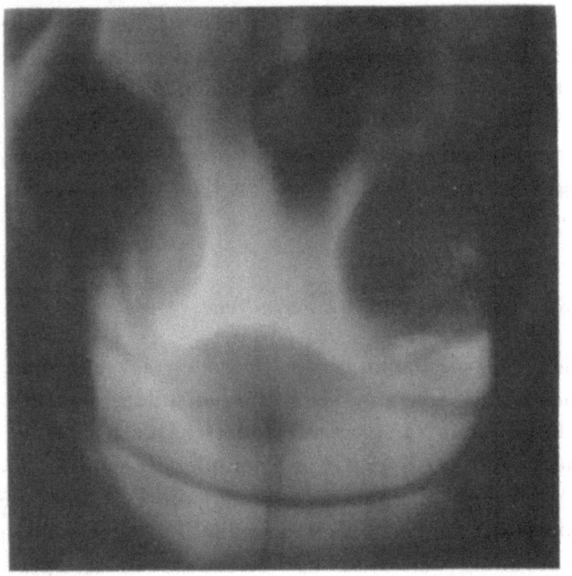

Abb. 132—134

Stein-Leventhal-Syndrom

27jähr. Patientin mit Oligomenorrhoe, primärer Sterilität, Hirsutismus

Tastbefund: Uterus normal groß, anteflektiert, beweglich, Ovarien vergrößert

Indikation: Größenbestimmung der Ovarien

Abb. 132: Auf dem *Übersichtsbild* starke Vergrößerung beider Ovarien. Ihr Umfang erscheint wesentlich größer als der Gebärmutterkörper. Die Oberfläche ist glatt

Abb. 133: Durchmesser der Ovarien nach dem *Tomogramm* in 6 cm Tiefe: Rechts 8,5 cm × 5,5 cm, links 8 cm × 6 cm. Vor dem rechten Ovar zieht ein Verwachsungsstrang zur Appendix

Abb. 134: Auf dem *Tomogramm* in 8 cm Tiefe werden die Schattenstrukturen des Uterus, der Tuben und der Ligamente regelrecht dargestellt

Verlauf: Bei der Laparotomie wird der typische Befund eines Stein-Leventhal-Syndroms erhoben. Es zeigen sich gut hühnereigroße graue Ovarien. Rechts besteht eine Verwachsung mit der Appendix. Resectio ovarii bds. und Appendektomie

Histologischer Befund: Beide Ovarien enthalten außer einer polyzystischen Rindenschicht mehrere kleine Dermoidzysten

Figs. 132—134

Stein-Leventhal's syndrome

Patient, 27, afflicted with oligomenorrhea, primary sterility, and hirsutism

Palpation finding: Uterus of normal size, anteflexed, movable, and ovaries enlarged

Indication: Determination of ovarian size

Fig. 132 is a *standard radiograph* showing strong enlargement ob both ovaries, their volume appearing to be much larger than that of the corpus uteri; smooth surface

Fig. 133 is a *tomogram*, 6 cm in depth, showing the diameters of the ovaries to be 8.5 cm × 5.5 cm on the right and 8 cm × 6 cm on the left; an adhesive chord is found to pass by the front side of the right ovary to extend up to the appendix

Fig. 134 is a *tomogram*, 8 cm in depth, showing in true scale the shadow structures of the uterus, tubes, and ligaments

Course: Laparotomy confirms the presence of a typical Stein-Leventhal's syndrome; the ovaries are of greyish coloration and hen-egg size; an adhesion with the appendix is identified on the right; resection of ovaries and appendectomy

Histological finding: Both ovaries contain polycystic cortical layers and several small dermoid cysts

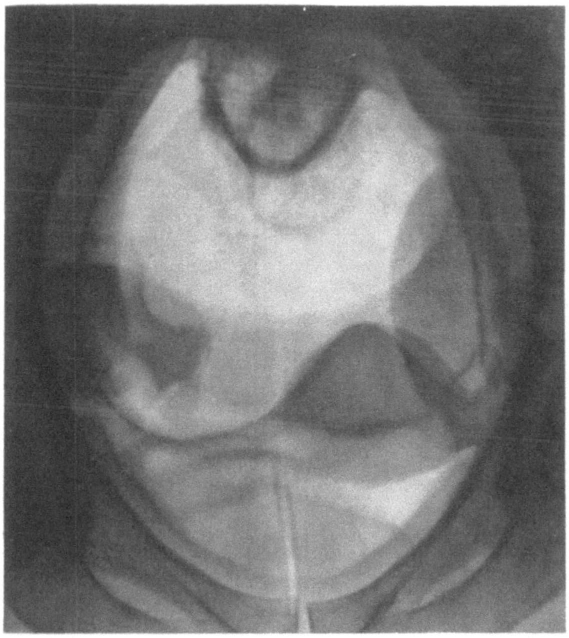

135

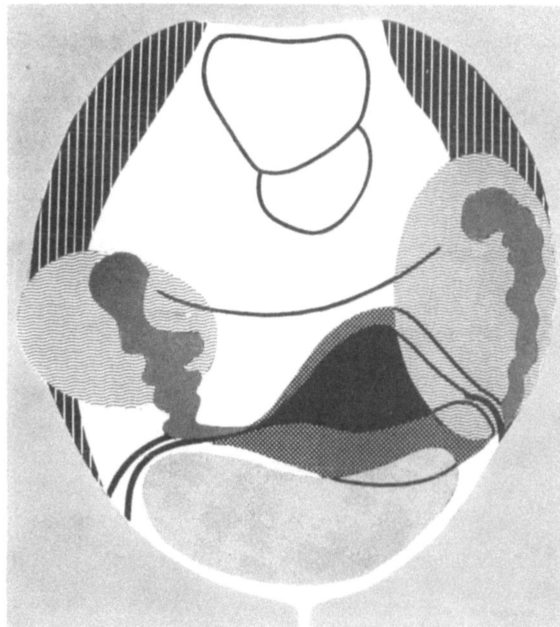

135 a

Abb. 135 und 136

Stein-Leventhal-Syndrom

33jähr. Patientin mit Oligomenorrhoe, primärer Sterilität, Hirsutismus, dringendem Kinderwunsch

Tastbefund: Uterus normal groß, anteflektiert, beweglich, Ovarien klein

Indikation: Größenbestimmung der Ovarien

Abb. 135: Auf dem *Übersichtsbild* Vergrößerung beider Ovarien, Sinistroposition des Uterus. Durchmesser der Ovarien nach dem *Tomogramm:*

Rechts 6 cm × 4 cm, links 6,5 cm × 4 cm

Bei der anschließenden *Salpingographie* erweisen sich beide Tuben als durchgängig

Verlauf: Laparotomie. Vor der Operation wird in Narkose untersucht. Auch dabei kann eine Vergrößerung der Ovarien nicht palpiert werden

Abb. 136: Nach Eröffnung der Bauchhöhle werden in Übereinstimmung mit dem Röntgenbefund deutlich vergrößerte Ovarien gefunden, deren Abmessungen mit den tomographisch ermittelten Werten exakt übereinstimmen. Resectio ovarii

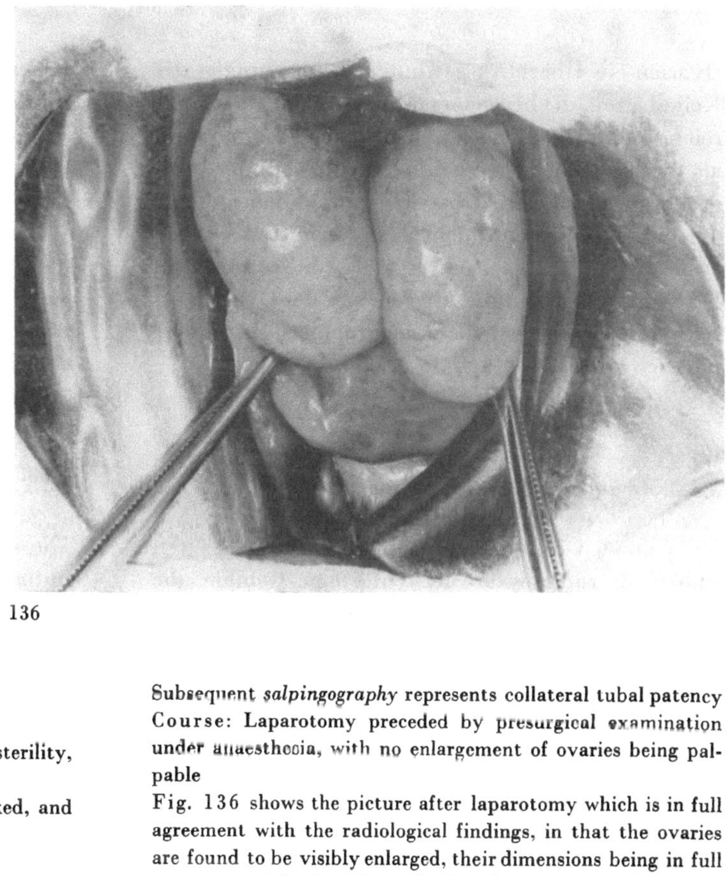

136

Figs. 135 and 136

Stein-Leventhal's syndrome

Patient, 33, afflicted with oligomenorrhea, primary sterility, and hirsutism; urgent desire for children

Palpation finding: Uterus of normal size, anteflexed, and movable; small ovaries

Indication: Assessment of ovarian size

Fig. 135 is a standard radiograph showing the two enlarged ovaries, with their diameters being 6 cm × 4 cm on the right and 6.5 cm × 4 cm on the left (values obtained from tomograms), sinistro-position of the uterus

Subsequent *salpingography* represents collateral tubal patency

Course: Laparotomy preceded by presurgical examination under anaesthesia, with no enlargement of ovaries being palpable

Fig. 136 shows the picture after laparotomy which is in full agreement with the radiological findings, in that the ovaries are found to be visibly enlarged, their dimensions being in full agreement with the values obtained from tomography; resection of ovaries

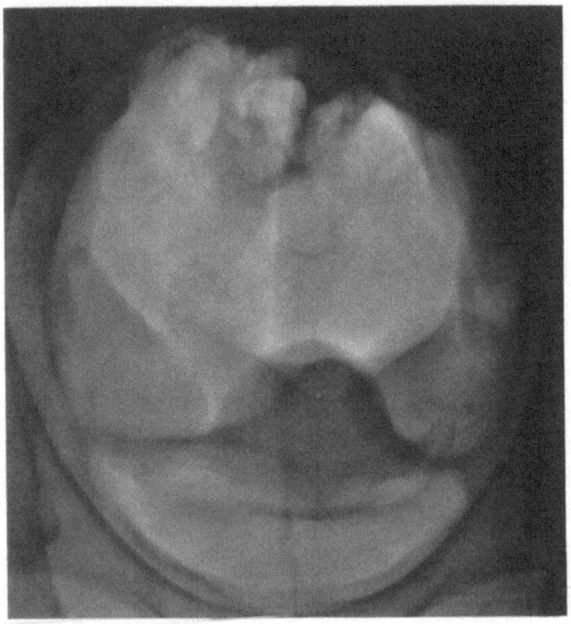

137

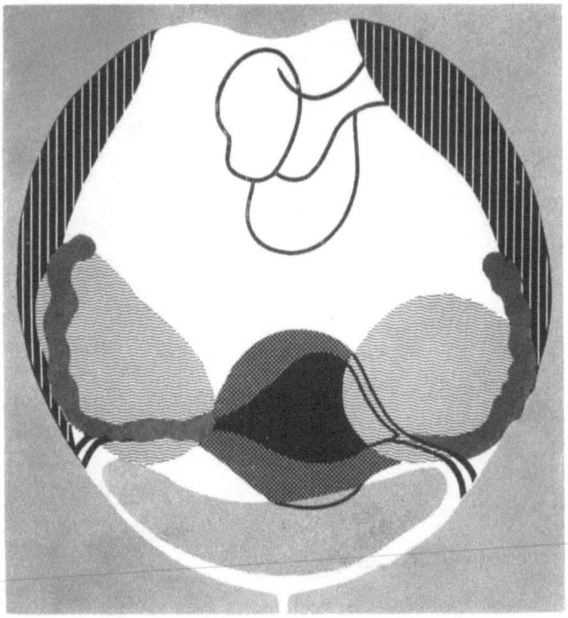

137a

Ovarien ein Überblick gewinnen. Abmessungen der Keimdrüsen, die besonders in Grenzfällen aufschlußreich sind, dürfen jedoch nur nach dem Tomogramm als verbindlich angesehen werden, weil der Vergrößerungsgrad auf Übersichtsaufnahmen infolge der Schrägprojektion nicht sicher ermittelt werden kann. Wenn Verwachsungen der Adnexe mit dem Darm bestehen und die Abgrenzung der Ovarien erschweren, erweist sich die Tomographie als besonders nützlich (Abb. 141—145).

5.3.2. *Gonadendysgenesie, Gonadenhypoplasie*

Die Gonaden imponieren in klassisch ausgeprägten Fällen als rudimentäre leistenförmige Gebilde, die nicht palpiert werden können, auf dem Röntgenbild jedoch zur Darstellung gelangen (Abb. 146 bis 148). Uterus und Tuben sind angelegt, bleiben aber auch im Erwachsenenalter hypoplastisch. Bei partiellen Formen des TURNER-Syndroms und Fällen mit geringer Ausprägung assoziierter Merkmale trägt die Pneumopelvigraphie zur Sicherung der Diagnose weitgehend bei. Die Ansprechbarkeit hypoplastischer Ovarien auf stimulierende Hormontherapie läßt sich ebenfalls durch die Pneumopelvigraphie beurteilen. Dafür ist eine zweite Untersuchung zum Größenvergleich notwendig (Abb. 149 und 150).

diograph by comparing uterus size with ovarian size. However, dimensions of the gonads, that are of great informative value mainly in borderline cases, should not be considered safe unless visualised by tomography, because due to oblique projection no safe determination is possible of the magnifying factor in standard radiographs. Tomography is found to be of particular usefulness in cases where the adnexa are adherent to the intestines, so that problems are added to the differentiation of the ovaries (Figs. 141 to 145).

5.3.2. *Gonodal dysgenesis, gonodal hypoplasia*

The classical appearance of the gonads is that of rudimentary structures which are not palpable, but may be demonstrated radiographically (Figs. 146 to 148). Uterus and tubes, while preformed, remain hypoplastic even in adult age. Pneumopelvigraphy can help essentially to achieve a consistent diagnosis of partial forms of TURNER's syndrome and of cases where associated characteristics are pronounced but little. Pneumopelvigraphy may be used also to assess the reactivity of hypoplastic ovaries to stimulation by hormone therapy, which, however, will require a second examination for dimensional comparison (Figs. 149 and 150).

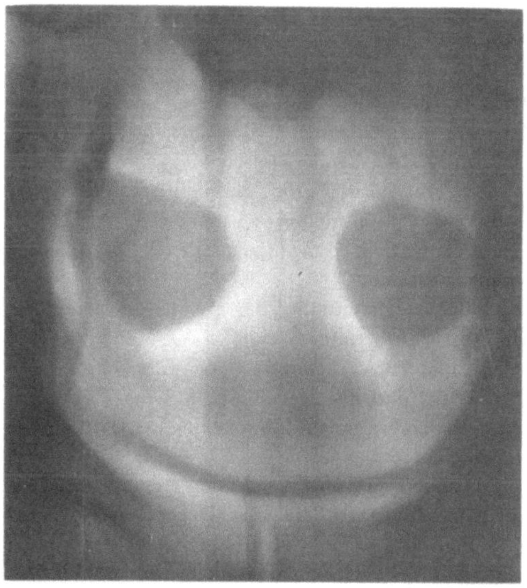

138

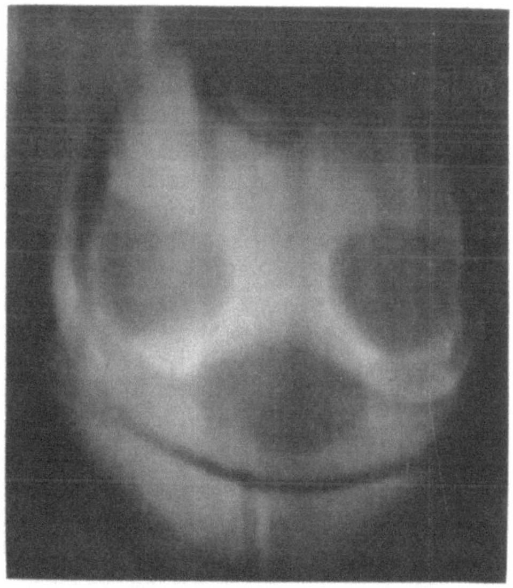

139

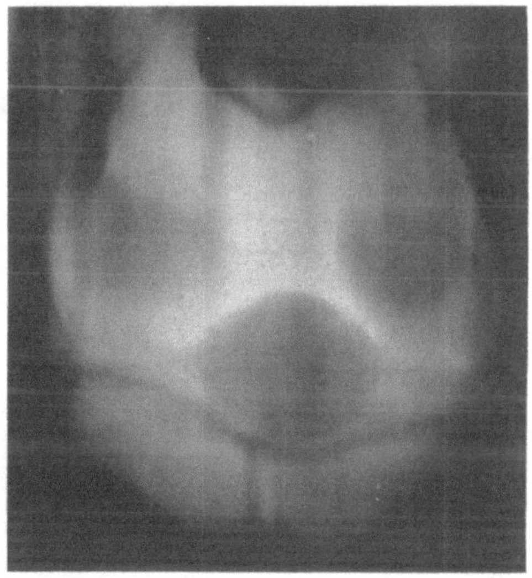

140

Abb. 137–140

Stein-Leventhal-Syndrom

23jähr. Patientin mit sekundärer Amenorrhoe, Hirsutismus, dringendem Kinderwunsch

Tastbefund: Uterus normal groß, anteflektiert, beweglich, Ovarien nicht vergrößert

Indikation: Größenbestimmung der Ovarien

Abb. 137: Auf dem *Übersichtsbild* Vergrößerung beider Ovarien, Durchmesser nach dem *Tomogramm:*
Rechts 5,5 cm × 4,5 cm, links 5 cm × 4 cm

Abb. 138–140: Die *Tomogramme* zeigen folgende Einzelheiten: In 5 cm Tiefe den ampullären Teil beider Tuben und die Ovarien (Abb. 138), in 6 cm Tiefe die Anheftungsstellen der Eileiter an den Fundusecken des Uterus (Abb. 139), in 7 cm Tiefe den Gebärmutterkörper, der die Harnblasenwand flach eindellt (Abb. 140)

Verlauf: Bei der Laparotomie werden hühnereigroße, graue Ovarien gefunden. Resectio ovarii

Figs. 137–140

Stein-Leventhal's syndrome

Patient, 23, afflicted with secondary amenorrhea and hirsutism; urgent desire for children

Palpation finding: Uterus of normal size, anteflexed, and movable; ovaries unenlarged

Indication: Assessment of ovarian size

Fig. 137 is a standard radiograph showing the two enlarged ovaries

Figs. 138–140 are *tomograms* showing the following details: the ampullary parts of the two tubes and the ovaries their diameters being 5.5 cm × 4.5 cm on the right and 5 cm × 4 cm on the left, 5 cm in depth (Fig. 138), the insertions of the oviducts to the fundic ends of the uterus, 6 cm in depth (Fig. 139), and the corpus uteri causing a slight depression of the urinary bladder wall, 7 cm in depth (Fig. 140)

Course: Laparotomy presents the ovaries in hen-egg size and grey coloration; resection of ovaries

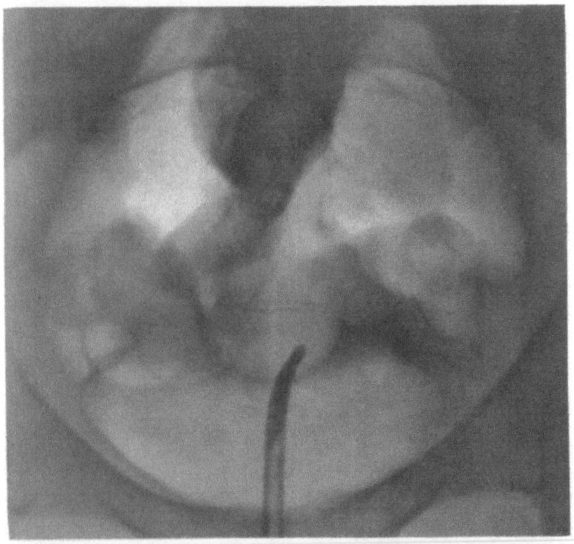

Abb. 141—145

Stein-Leventhal-Syndrom

29jähr. Patientin mit Oligomenorrhoe, primärer Sterilität, Hirsutismus, dringendem Kinderwunsch

Tastbefund: Uterus normal groß, anteflektiert, linkes Ovar hühnereigroß, Verdacht auf mehrere Zysten des rechten Ovars. Bei zwei späteren Untersuchungen wird keine Vergrößerung der Ovarien mehr getastet

Indikation: Größenbestimmung der Ovarien, Klärung des wechselnden Palpationsbefundes

Abb. 141: Multiple Verwachsungen beider Ovarien und Tuben mit dem Darm und der Harnblase. Auf der *Übersichtsaufnahme* ist deshalb eine genaue Abgrenzung der Ovarien und Tuben nicht möglich

Abb. 142—144: Die *Tomogramme* in 6 cm, 7 cm und 8 cm Tiefe zeigen beide Ovarien vergrößert. Der Durchmesser beträgt rechts 5 cm × 4 cm, links 6 cm × 4 cm. Im Bereich der Adnexe bestehen zahlreiche Verwachsungsstränge. Bei der anschließenden *Salpingographie* wird beiderseits ein ampullärer Tubenverschluß nachgewiesen

A = Corpus uteri; B = rechtes Ovar; C = linkes Ovar; D = rechte Tube; E = Rectum; → = Verwachsungsstränge

Verlauf: Laparotomie. Es finden sich große graue Ovarien und zahlreiche Verwachsungsstränge. Salpingolyse rechts, Tubenresektion und Stomatoplastik links

Abb. 145: Operationsfoto

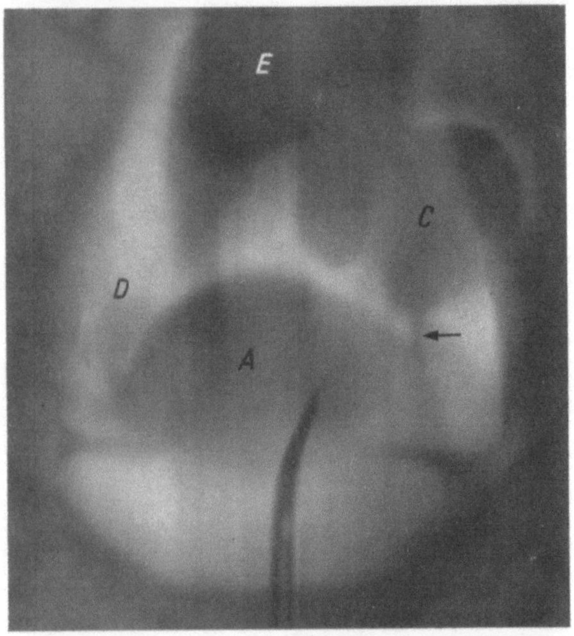

Figs. 141—145

Stein-Leventhal's syndrome

Patient, 29, afflicted with oligomenorrhea, primary sterility, and hirsutism; urgent desire for children

Palpation finding: Uterus of normal size and anteflexed; left ovary of hen-egg size; several cysts suspected in right ovary; no ovarian enlargement is palpated any longer in two follow-up examinations

Indication: Assessment of ovarian size; elucidation of deviating palpation findings

Fig. 141 is a ***standard radiograph*** which does not enable any precise delimination of the ovaries and tubes, because of multiple adhesions of either ovary and tube with the intestine and urinary bladder

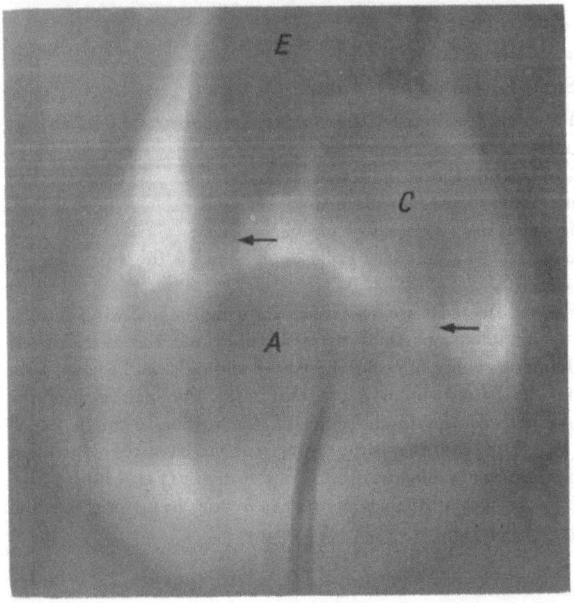

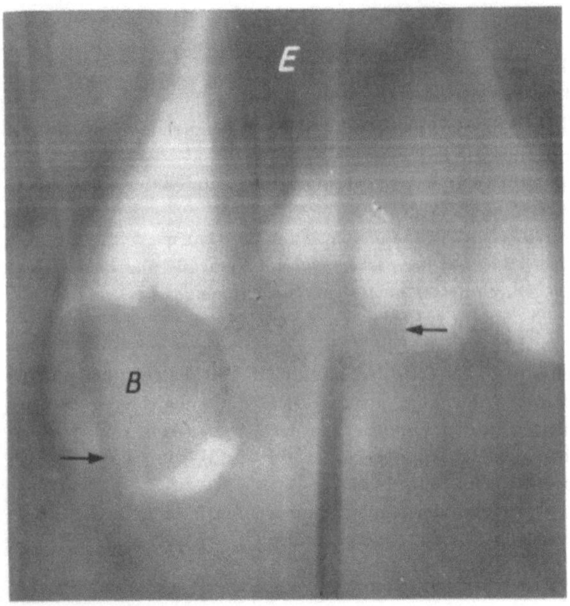

Figs. 142–144 are *tomograms*, 6 cm, 7 cm, and 8 cm in depths, showing both ovaries enlarged, the diameters being 5 cm × 4 cm on the rigth and 6 cm × 4 cm on the left; numerous adhesive chords are visualised in the adnexal region; *salpingography* is added to confirm collateral ampullary tubal obstruction
A = corpus uteri; B = right ovary; C = left ovary; D = right tube; E = rectum; → = adhesive chords
Course: Laparotomy reveals large grey ovaries and numerous adhesive chords; salpingolysis on the right; salpingectomy and stomatoplasty on the left
Fig. 145: Photograph of operation

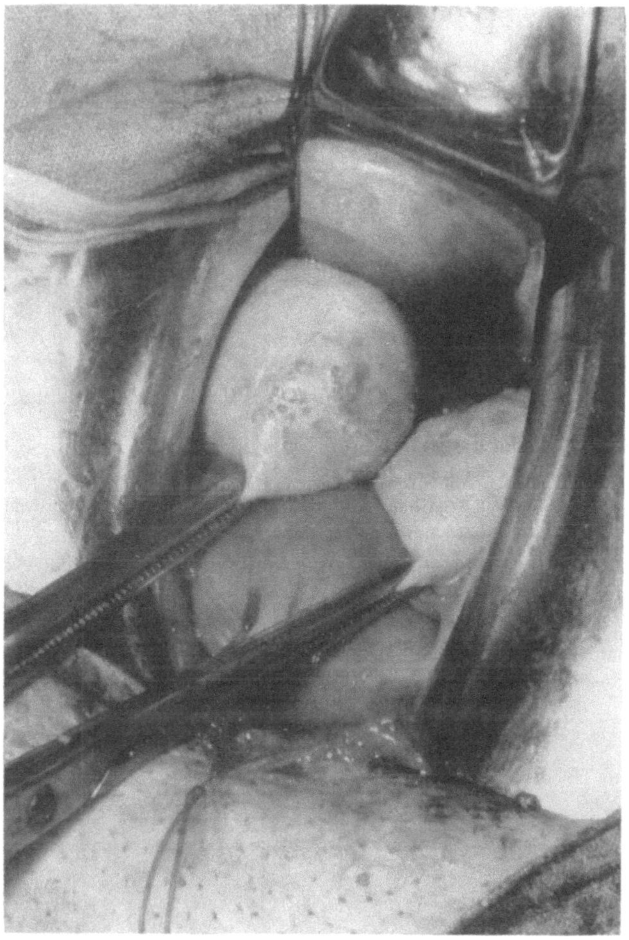

145

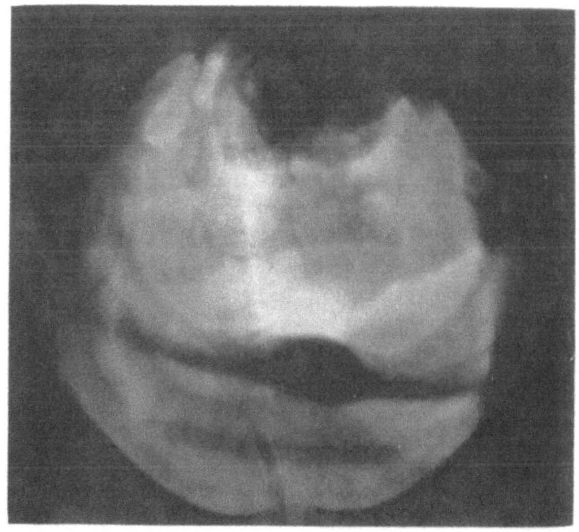

146

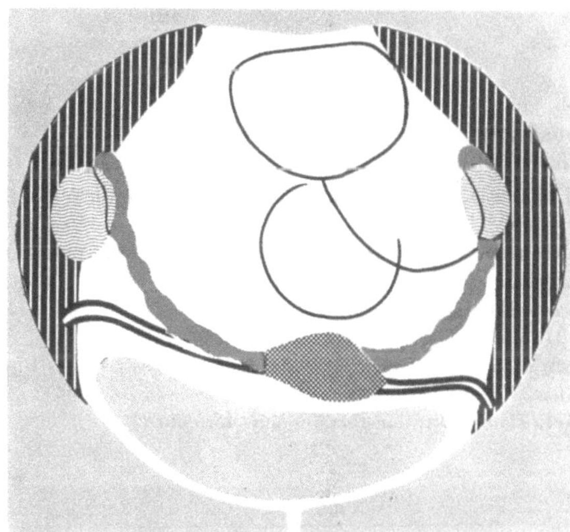

146a

Abb. 146
Gonadendysgenesie
Turner-Syndrom

25jähr. Patientin mit primärer Amenorrhoe, Kleinwuchs, zahlreichen Pigmentnaevi
Tastbefund: Hypoplasie der Vulva und Vagina, Uterus als fingerkuppengroße Resistenz tastbar, Adnexe nicht zu beurteilen
Chromosomales Geschlecht: ♀
Indikation: Darstellung der Ovarien
Abb. 146: Hypoplasie des Uterus, hochgradige Hypoplasie der Ovarien, die als flache Vorwölbungen auf beiden Seiten im Becken sichtbar sind. Tuben und Genitalligamente regelrecht angelegt
Verlauf: Substitutionstherapie mit Hormonen

Fig. 146
Gonadal dysgenesis
Turner's syndrome

Patient, 25, afflicted with primary amenorrhea, nanosoma, and numerous pigmented novi
Palpation finding: Hypoplasia of vulva and vagina; uterus palpable as a resistance of fingertip-size; adnexa beyond assessment
Chromosomal sex: ♀
Indication: Visualisation of ovaries
Fig. 146: Hypoplasia of the uterus; severe hypoplasia of the ovaries visible as flat protrusions on either side in the pelvis: tubes and genital ligaments formed properly
Course: Substitution therapy, using hormones

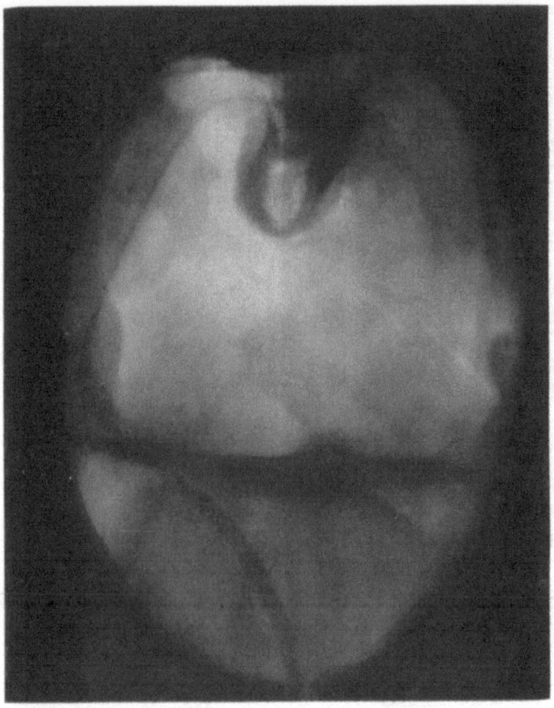

147

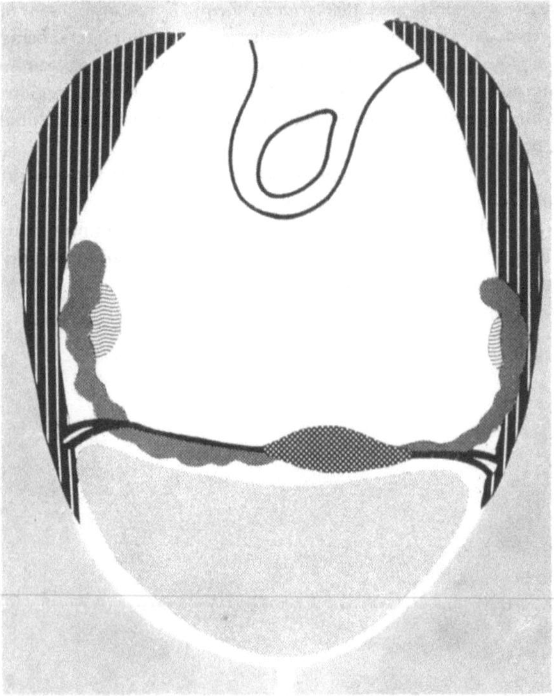

147 a

Abb. 147
Gonadendysgenesie
Turner-Syndrom

20jähr. Patientin mit primärer Amenorrhoe, infantilem Habitus, kurzem breitem Hals
Tastbefund: Fingerkuppengroßer Uterus, Adnexe nicht zu beurteilen
Chromosomales Geschlecht: ♂
Indikation: Darstellung der Gonaden
Abb. 147: Hochgradige Hypoplasie des Uterus und der Gonaden
Verlauf: Substitutionstherapie mit Hormonen

Fig. 147
Gonadal dysgenesis
Turner's syndrome

Patient, 20, afflicted with primary amenorrhea; infantile habitus, short and broad neck
Palpation finding: Uterus of fingertip size; adnexa beyond assessment
Chromosomal sex: ♂
Indication: Visualisation of the gonads
Fig. 147: Severe hypoplasia of the uterus and gonads
Course: Substitution therapy, using hormones

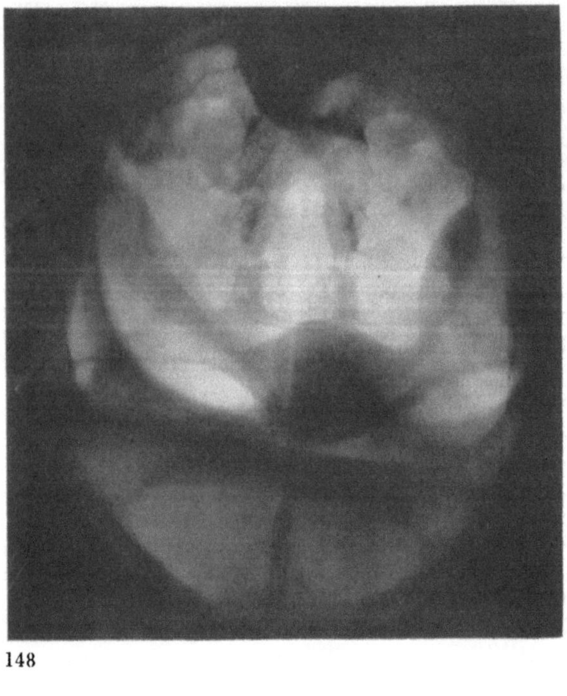

148

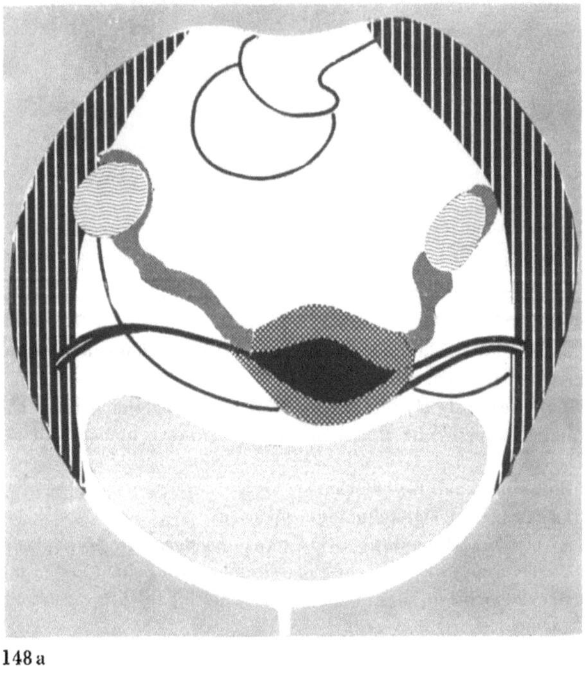

148 a

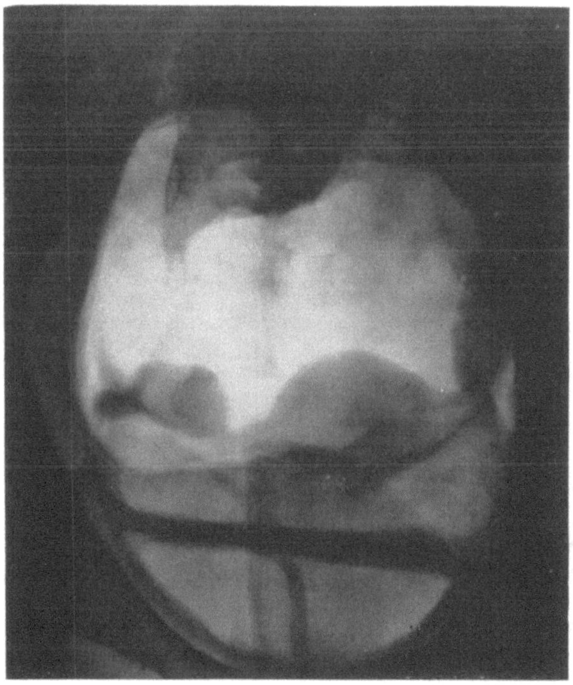

149

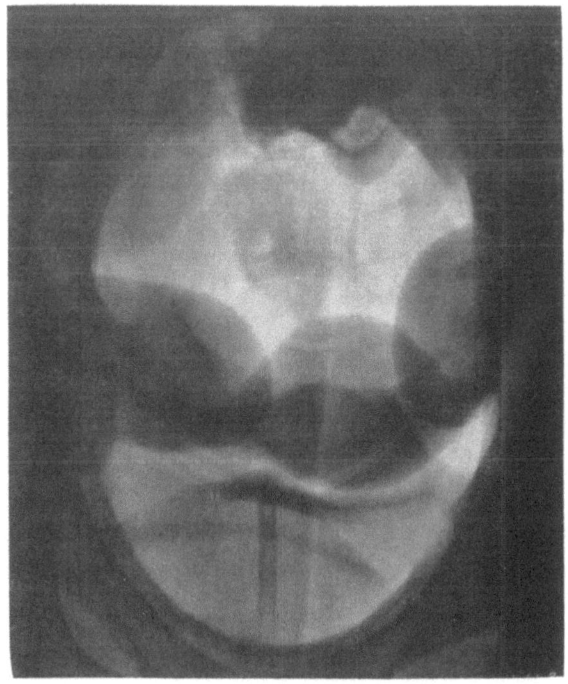

150

Abb. 149 und 150

Gonadenhypoplasie

20jähr. Patientin mit primärer Amenorrhoe

Tastbefund: Uterus hypoplastisch, gestreckt, Adnexe unauffällig

Chromosomales Geschlecht: ♀

Indikation: Darstellung der Ovarien

Abb. 149: Hypoplasie der Ovarien, geringe Hypoplasie des Uterus, Tuben unauffällig

Verlauf: Probelaparotomie. Es werden langgestreckte, weißliche, derbe Ovarien von der Größe eines Fingerendgliedes gefunden. Teilexzision zur geweblichen Untersuchung

Histologischer Befund: Eianlagen vorhanden, überwiegend Primärfollikel, vereinzelt Sekundärfollikel, kein Corpus luteum

Abb. 150: Untersuchung nach Hormontherapie mit FSH. Die Größe der Ovarien hat unter der stimulierenden Hormonwirkung beträchtlich zugenommen. Ihr Volumen ist annähernd auf das 5fache angestiegen. Palpatorisch konnte diese Vergrößerung der Ovarien jedoch nicht festgestellt werden

Figs. 149 and 150

Gonadal hypoplasia

Patient, 20, afflicted with primary amenorrhea

Palpation finding: Uterus hypoplastic and stretched; adnexa unpathological

Chromosomal sex: ♀

Indication: Visualisation of the ovaries

Fig. 149: Hypoplasia of the ovaries; slight hypoplasia of the uterus; tubes unpathological

Course: Exploratory laparotomy reveals longish, whitish, hard ovaries of the size of a distal phalanx, partial biopsy

Histological finding: Ovaries preformed, mainly primary follicles, few secondary follicles, absence of corpus luteum

Fig. 150: Examination following hormonotherapy, using FSH, reveals considerable growth of ovaries under stimulating hormone action, their volume having grown almost by the factor of five; this enlargement, however, was not assessable by palpation

Abb. 148

Gonadendysgenesie

24jähr. Patientin mit primärer Amenorrhoe

Tastbefund: Uterus hypoplastisch, spitzwinklig anteflektiert, Adnexe unauffällig

Chromosomales Geschlecht: ♀

Indikation: Darstellung der Ovarien

Abb. 148: Hypoplasie des Uterus, Hypoplasie der Ovarien. Es handelt sich um rudimentäre spindelförmige Keimdrüsenanlagen

Verlauf: Substitutionstherapie mit Hormonen

Fig. 148

Gonadal dysgenesis

Patient, 24, afflicted with primary amenorrhea

Palpation finding: Hypoplasia of the uterus which is of acute angle shape and anteflexed; adnexa unpathological

Chromosomal sex: ♀

Indication: Visualisation of the ovaries

Fig. 148: Hypoplasia of the uterus and ovaries; rudimentary, spindle-shaped formation of gonads

Course: Substitution therapy, using hormones

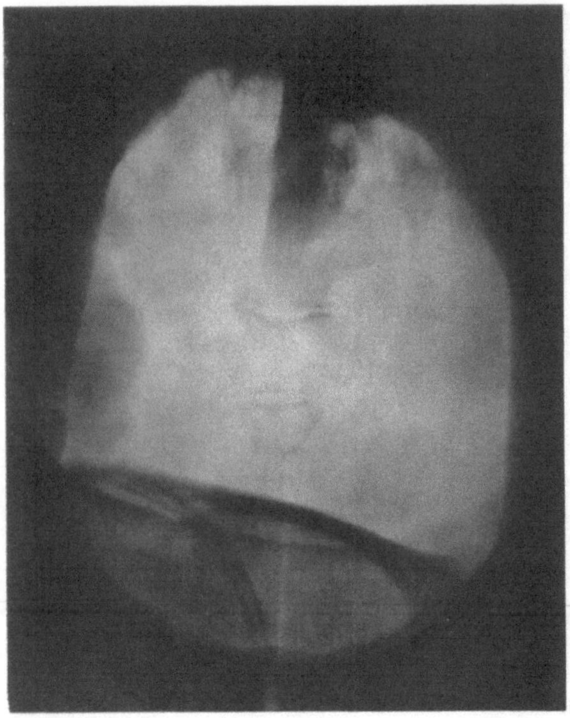

151

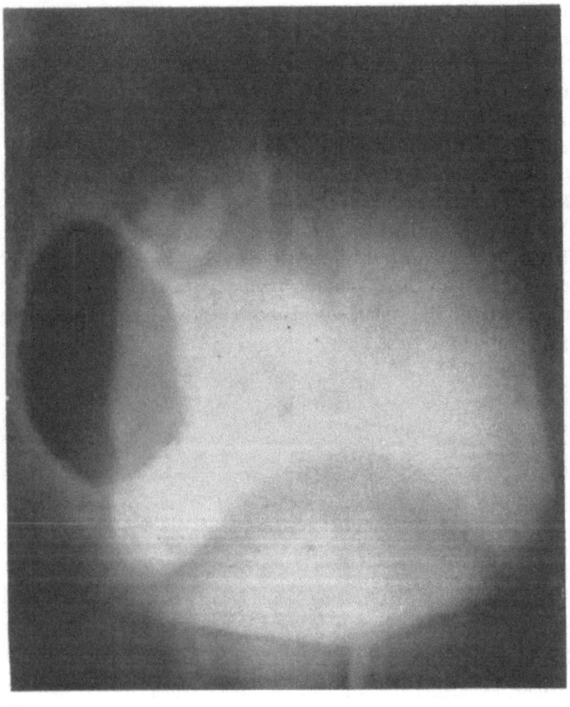

152

Abb. 151—152

Pseudohermaphroditismus masculinus

Testikuläre Feminisierung

31jähr. Patientin mit primärer Amenorrhoe

Tastbefund: Äußeres Genitale unauffällig. Vagina 8 cm lang, blind endend, Fehlen der Portio, kein Uterus und keine Adnexe palpabel. In der linken Leistenbeuge ist eine Keimdrüsenanlage tastbar

Chromosomales Geschlecht: ♂

Nebenbefund: Nierenaplasie links

Indikation: Darstellung des inneren Genitales

Abb. 151: Die Mitte des kleinen Beckens erscheint leer, Uterus und Eileiter fehlen. Rechts ist ein ovalgeformter Schatten sichtbar, dessen Konturen etwas unregelmäßig erscheinen

Abb. 152: Im *Tomogramm* erkennt man die gebuckelte Oberfläche besonders deutlich. Es handelt sich um die rechtsseitige Keimdrüse, deren Durchmesser nach dem Tomogramm 7 cm mal 5 cm beträgt. Die linksseitige Gonadenanlage ist im Leistenkanal gelegen (beiderseits retinierte Hoden). Auf Grund der Vergrößerung und der gebuckelten Oberfläche der retinierten rechten Keimdrüse besteht Verdacht auf das Vorliegen tubulärer Adenome

Verlauf: Auf Wunsch der Patientin wird ein operativer Eingriff nicht vorgenommen

Figs. 151 and 152

Male pseudohermaphroditism

Testicular feminisation

Patient, 31, afflicted with primary amenhorrhea

Palpation finding: External genitals unpathological; vagina 8 cm in length with blind end; absence of portio; uterus and adnexa not palpable; gonadal preformation palpable in left groin

Chromosomal sex ♂

Secondary finding: Nephroaplasia, left

Indication: Visualisation of internal genital

Fig. 151: Centre of minor pelvis seems to be empty, with uterus and oviducts being absent; oval shadow with somewhat irregular contours visible on the right

Fig. 152 is a *tomogram* showing clearly gibbous surface of the right gonad, its diameter being 7 cm × 5 cm by tomographic determination; left gonad is situated in the inguinal canal (retained testicles on either side); enlargement and gibbous surface of retained right gonad supports suspicion of tubular adenomas

Course: No operation is performed on a request by the patient

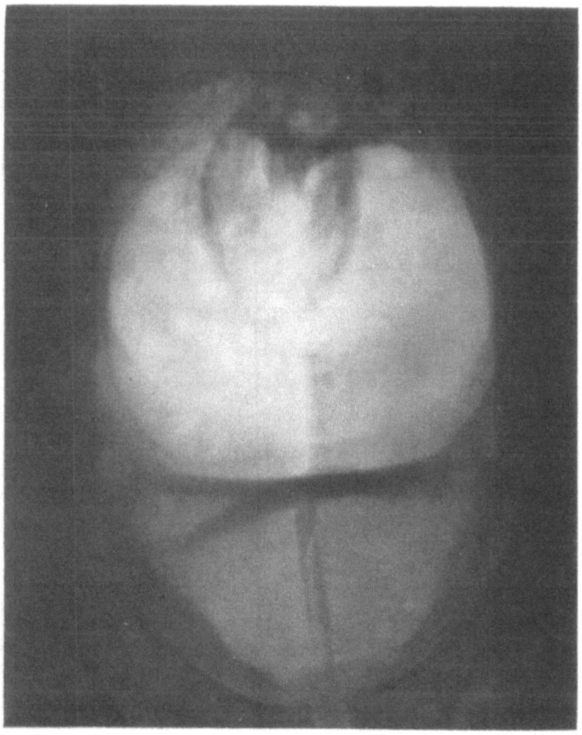

153

Abb. 153
Pseudohermaphroditismus masculinus
14jähr. Patientin ohne Menarche
Tastbefund: Kleiner Introitus vaginae, sondierbare, sehr kurze Vagina, rektal kein Uterus palpabel, im linken Leistenkanal mandelgroße Keimdrüsenanlage.
Chromosomales Geschlecht: ♂
Indikation: Darstellung des inneren Genitales
Abb. 153: Innerhalb des Cavum peritonei pelvis sind Keimdrüsenanlagen nicht nachweisbar. Aplasie des Uterus und der Tuben

Fig. 153
Male pseudohermaphroditism
Patient, 14, without menarche
Palpation finding: Small vaginal introitus; vagina very short but explorable; no rectal palpability of the uterus; presence of gonadal preformation of almond size in the left inguinal canal
Chromosomal sex: ♂
Indication: Visualisation of internal genital
Fig. 153: No gonadal preformations are recordable from within the cavum peritonei pelvis; aplasia of the uterus and tubes

5.3.3. *Intersexualität*

Zur Differentialdiagnose der Intersexformen ist der morphologische Genitalbefund von großer Bedeutung. Kennt man neben dem äußeren Genitale auch die inneren Strukturen, so läßt sich das Urteil präzisieren. Bei der Vielfalt der Mißbildungsformen und infolge der zahlreichen anatomischen Varianten im Bereich der Urogenitalöffnung bleiben Tastbefund, Katheterisierung, Spekulumuntersuchung und Endoskopie in ihrer Aussage häufig begrenzt. Unter diesem Aspekt stellt die Pneumopelvigraphie eine Bereicherung der Untersuchungsmethoden dar. Sie gibt insbesondere Aufschluß über die Derivate der MÜLLERschen Gänge und die Gonaden (Abb. 151 bis 159).

5.3.3. *Intersexuality*

The morphological genital finding is of greatest importance to a differential diagnosis of intersexual forms. Knowledge not only of the external genital but also of the internal structure is a precondition for more accuracy in assessment. The variety of possible malformations and anatomic variants in the region of the urogenital opening is such that narrow upper limits are often imposed upon the informative value of palpation, catheterisation, speculum examination, and endoscopy. Viewed from this angle, pneumopelvigraphy has something to add to the methods of examination. Information is obtainable, in particular, about the derivatives of MÜLLER's ducts and about the gonads (Figs. 151 to 159).

5.3.4. *Uterovaginale Mißbildungen*

Von den Entwicklungsstörungen der MÜLLERschen Gänge sind Mißbildungen, welche die Gebärmutter betreffen, im Pneumopelvigramm gut darzustellen, weil die Serosafläche des Uterus vom Gas allseitig umflossen wird. *Hypoplasie*, *Aplasie* und *Doppelbildungen des Uterus* ergeben charakteristische Bilder (Abb. 160—169). *Bikornität* läßt sich nicht nur bei symmetrischer Anlage (Abb. 160—169), sondern auch bei Asymmetrie und rudimentären Nebenhör-

5.3.4. *Uterovaginal malformations*

These defects in the development of MÜLLER's ducts which are malformations with bearings on the uterus can be demonstrated readily in the pneumopelvigram, since the serosa of the uterus will be encircled entirely by the flow of insufflated gas. Characteristic radiographic patterns are obtained from *hypoplasia*, *aplasia*, and *diplogenesis of the uterus* (Figs. 160—169). *Bicornuation* can be identified not only when preformed symmetrically (Figs.

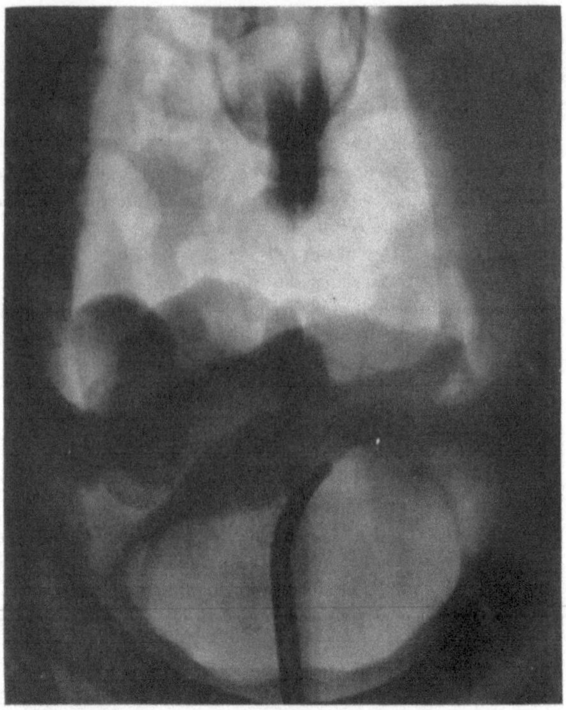

154

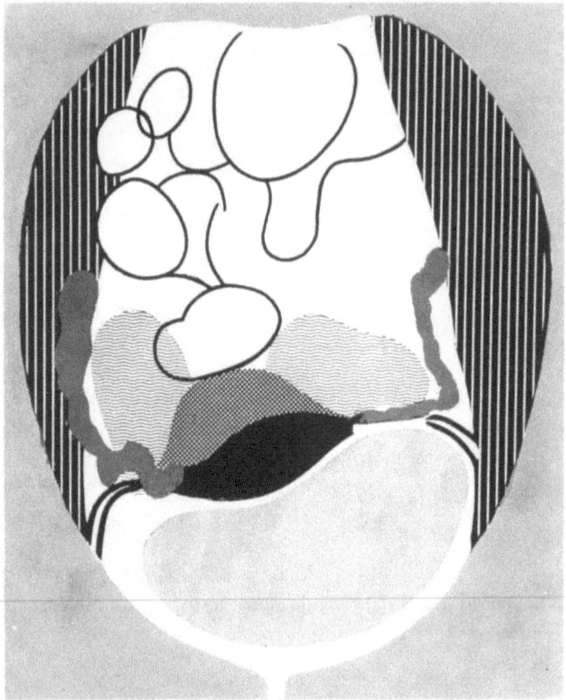

154a

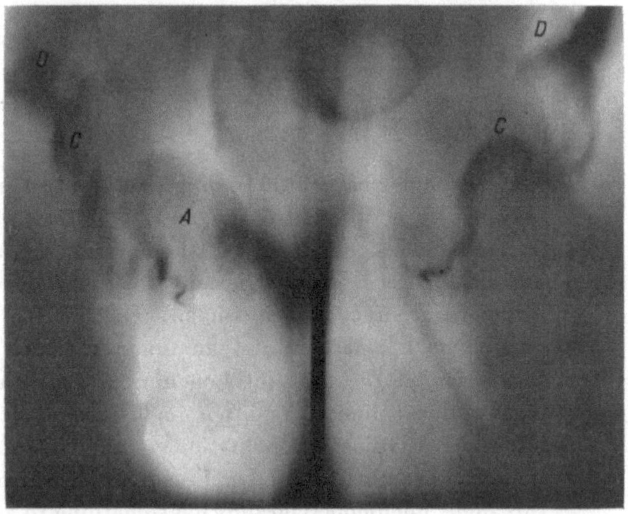

155

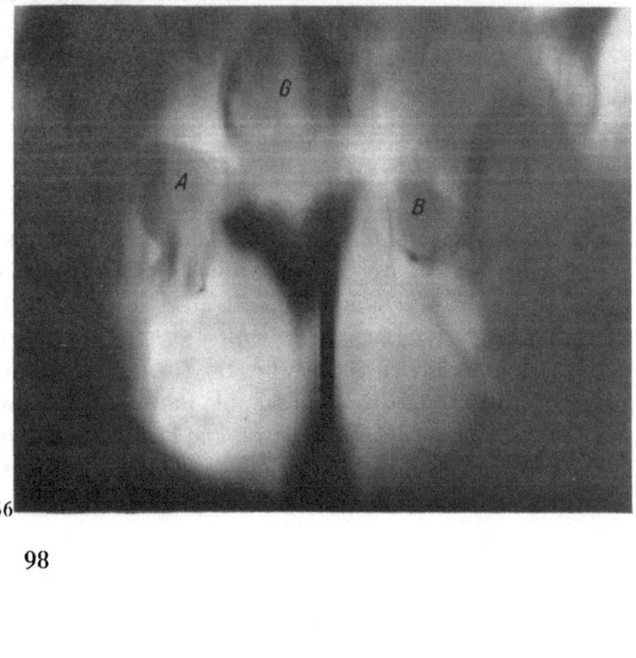

156

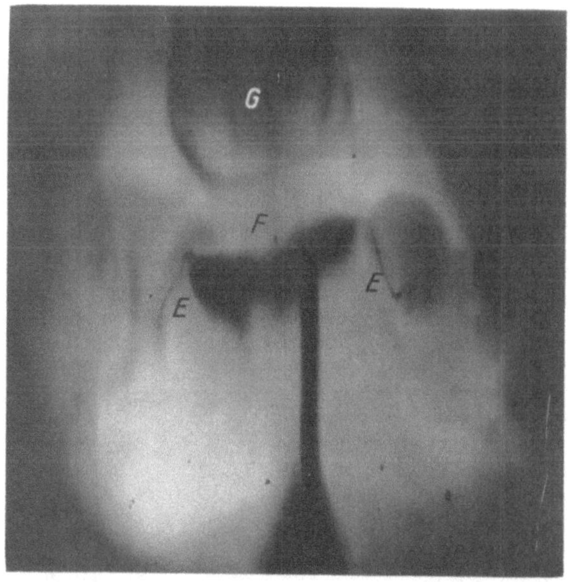

157

Abb. 154—159
Pseudohermaphroditismus femininus

22jähr. Patientin mit männlich gerichteter Psyche. Jünglinghafter Habitus, männliche Stimme. Klitorishypertrophie, hypoplastische Mammae, vereinzelt schwache Menstruationen
Tastbefund: Uterus gestreckt, Gonaden nicht sicher zu beurteilen
Chromosomales Geschlecht: ♀
Indikation: Kombination mit *Hysterosalpingographie* zur Darstellung des inneren Genitales
Abb. 154: Auf der *Übersichtsaufnahme* projizieren sich Uterus und Gonaden aufeinander
Abb. 155—159: Nach zusätzlicher *Hysterosalpingographie* sind auf den *Tomogrammen* in 3 cm—7 cm Tiefe folgende Einzelheiten zu erkennen: Größendifferenz der Keimdrüsen, Durchmesser rechts 4 cm × 2,5 cm, links 2,5 cm × 1,5 cm, Uterus arcuatus, normal angelegte durchgängige Tuben, weiblich determinierte innere Genitalstrukturen
A = rechtes Ovar; B = linkes Ovar; C = Ampulla tubae uterinae; D = in die Bauchhöhle eingeflossenes Kontrastmittel; E = Isthmus tubae uterinae; F = Corpus uteri; G = Rectum

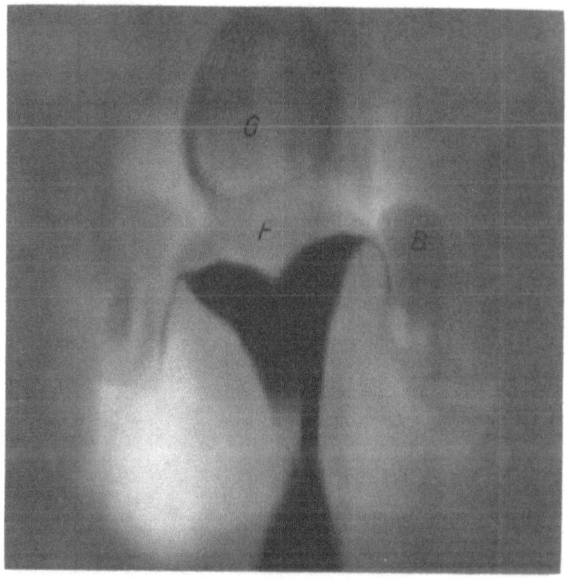

158

Figs. 154—159
Female pseudohermaphroditism

Patient, 22, male-oriented psychological state, adolescent habitus, male voice, hypertrophy of the clitoris, hypoplasia of the breast, scattered, poor menstruation
Palpation finding: Uterus stretched; no safe assessment of gonads
Chromosomal sex: ♀
Indication: Combination with *hysterosalpingography* to visualise internal genital
Fig. 154 is a *standard radiograph* showing uterus and gonads superimposed
Figs. 155—159 are *tomograms*, 3 cm to 7 cm in depths, taken after additional *hysterosalpingography* and showing the following details; difference between gonadal sizes, diameters being 4 cm × 2.5 cm on the right and 2.5 cm × 1.5 cm on the left; uterus arcuatus; tubes formed normally and patent; internal genital structures with female derermination
A = right ovary; B = left ovary; C = ampulla tubae uterinae; D = contrast medium flown into peritoneal cavity; E = isthmus tabae uterinae; F = corpus uteri; G = rectum

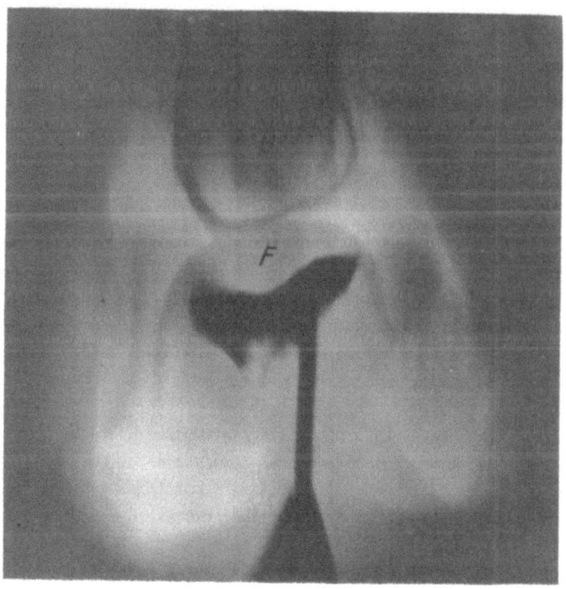

159

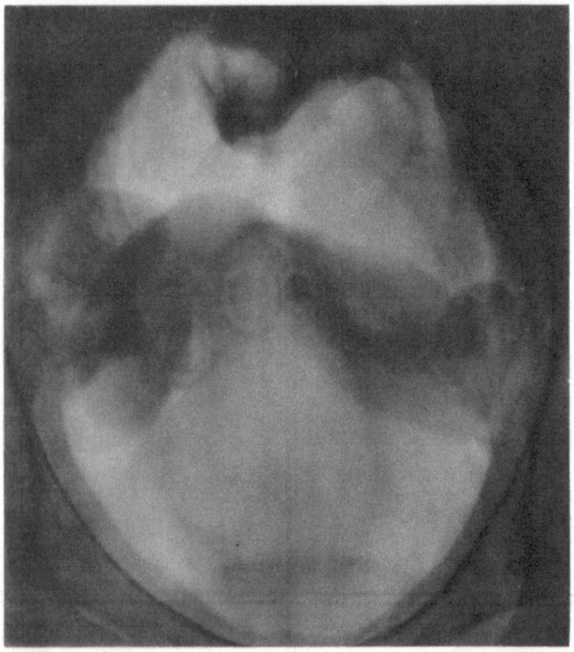

160

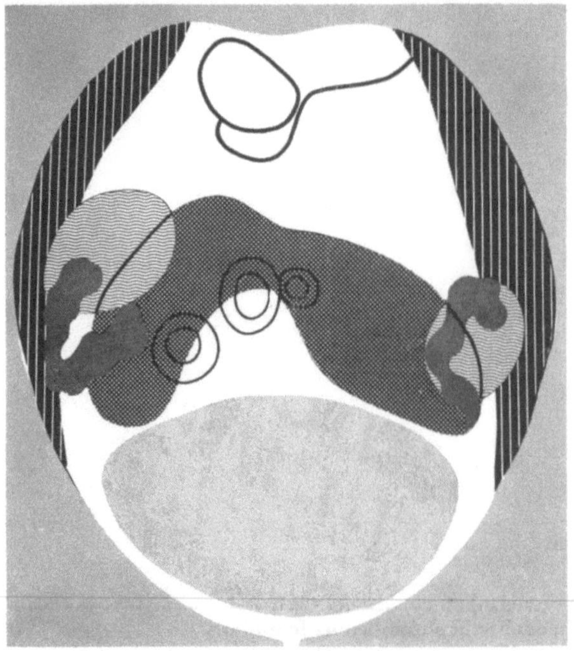

160 a

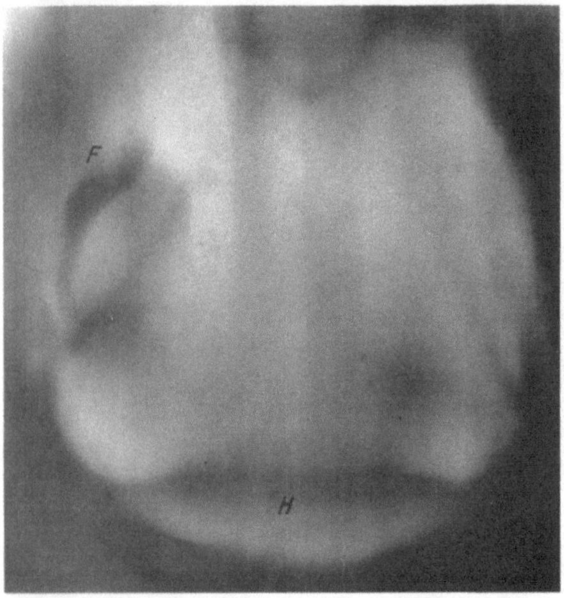

161

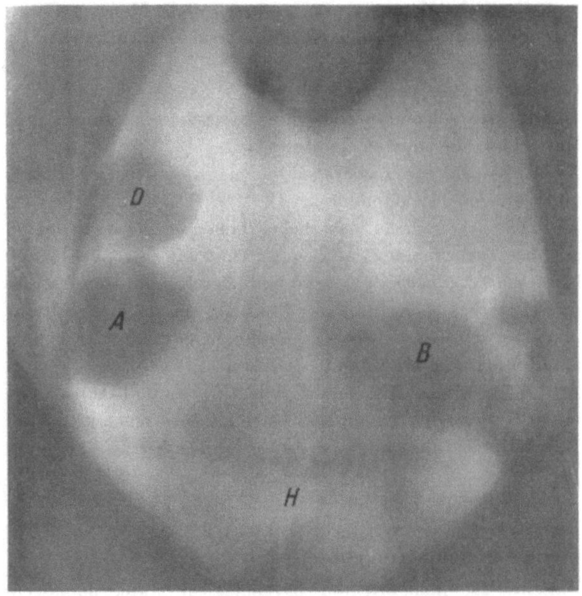

162

Abb. 160–166

Uterus bicornis

23jähr. Patientin mit primärer Sterilität und dringendem Kinderwunsch

Tastbefund: Uterus plump, anteflektiert, beweglich, Verdacht auf Bikornität, Adnexe unauffällig

Indikation: Darstellung des inneren Genitales und zusätzliche *Salpingographie* zur Beurteilung der Tubendurchgängigkeit

Abb. 160: Uterus bicornis mit symmetrischen, stark divergierenden Hörnern. Auf der *Übersichtsaufnahme* sind in Beckenmitte die ringförmigen Schatten von 3 zur Dosismessung ins Scheidengewölbe eingelegten Kugelkondiometern sichtbar

Abb. 161–165: Die *Tomogramme* zeigen folgende Details: In 5 cm Tiefe die rechte Tube mit Infundibulum, Isthmus und Anschluß an die Spitze des rechten Uterushorns (Abb. 161), in 6 cm und 7 cm Tiefe das rechte Ovar, darunter das rechte Uterushorn und auf der linken Seite die bogenförmig verlaufende Tube (Abb. 162 und 163), in 8 cm Tiefe beide Uterushörner und die linke Tube (Abb. 164), in 9 cm Tiefe das linke Ovar und die sattelförmige Verschmelzung beider Uterushörner im Zervixbereich (Abb. 165)

Hysterosalpingographie: Uterus bicornis unicollis

A = rechtes Uterushorn; B = linkes Uterushorn; C = Vereinigung der Uterushörner; D = rechtes Ovar; E = linkes Ovar; F = rechte Tube; G = linke Tube; H = Harnblase; I = Rectum

Verlauf: STRASSMANNsche Operation

Abb. 166: Das Operationsfoto zeigt die beiden Uterushörner von Kugelzangen gefaßt, darüber die Ovarien

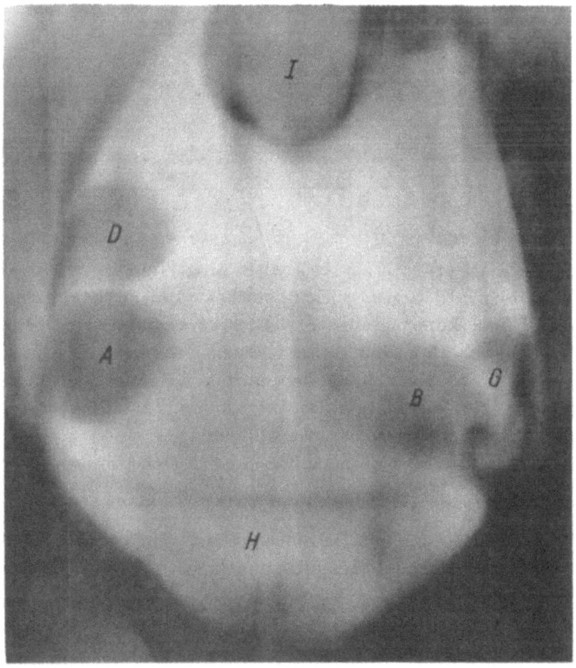

163

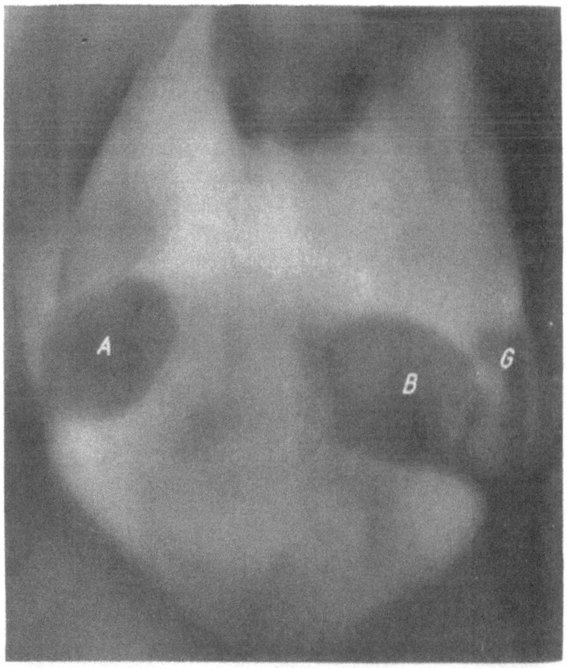

164

Figs. 160—166
Uterus bicornis

Patient, 23, with primary sterility and urgent desire for children
Palpation finding: Uterus dumpy, anteflexed, and movable, suspect of bicornuation; adnexa unpathological
Indication: Visualisation of internal genital and additional salpingography to assess tubal patency
Fig. 160 is a *standard radiograph* showing the uterus bicornuated with symmetrical and strongly divergent cornua as well as, in the centre of the pelvis, the annular shadows of three ball condiometers inserted in the vaginal fornix for dosimetry
Figs. 161—165 are *tomograms* showing the following details; right tube with infundibulum, isthmus, and attachment to the tip of the right uterine cornu visible in a depth of 5 cm (Fig. 161); right ovary with right uterine cornu underneath and arciform tube on the left visible in depths of 6 cm and 7 cm (Figs. 162 and 163); the two uterine cornua and the left tube, 8 cm in depth (Fig. 164); the left ovary and the saddle-shaped fusion of the two uterine cornua in the cervical region, 9 cm in depth (Fig. 165)
Hysterosalpingography: Uterus bicornis unicollis
A = right uterine cornu; B = left uterine cornu; C = fusion of the uterine cornua; D = right ovary; E = left ovary; F = right tube; G = left tube; H = urinary bladder; I = rectum
Course: STRASSMANN's operation
Fig. 166 is a photograph taken of the operation and showing the two uterine cornua, gripped by the bullet forceps, and the ovaries above

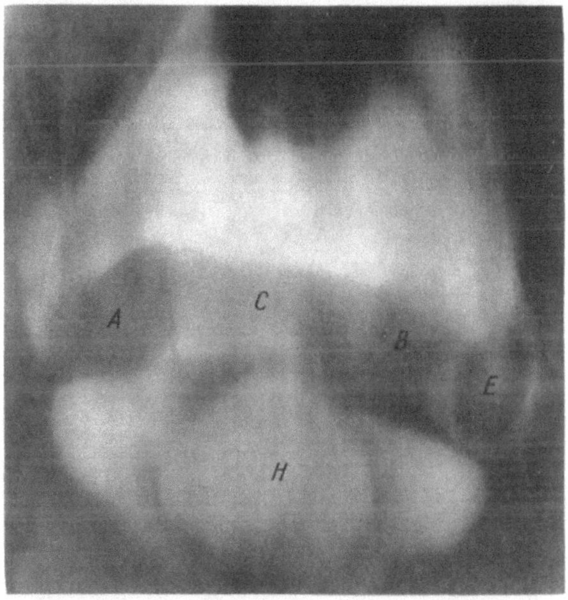

165

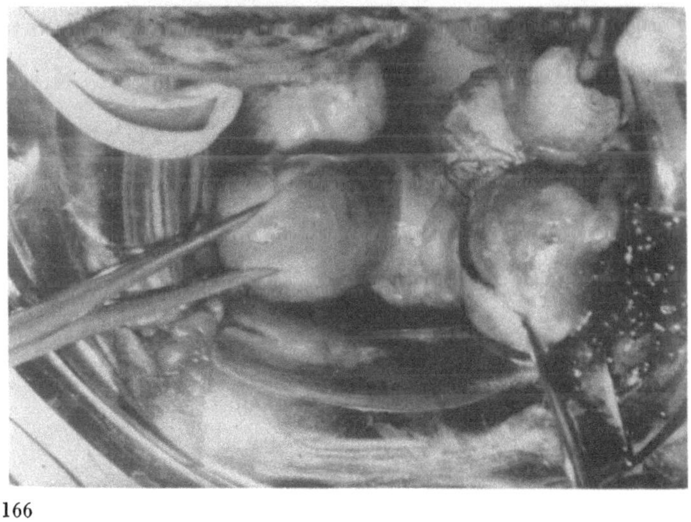

166

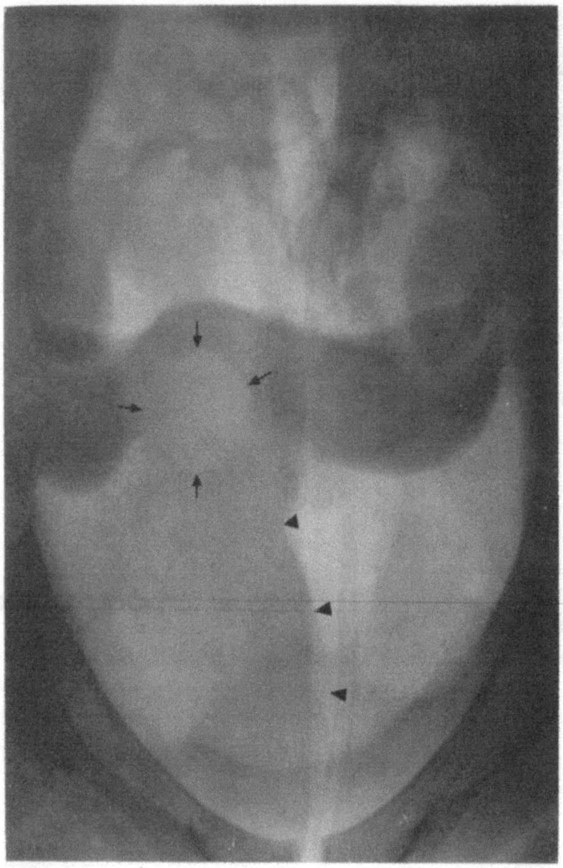

167a

Abb. 167–169

Uterus bicornis

14jähr. Patientin mit paravaginalem Abszeß unklarer Genese

Tastbefund: Uterus nicht palpabel, Adnexe unauffällig, rektal fingerkuppengroßer, beweglicher retroflektierter Uterus

Im Urogramm ist keine rechte Niere nachweisbar

Indikation: Darstellung des inneren Genitales zum Ausschluß einer Ausbreitung der Abszeßbildung im Beckenraum und zum Nachweis eventueller Mißbildungen

Abb. 167: Uterus bicornis mit symmetrischen Hörnern

a) Paravaginaler Abszeß (◄) mit kleiner Gaskuppel (←)

b) Nach Eröffnung und Lokalbehandlung des Abszesses 7 Monate später keine Verschattung mehr

Abb. 168 und 169: Die *Tomogramme* zeigen folgende Einzelheiten: In 6 cm Tiefe die beiden Ovarien, Teile beider Tuben und das rechte Uterushorn, in 8 cm Tiefe die Vereinigung der Hörner im Zervixbereich. Im Cavum peritonei nach Abschluß der Behandlung keine Verschattungen, die auf die Abszeßbildung bezogen werden können

A = Uterushörner; B = Vereinigung der Uterushörner; C = Ovarien, D = Tuben

Verlauf: Vaginale Eröffnung und Lokalbehandlung des Abszesses. Nach Abheilung Laparotomie zur Exploration des Beckenraumes. Bestätigung des Röntgenbefundes

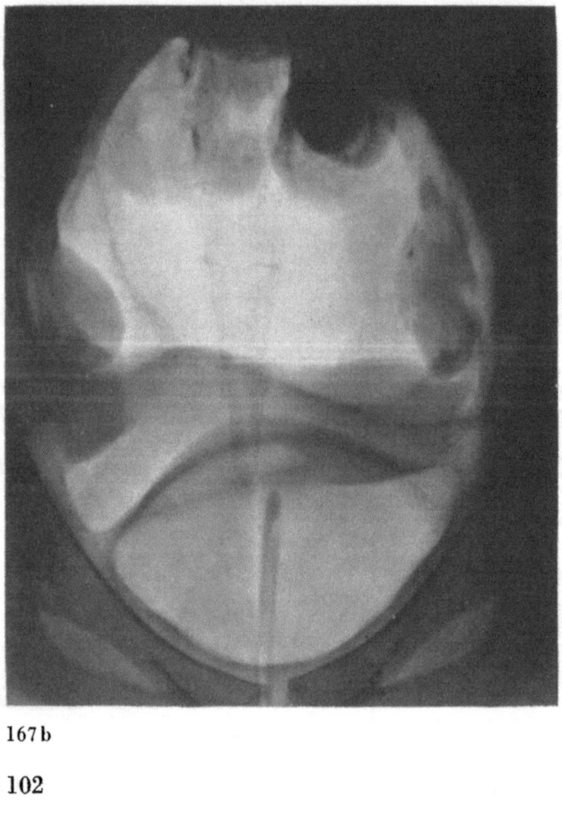

167b

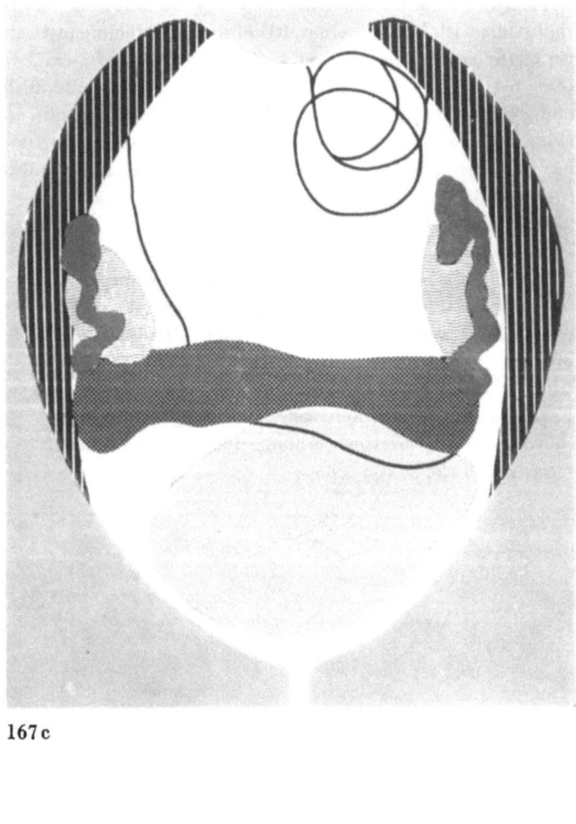

167c

Figs. 167—169
Uterus bicornis

Patient, 14, with paravaginal abscess of obscure genesis
Palpation finding: Uterus not palpable; adnexa unpathological; rectal palpability of movable retroflexed uterus of fingertip size
No right kidney detectable by urography
Indication: Visualisation of internal genital to rule out proliferation of suppuration in pelvic cavity and to elucidate presence of malformations
Fig. 167: Uterus bicornis with symmetrical cornua

a) Paravaginal abscess (◄) with small gas bubble (←)

b) incision and local treatment of the abscess, with no shadow after seven months

Figs. 168 and 169 are *tomograms* showing the following details: both ovaries, parts of either tube, and right cornu, 6 cm in depth; fusion of cornua in the cervical region, 8 cm in depth; no shadows applicable to suppuration are found in the peritoneal cavity after completion of treatment
A = uterine cornua; B = fusion of uterine cornua; C = ovaries; D = tubes
Course: Vaginal incision and local treatment of the abscess: after healing, laporotomy to explore pelvic cavity; confirmation of radiological findings

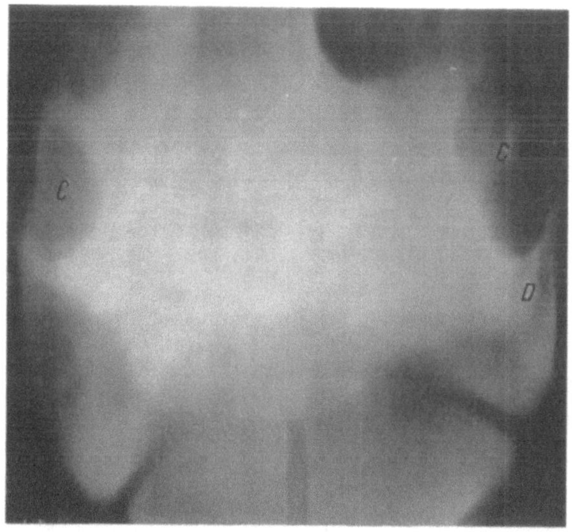

168

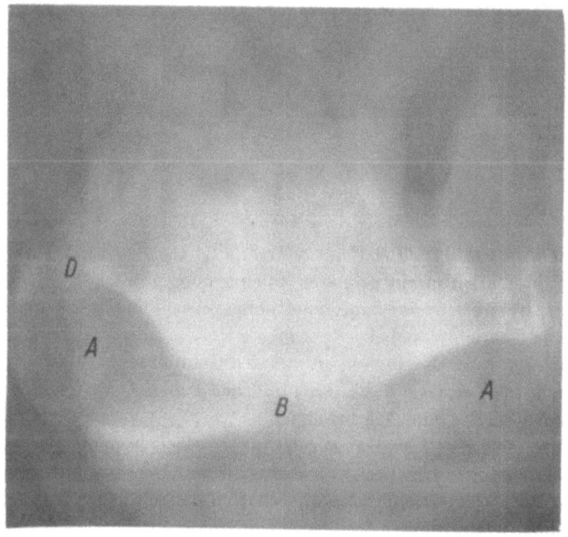

169

nern erkennen (Abb. 184—187). Sind Doppelbildungen mit Gynatresien vergesellschaftet, so ist die Kombination von Pneumopelvigraphie und Hysterosalpingographie in manchen Fällen besonders aufschlußreich. Wird bei *Aplasia vaginae* eine künstliche Scheidenbildung geplant, kann man sich mit Hilfe des Pneumoperitoneum über die morphologische Beschaffenheit der übrigen inneren Genitalien praeoperativ genau informieren und auf diese Weise die operative Korrekturmöglichkeit im Einzelfall von vornherein besser beurteilen (Abb. 170 bis 183). Läßt sich infolge Atresie der Vagina bzw. ihres kaudalen Abschnittes der Verdacht auf Haematometra, Haematosalpinx oder Haematokolpos im kranialen Teil der Vagina nicht genügend sichern, so ermöglicht die Pneumopelvigraphie entscheidende Aussagen für die Diagnose (Abb. 188—191).

160—169), but also in cases of asymmetrical preformation and in the presence of additional rudimentary cornua (Figs. 184—187). In certain cases where diplogenesis is associated with gynatresia, much information can be obtained by a combination of pneumopelvigraphy with hysterosalpingography. In cases of *vaginal aplasia* where colpopoiesis is intended, the pneumoperitoneum may yield detailed presurgical information about the morphological conditions of the other internal genitals for better assessment of the possibilities given for surgical correction in the case concerned (Figs. 170—183). Consistent information to secure diagnosis may be obtained by pneumopelvigraphy, particularly in cases where suspicion of hematometra, hematosalpinx or hematocolpos cannot be sufficiently backed with reference to the cranial part of the vagina because of atresia of the vagina or its caudal part (Figs. 188—191).

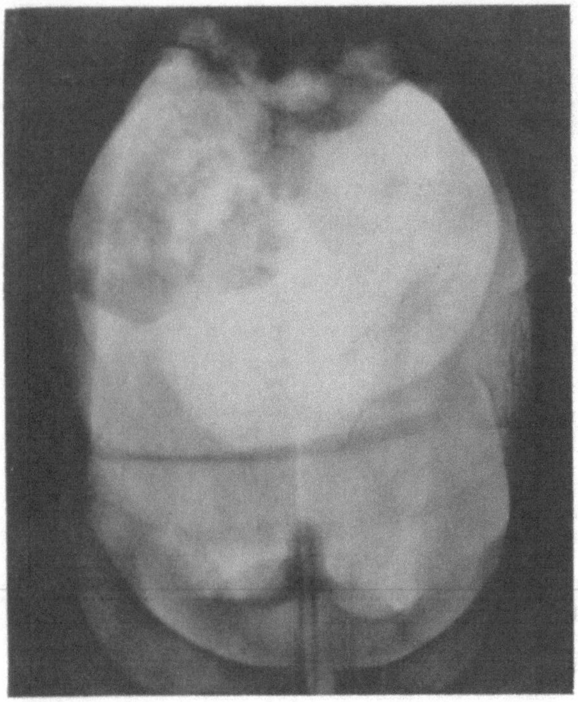

170

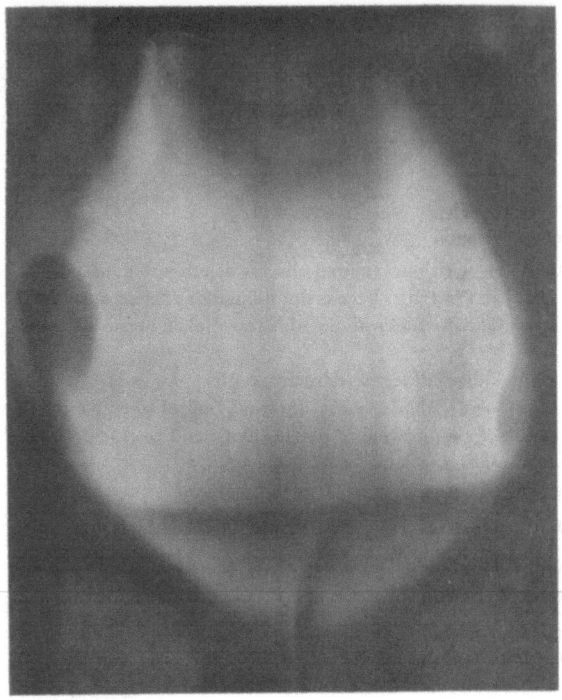

171

Abb. 170 und 171

Aplasia vaginae et uteri

18jähr. Patientin mit primärer Amenorrhoe

Tastbefund: Keine Scheidenöffnung, rektal kein Uterus und keine Ovarien palpabel

Indikation: Darstellung des inneren Genitales

Abb. 170: Aplasie des Uterus und der Tuben. Querstehende Bauchfellfalte ohne Verdickungen

Abb. 171: Das *Tomogramm* zeigt in 5 cm Tiefe hypoplastische Ovarien (rechts > links) an der seitlichen Beckenwand, die auf der *Übersichtsaufnahme* im Schatten des seitlichen Weichteilmantels verborgen bleiben

Figs. 170 and 171

Aplasia vaginae et uteri

Patient, 18, with primary amenorrhea

Palpation finding: No vaginal entrance; no rectal palpability of uterus nor ovaries

Indication: Visualisation of internal genital

Fig. 170: Aplasia of the uterus and tubes; transverse peritoneal fold without thickening

Fig. 171 is a *tomogram*, 5 cm in depth, showing hypoplastic ovaries (right > left) on the side wall of the pelvis, not detectable from the *standard radiograph* where they remain concealed by lateral soft-part shadow

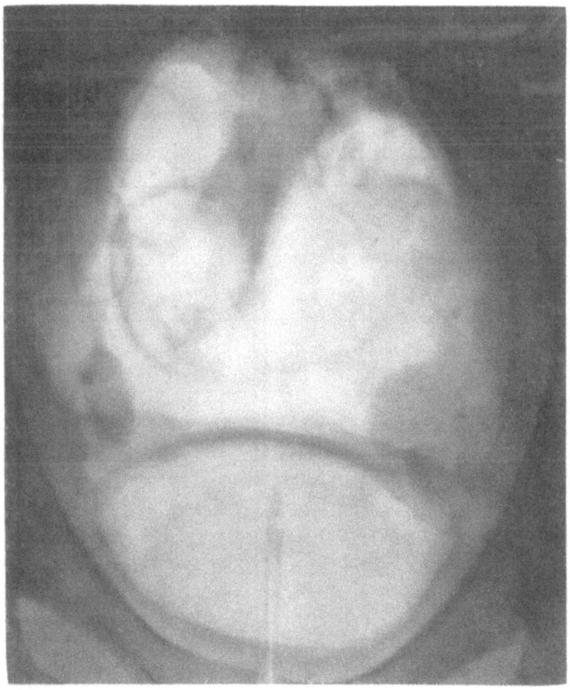

172

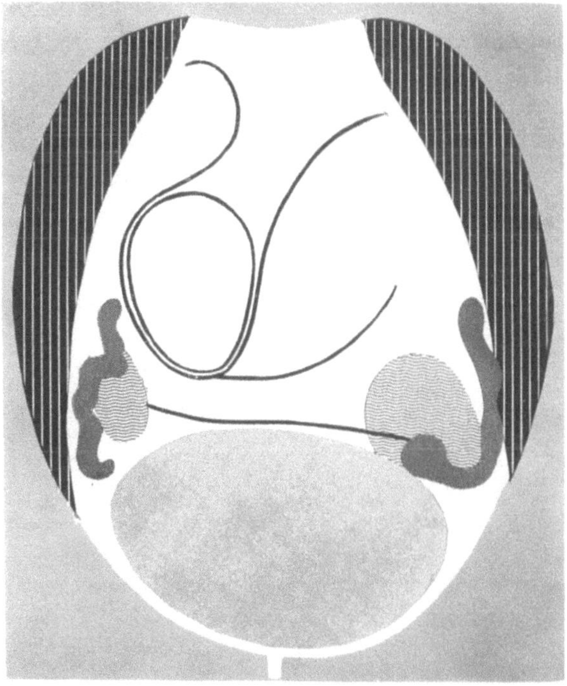

172 a

Abb. 172 und 173
Aplasia vaginae et uteri

17jähr. Patientin mit primärer Amenorrhoe
Tastbefund: Keine Scheidenöffnung. Rektal wird eine querstehende Spange gefühlt
Indikation: Darstellung des inneren Genitales
Abb. 172: Aplasie des Uterus, Hypoplasie der Ovarien (rechts < links). Beide Tuben sind angelegt. Sie laufen in eine quergestellte Bauchfellfalte ein
Abb. 173: Auf dem *Tomogramm* in 4 cm Tiefe ist die rechte Tube dargestellt. Links knopfförmige Verschattung unterhalb des Ovars durch gewundenen Tubenverlauf
Verlauf: Operative Scheidenbildung aus dem Colon sigmoideum. Bei der Laparotomie wird der Röntgenbefund bestätigt. Beide Tuben setzen sich in einen quer verlaufenden Gewebestrang fort. Eine Uterusanlage fehlt

Figs. 172 and 173
Aplasia vaginae et uteri

Patient, 17, with primary amenorrhea
Palpation finding: No vaginal entrance; rectal palpability of transverse clasp
Indication: Visualisation of internal genital
Fig. 172: Aplasia of the uterus; hypoplasia of the ovaries (right < left); both tubes are preformed and extend into a transverse peritoneal fold
Fig. 173 is a *tomogram*, 4 cm in depth, showing the right tube and umbonate shadow beneath ovary cast by curviform tube;
Course: Surgical colpopoiesis from colon sigmoideum; radiological findings are confirmed by laparotomy; both tubes are continued in a transverse tissue chord; absence of uterus preformation

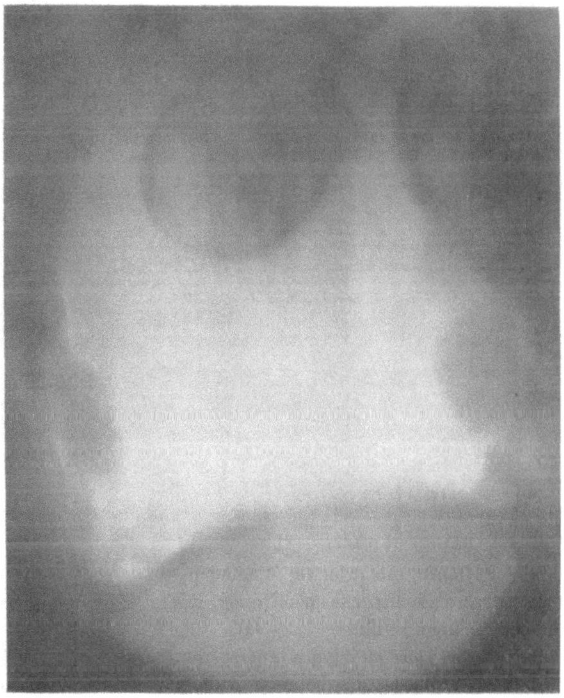

173

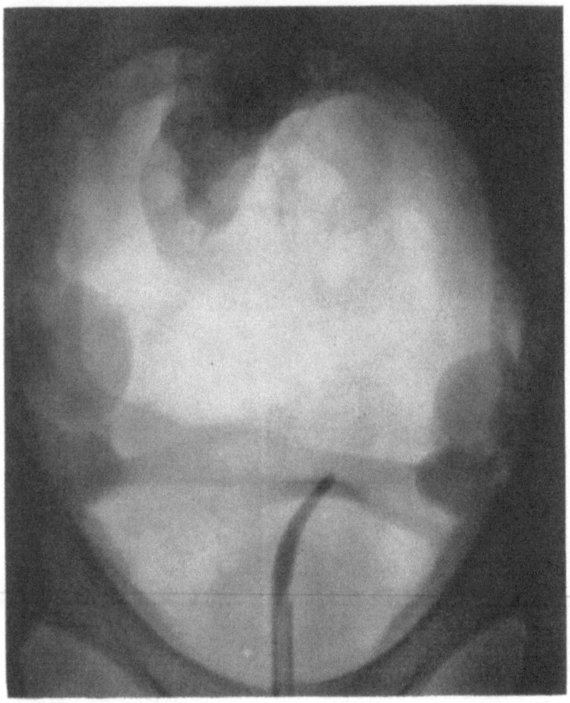

174

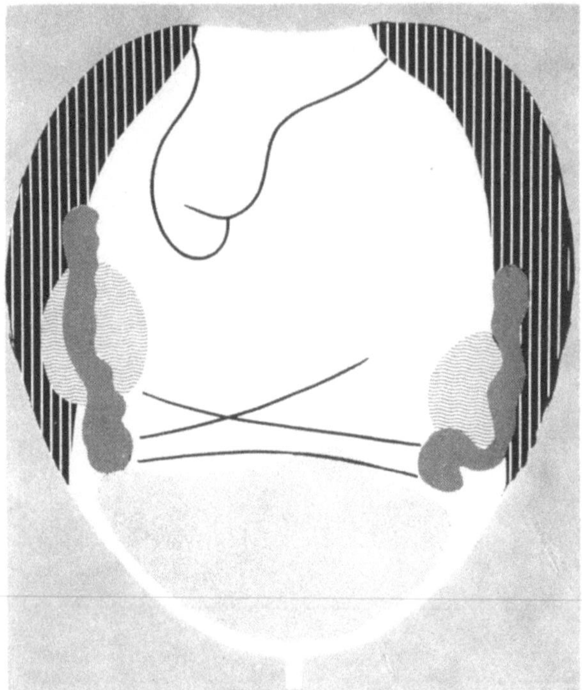

174a

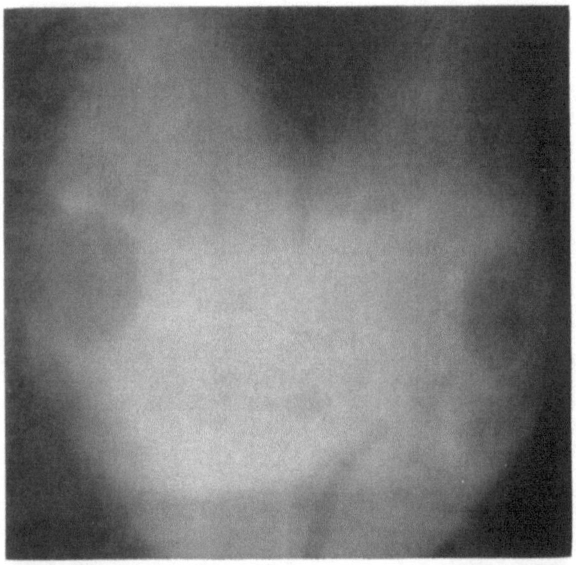

175

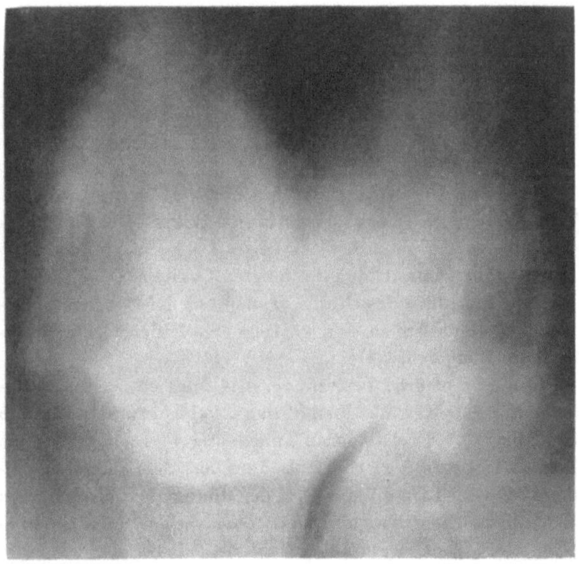

176

Abb. 174–176

Aplasia vaginae et uteri

20jähr. Patientin mit primärer Amenorrhoe

Tastbefund: Keine Scheidenöffnung. Rektal wird eine querstehende Spange gefühlt

Indikation: Darstellung des inneren Genitales

Abb. 174: Aplasie des Uterus, Hypoplasie der Ovarien (rechts > links). Beide Tuben sind angelegt. Sie werden als knopfförmige Verschattungen am unteren Pol der Ovarien abgebildet und laufen in eine quergestellte Bauchfellfalte ein

Abb. 175 und 176: *Tomogramme* in 5 cm und 6 cm Tiefe

Verlauf: Operative Scheidenbildung aus dem Colon sigmoideum. Bei der Laparotomie wird der Röntgenbefund bestätigt. Beide Tuben setzen sich in einen quer verlaufenden Gewebestrang fort. Eine Uterusanlage fehlt

Figs. 174–176

Aplasia vaginae et uteri

Patient, 20, with primary amenorrhea

Palpation finding: No vaginal entrance; rectal palpability of transverse clasp

Indication: Visualisation of internal genital

Fig. 174: Aplasia of the uterus; hypoplasia of the ovaries (right > left); both tubes are preformed and visualised at the lower pole of the ovaries as umbonate shadows that extend into a transverse peritoneal fold

Figs. 175 and 176 are *tomograms*, 5 cm and 6 cm in depths:

Course: Surgical colpopoiesis from colon sigmoideum; radiological findings confirmed by laparotomy; both tubes are continued in a transverse tissue chord; absence of uterus preformation

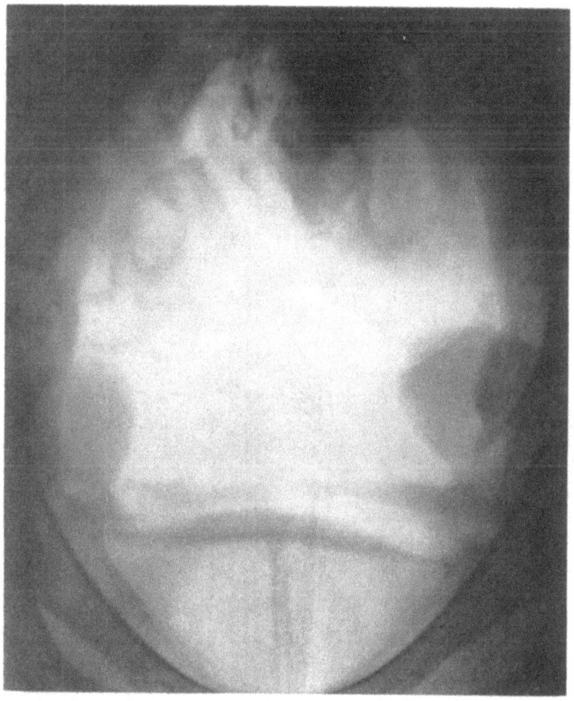

177

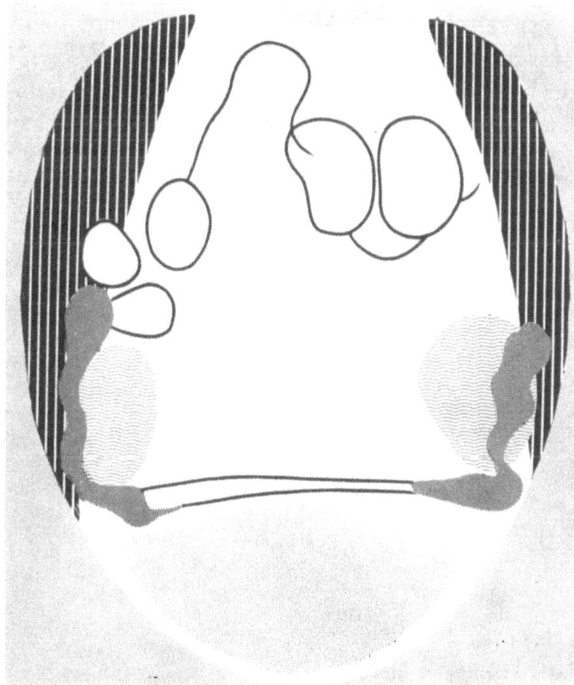

177a

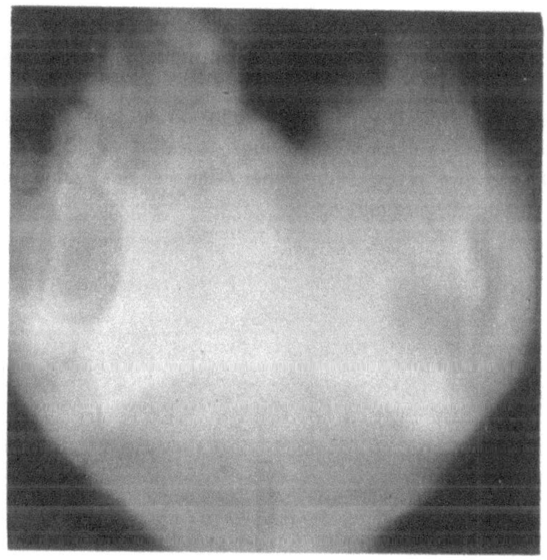

178

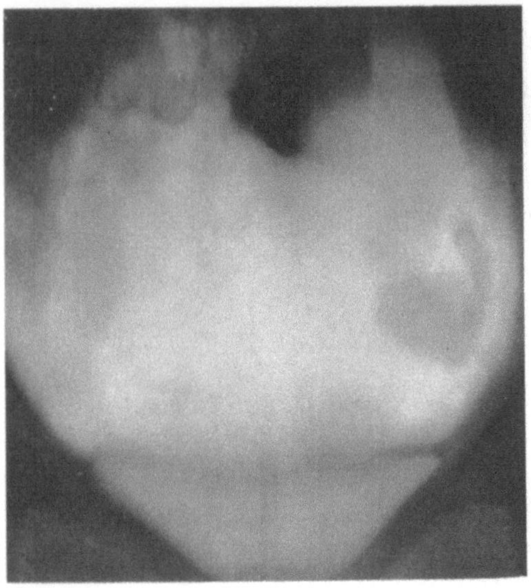

179

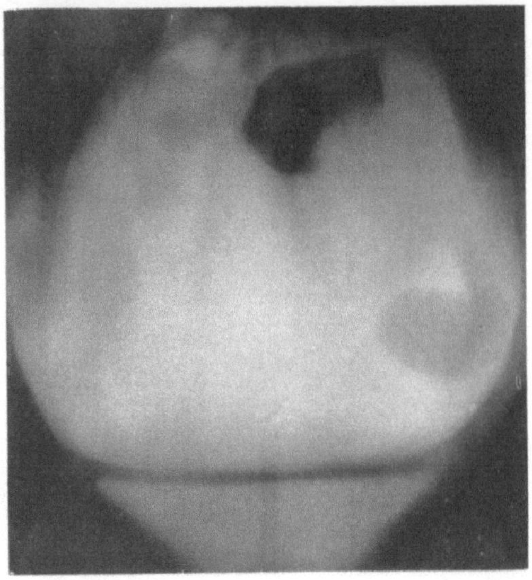

180

Abb. 177—180

Aplasia vaginae et uteri

17jähr. Patientin mit primärer Amenorrhoe

Tastbefund: Flache rudimentäre, für die Fingerkuppe eingängige Scheidengrube. Rektal zwei dünne, quer verlaufende Stränge palpabel, kein Uterus, keine Ovarien zu tasten

Indikation: Darstellung des inneren Genitales

Abb. 177: Aplasie des Uterus. Ovarien und Tuben sind regelrecht. Anstelle des Uterusschattens wird eine querstehende schmale Bauchfellfalte abgebildet, in deren seitlicher Basis sich die beiden Tubenschatten verlieren

Abb. 178—180: Der gewundene Verlauf der Eileiter ist auf den *Tomogrammen* in 3 cm, 5 cm und 7 cm Tiefe deutlich von den Ovarien zu unterscheiden.

Abb. 178 zeigt eine Harnansammlung im Blasenscheitel (vgl. Abb. 26)

Verlauf: Operative Scheidenbildung aus dem Colon sigmoideum. Bei der Laparotomie zeigt sich, daß die Tuben in einen soliden Gewebestrang übergehen, der sich im kleinen Becken querstehend vereinigt

Figs. 177—180

Aplasia vaginae et uteri

Patient, 17, with primary amenorrhea

Palpation finding: Flat rudimentary vaginal groove accessible only to the fingertip; rectal palpability of two thin transverse chords; no uterus nor ovaries palpable

Indication: Visualisation of internal genital

Fig. 177: Aplasia of the uterus; ovaries and tubes normal; a transverse, narrow peritoneal fold is projected instead of the uterus shadow, with the two tube shadows fading into its lateral base

Figs. 178—180 are *tomograms*, 3 cm, 5 cm, and 7 cm in depths, showing clearly the curvatures of the oviducts and their demarcation from the ovaries

Fig. 178 shows an accumulation of urine in the fundus of the bladder (see Fig. 26)

Course: Surgical colpopoiesis from colon sigmoideum; laparotomy shows the tubes to be continued by solid tissue chords that grow together transversally inside the minor pelvis

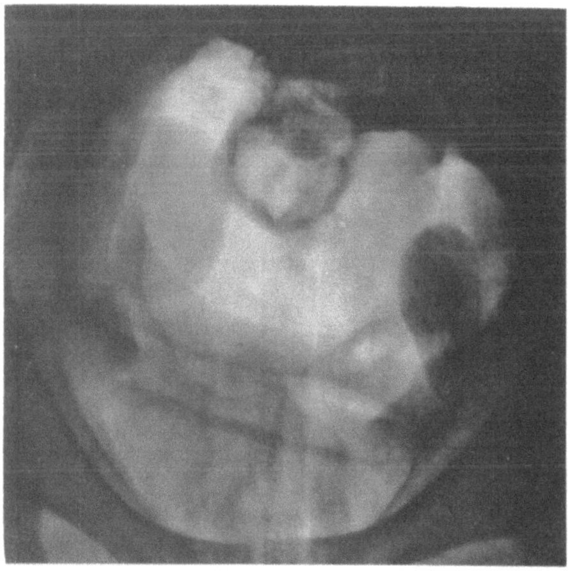

181

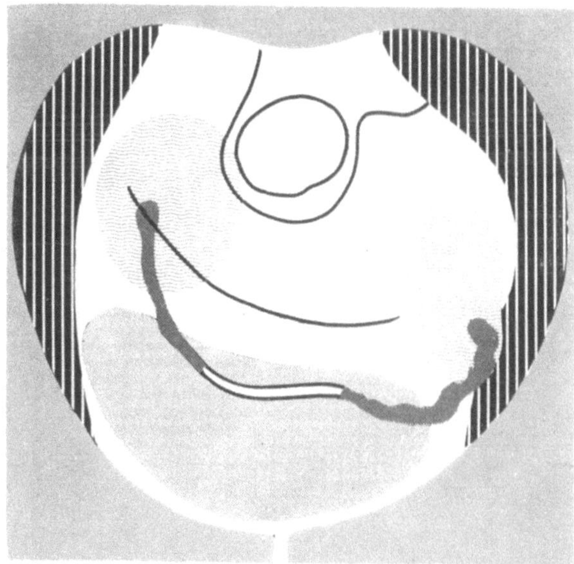

181 a

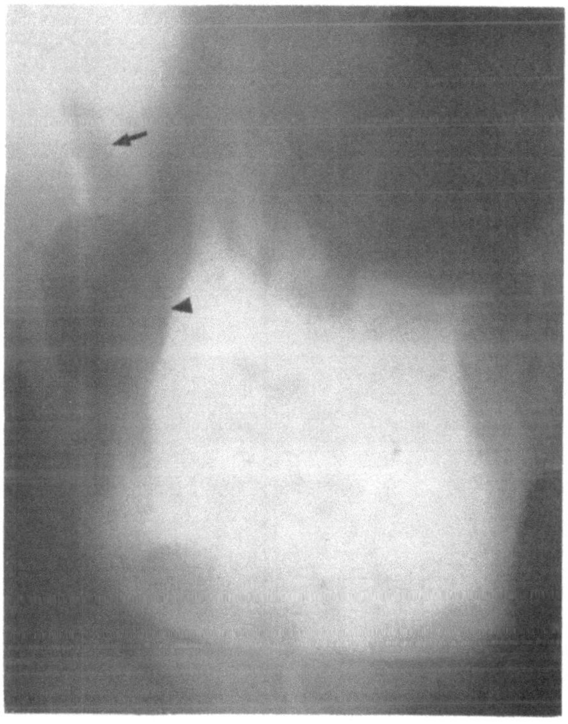

182

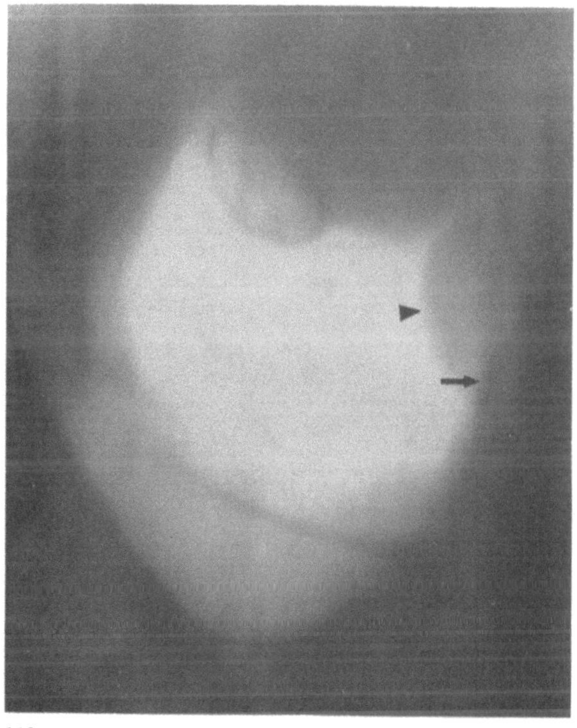

183

Abb. 181—183

Aplasia vaginae et uteri

16jähr. adipöse Patientin mit primärer Amenorrhoe

Tastbefund: Keine Scheidenöffnung. Rektal bohnengroßer Knoten in Beckenmitte tastbar, Adnexe nicht palpabel

Indikation: Darstellung des inneren Genitales

Abb. 181: Aplasie des Uterus. Ovarien und Tuben normal angelegt. Quergestellte Bauchfellfalte ohne Verdickung

Abb. 182 und 183: Die *Tomogramme* in 6 cm und 8 cm Tiefe zeigen die Ovarien (▸) und die Eileiter (→)

Figs. 181—183

Aplasia vaginae et uteri

Patient, 16, afflicted with adiposity and primary amenorrhea;

Palpation finding: No vaginal entrance; rectal palpability of bean-size node in centre of pelvis; adnexa not palpable

Indication: Visualisation of internal genital

Fig. 181: Aplasia of the uterus; normal preformation of ovaries and tubes; transverse peritoneal fold without thickening

Figs. 182 and 183 are *tomograms*, 6 cm and 8 cm in depths, showing the ovaries (▸) and the oviducts (→)

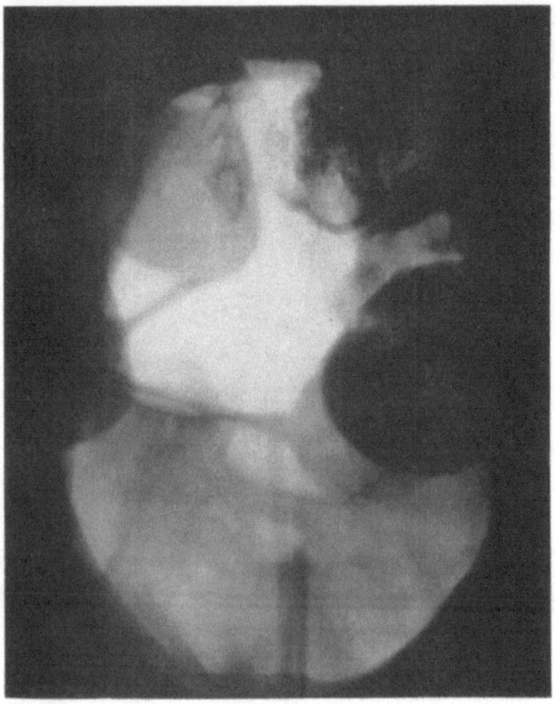

184

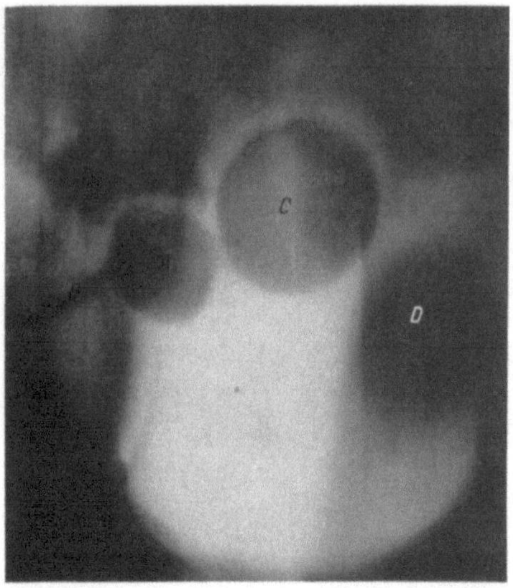

185

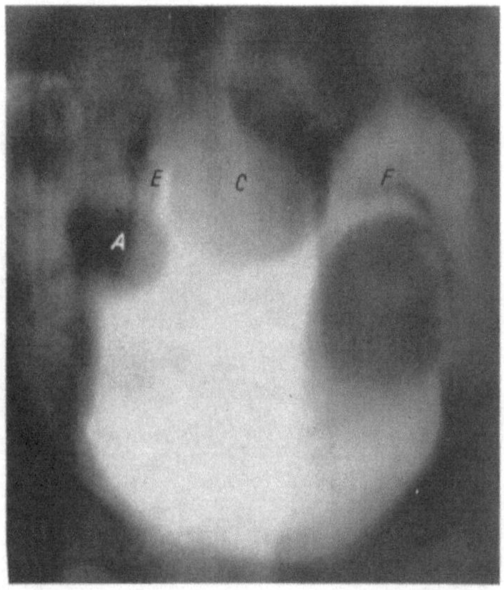

186

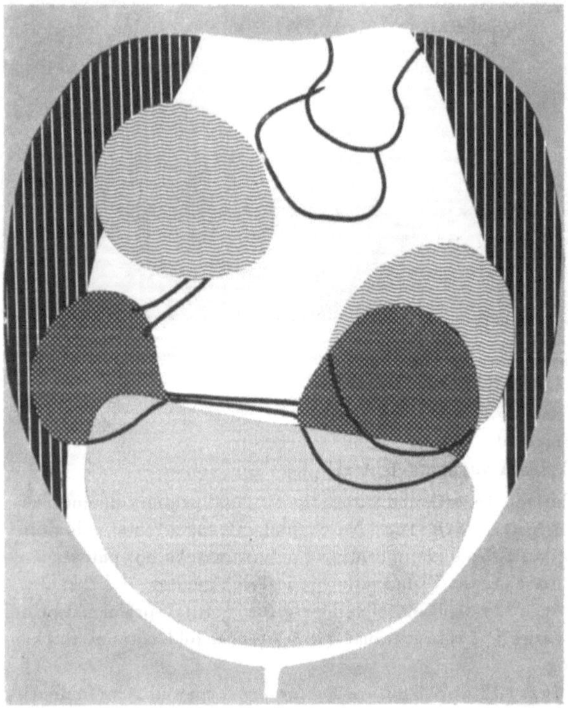

184a

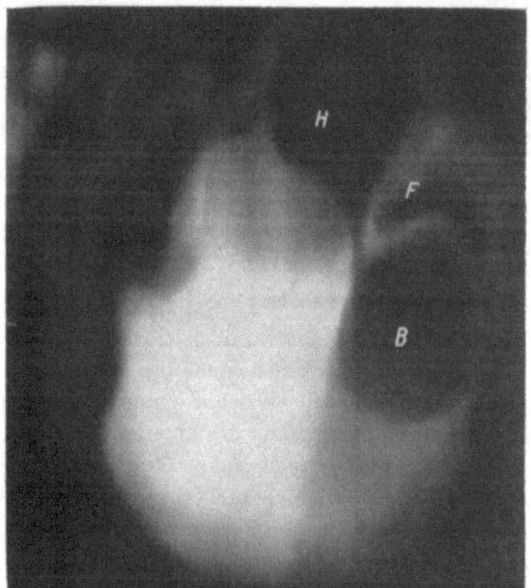

187

Abb. 184—187

Hypoplasia vaginae, Uterus bicornis rudimentarius

19jähr. Patientin mit primärer Amenorrhoe. Seit 6 Jahren bestehen in monatlichen Intervallen krampfartige Schmerzen im Unterleib

Tastbefund: Rudimentäre, 2 cm lange Vagina sondierbar, hypoplastischer Uterus, sinistroponiert, rechts weiche Resistenz palpabel, die nicht genau abgegrenzt werden kann

Indikation: Darstellung des inneren Genitales

Abb. 184: Das *Übersichtsbild* zeigt auf beiden Seiten des kleinen Beckens je zwei Rundschatten, die den Ovarien und zwei atretischen Uterushörnern entsprechen. Letztere werden durch eine schmale Bauchfellfalte verbunden. Das linke Horn erscheint wesentlich größer als das rechte

Abb. 185—187: Nach den *Tomogrammen* in 4 cm—8 cm Tiefe lassen sich außerdem die Tuben differenzieren, welche die Ovarien umfassen

A = rechtes Uterushorn; B = linkes Uterushorn; C = rechtes Ovar; D = linkes Ovar; E = rechte Tube; F = linke Tube; G = Lig. teres uteri; H = Rectum und Colon sigmoideum

Verlauf: Laparotomie. Bestätigung des Röntgenbefundes. Entleerung einer Haematometra und Haematosalpinx aus dem atretischen linken Uterushorn, Salpingektomie links. Schaffung einer Verbindung zwischen linkem Uterushorn und Scheidenrudiment. In einer zweiten Sitzung ist die Implantation der rechten Tube in das linke Uterushorn vorgesehen

Figs. 184—187

Hypoplastic vagina, bicornuate rudimentary uterus

Patient, 19, afflicted with primary amenorrhea and reporting spasmic pain in the hypogastrium to have occured in monthly intervals for six years

Palpation finding: Rudimentary vagina, 2 cm in length; hypoplastic uterus in sinistro-position; on the right palpability of soft resistance which is not safely demarcable

Indication: Visualisation of internal genital

Fig. 184 is a *standard radiograph* showing two round shadows on either side of the minor pelvis which are cast apparently by the ovaries and two atresic uterine cornua; the latter being connected with each other by a narrow peritoneal fold; the left cornu appears to be much larger than the right one

Figs. 185—187 are *tomograms*, 4 cm to 8 cm in depths, facilitating differentiation of the tubes which encircle the ovaries

A = right uterine cornu; B = left uterine cornu; C = right ovary; D = left ovary; E = right tube; F = left tube; G = lig. teres uteri; H = rectum and colon sigmoideum

Course: Laparotomy; confirmation of radiological findings; discharge of a hematometra and hematosalpinx from the atresic left uterine cornu; salpingectomy on the left; anastomosis between left uterine cornu and rudimentary vagina; second operation envisaged to implant the right tube into the left uterine cornu

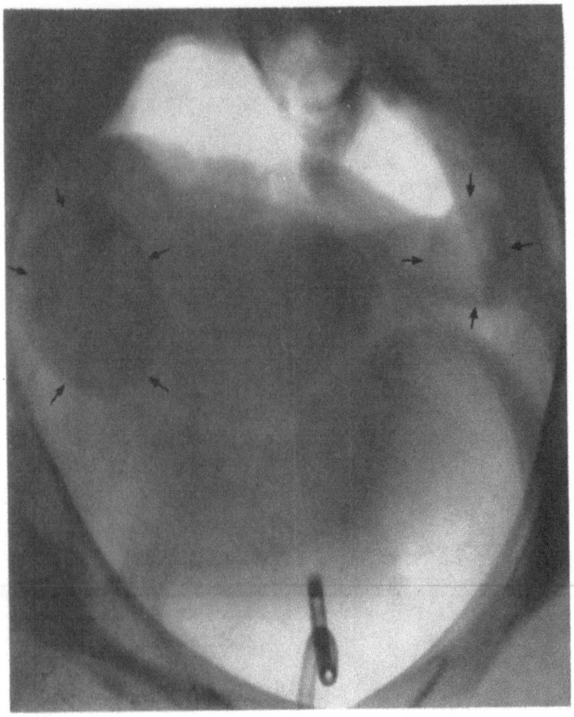

188

Abb. 188–191

Partielle Aplasie der Vagina, Haematokolpos

18jähr. Patientin mit primärer Amenorrhoe und Schmerzen im Unterbauch in 3–4wöchigen Intervallen

Tastbefund: Flache rudimentäre, 1 cm tiefe Scheidengrube. Rektal wird eine mandarinengroße weiche Resistenz rechts im kleinen Becken palpiert

Indikation: Darstellung des inneren Genitales, Verdacht auf Haematometra

Abb. 188: Die *Übersichtsaufnahme* zeigt eine großflächige Verschattung des mittleren Beckenraumes. Innerhalb dieses Schattens lassen sich die beiden Ovarien differenzieren (→)

Abb. 189–191: Die *Tomogramme* in 3 cm, 5 cm und 7 cm Tiefe ermöglichen eine Differenzierung des (nicht vergrößerten) Uterus, der Ovarien (rechts > links), der Tuben und der Genitalligamente. Außerdem wird in der Umgebung der Cervix uteri eine ausgedehnte pathologische Verschattung abgebildet. Diese erstreckt sich mit einem spindelförmigen Ausläufer nach ventral zwischen Uterus und Harnblase und imprimiert die Harnblasenwand (Abb. 189 u. 190). Nach dorsal erweitert sich das Schattengebilde im Douglasschen Raum (Abb. 191). Form und Lage dieser Verschattung erwecken den Verdacht auf Haematokolpos im Bereich des kranialen Scheidenabschnittes (Fornix vaginae) bei Atresie des kaudalen Vaginalabschnittes

Verlauf: Operation, Umschneidung des Introitus, Inzision des Haematokolpos, der infolge Atresie des kaudalen Vaginalabschnittes äußerlich nicht sichtbar oder tastbar ist, Vernähungen der Wundränder mit dem Introitus, keine Haematometra

Figs. 188–191

Partial aplasia of the vagina, hematocolpos

Patient, 18, with primary amenorrhea and reporting pain in the lower abdomen to occur in intervals of three to four weeks

Palpation finding: Flat rudimentary vaginal groove, 1 cm in depth; rectal palpability of a mandarine-size soft resistance in the right half of the minor pelvis

Indication: Visualisation of internal genital for suspicion of hematometra

Fig. 188 is a *standard radiograph* showing large, massive shadow in the central space of the pelvis within which the two ovaries can be differentiated (→)

Figs. 189–191 are *tomograms*, 3 cm, 5 cm, and 7 cm in depths, that facilitate differentiation of the (unenlarged) uterus, the ovaries (right > left), the tubes, and the genital ligaments; in addition, visualisation of expanded pathological shadow near the cervix uteri of which a spindle-shaped branch is found to extend ventrally between the uterus and urinary bladder and to indent the latter's wall (Figs. 189 and 190); the shadow grows larger in dorsal direction in Douglas' pouch (Fig. 191); shape and position of this shadow support suspicion of hematocolpos in the cranial region of the vaginal fornix, with the caudal region of the vagina being atresic

Course: Operation, peritomisation of the introitus; incision of the hematocolpos which is neither visible externally nor palpable due to atresia of the caudal vaginal portion; suturing of the wound edges and uniting them with the introitus; no hematometra

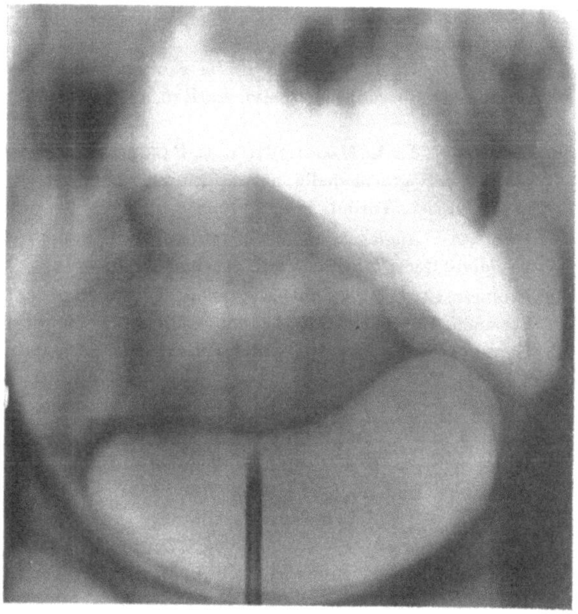

189

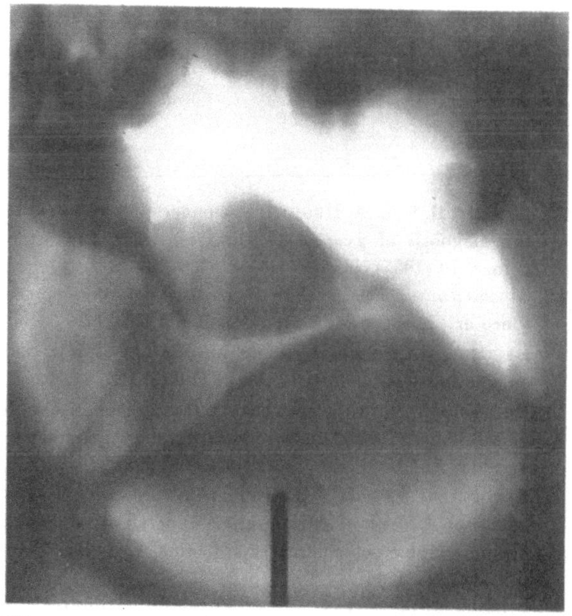

190

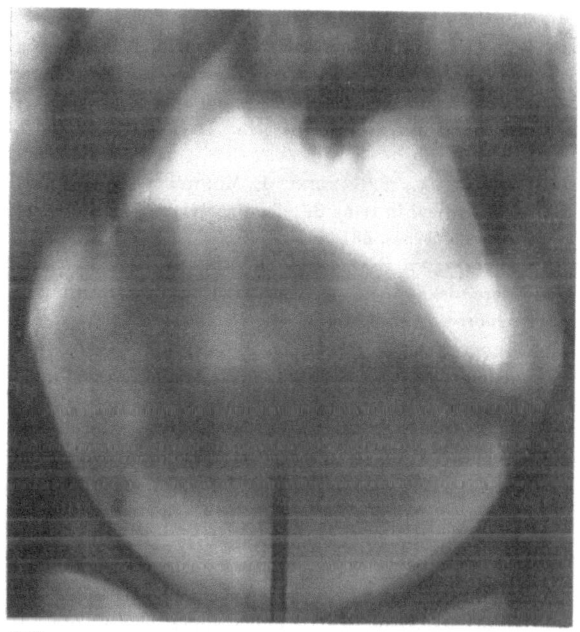

191

Literatur References

1. Abrams, B. S., u. A. Hughes: Pneumography as an aid in the diagnosis of gynecologic diseases. Amer. J. Obstet. Gynec. 70 (1955), 1115
2. Alessandrini, P.: Il valore diagnostico del pneumoperitoneo artificiale. Radiol. med. Milan 7 (1920), 179
3. Beclere, G.: Pneumopéritoine, insufflation et injection opaque intra-utérine. Paris méd. 1 (1928), 109
4. Belluci, M., u. A. Parentela: I tema di tecnica e di questi diagnostici sulla pneumoginecografia o pneumopelvigrafia. Ann. Ital. chir. 16 (1959), 488
5. Bétouliéres, P., M. Pélissier, L. Beltrando, R. Paleirac u. J. Candon: Stratigraphie et agran dissement en pneumographie pelvienne chez la femme. J. Radiol. Electrol. 36 (1955), 94
6. Birarelli, B., u. L. Tinelli: Possibilitâ e limiti della pneumoginecografia. Minerva Med. 51 (1960), 1460
7. Blandamura, M. u. P. Bellomo: La ginecografia. Indagine necessaria per l'indicazioni alla terapia chirurgica delle policistosi ovariche. Atti Soc. Ostet. Ginec. 10 (1961), 131
8. Blandamura, M., P. Bellomo, M. Cammisa, u. G. C. Gormanni: Saggio di pelvigrafia gassosa nelle affezioni uteroovariche. La Rad. Med. 47 (1961), 975
9. Böck, G.: Farbige Röntgenbilder im Dienst der Dosisverminderung bei Aufnahmen im Gonadenbereich. Fortschr. Röntgenstr. 107 (1967), 799
10. Böck, G., K. Richter, B. Kankelwitz u. W. Krug: Anwendungsmöglichkeiten der Chromogenentwicklung und Blauverstärkung von Röntgenaufnahmen bei Untersuchungen im Gonadenbereich. Dtsch. Ges.wesen 23 (1968), 1
11. Bompiani, A., S. Gandini, E. Moneta u. E. Zanetti: Alcuni rilievi in tema di pneumopelvigrafia. Ann. Ostet. Ginec. 86 (1964), 881
12. Bompiani, A., S. Gandini, E. Moneta u. E. Zanetti: Valore della pneumopelvigrafia nella diagnostica delle amenorree. Ann. Ostet. Ginec. 86 (1964), 889
13. Bompiani, A., A. Moneta u. S. Gandini: Apporto della pneumopelvigrafia allo studio delle malformaziona muelleriane in sogetti con aplasia vaginale congenita. Nunt. radiol. Firenze 28 (1962), 871
14. Bompiani, A., u. L. Rigat: Sul contributo della pneumopelvigrafia alla diagnosi delle malformazioni dell'apparato genitale interno femminile et allo studio della sindrome di Stein-Leventhal. Ann. Ostet. Ginec. 80 (1958), 114
15. Bompiani, A., u. L. Rigat: La pneumopelvigraphie dans l'étude des dysplasies utéro-ovariennes. Gynéc. prat. 10 (1959), 413
16. Bossi, R., P. Fabris u. E. Dormia: Il pelvipneumoperitoneo associato alla cistroparietografia gassosa indagine complementare, preoperatoria, in urologia. Arch. it. urol. 35, (1962), 460
17. Borghi, A., L. dalla Palma, C. Cavina, M. de Simone u. G. Giusti: Emploi de la pneumogynécographie pour le diagnostic endocrinologique. Contribution à l'étude des aménorrhées primaires et des hirsutismes "simples". Presse méd. 69 (1961), 400
18. Braibanti, T.: Pneumostratipelvigrafia. Ann. Radiol. Diagn. 33 (1960), 1
19. Braibanti, T.: La constrastografia gassosa nella esplorazione degli organi della pelvi. La Rad. méd. 47 (1961), 975
20. Braibanti, T., B. Maggipinto u. C. Pazienza: La pneumostratipelvigrafia nella pratica ginecologica. Ed. Minerva Medica, Torino, 1962
21. Breit, A.: Angiographie der Uterustumoren und ihrer Rezidive. Georg Thieme-Verl., Stuttgart, 1967
22. Bublitz, G.: Die Pelvipneumographie: Technik und Indikationen. Röntgenpraxis 21 (1968), 175
23. Buffetaut, M.: La gynécographie. Rev. méd. Normandes 3 (1961), 293
24. Buffetaut, M.: Iconographie médicale du praticien. La gynécographie. Sem. Hôp. Paris 61 (1956), 6
25. Buice, J. W., u. D. M. Gould: Abdominal and pelvic pneumography. Radiology 69 (1957), 704
26. Busingo, O.: La pneumostratigrafia degli organi pelvici. Atti III. Congr. Elettrocardiologi Cultura Latina e 18. Congr. SIRM, Roma, 1954 Ed. Min. Med., Torino, 1954
27. Cammisa, M.: Contributo alla tecnica ginecografica gassosa. La Rad. Méd. 47 (1962), 975
28. Capua, A., u. Cammisa, M.: Anatomia e semeiotica radiologica degli organi dello scavo pelvico della donna analizzati mediante pneumopelvigrafia. Journ. Belge Radiol. 47 (1964), 321
29. Carnevali, G., V. Lucarelli u. P. Parachi: Possibilità e limiti della radiologia nella diagnostica delle metastasi pelviche e delle infiltratzioni parametrali da carcinoma uterino. Radiol. méd. 42 (1956), 113
30. Carnevali, G., V. Lucarelli u. P. Parachi: Il pneumoperitoneo nella diagnostica ginecologica. Radiol. med. Milan. 41 (1955), 721
31. Carnevali, G., V. Lucarelli u. P. Parachi: La pneumopelvigrafia nella diagnosi dei tumori ginecologici. Casa Ed. Renzo Cortina, Pavia, 1957
32. Case, J. T.: A review of three years work and articles on pneumo-peritoneum. Amer. J. Roentgenol. 8 (1921), 714
33. Cavina, C.: Le pneumoginecografia nella patologia tumorale ovarica con sintomatologia endocrinologica. La Rad. Méd. 47 (1961), 646
34. Chatton, P., A. Lévy, M. Pélissier, P. Barjon u. L. Beltrando: La gynécographie dans le syndrome de Turner. J. Radiol. Electrol. 37 (1956), 448
35. Clark, K. C.: Positioning in radiography, 8th Edition, Ilford Limited London, 1964
36. Coliez, R.: Le pneumopéritoine artificiel en radiodiagnostic. Thése doctorat en Médicine, Paris, 1920
37. Costa, M. u. M. di Lorenzo: La pneumopelvigrafia in endocrinologia. Rev. Radiol. 1 (1961), 427
38. Dalla Palma, L., u. C. Cavina: Quadri pneumoginecografici di interesse endocrinologico. La Rad. Méd. 45 (1959), 791
39. Dalla Palma, L., u. C. Cavina: La pneumoginecografia nella diagnostica differenziale delle aménorree primarie. La Rad. Méd. 47 (1961), 463, 976
40. Dalla, Palma, L., u. C. Cavina: Le disgenesis gonadiche. Aspetti pneumoginecografici. Riv. Radiol. 2 (1962), 236
41. Dalla Palma, L., u. C. Cavina: L'apporto diagnostico della pneumopelvigrafia in campo endocrinologico. Journ. Belge Radiologie 47 (1964), 375
42. Daves, M. L., W. C. Diner u. G. H. Brenner: Pelvic pneumography. Amer. J. Roentgenology 92 (1964), 390

43. DECKER, A.: Arteficial pneumoperitoneum by cul-de-sac puncture. New technique for pelvic pneumograms. N. Y. St. J. Med. 46 (1946), 314
44. DURANDO, G. u. M. MACCINI: L'associazione celioscopia e pneumoginecografia nella diagnostica ginecologica. Minerva Ginec. 10 (1958), 187
45. DOLAN, P. A.: Lymphography. Brit. J. Radiol. 37 (1964), 405
46. DYROFF, R.: Die Deutung des gynäkologischen Pneumoperitoneums. Dtsch. med. Wschr. 60 (1924), 572
47. EDWARDS, E. M. u. K. E. EVANS: Pelvic pneumography in the STEIN-LEVENTHAL-syndrome. Brit. J. Radiol. 36 (1963), 46
48. FACCINI, M. u. G. NOCCA: Il pneumoperitoneo. Arch. Chir. Ortop. Med. 22 (1956)
49. FOCHEM, K.: Einführung in die geburtshilfliche und gynäkologische Röntgendiagnostik. Georg Thieme Verl. Stuttgart, 1967
50. FOURNIER, M., G. BOSSI, L. PIANA u. M. ARGEME: Étude pelvigraphique des ovaires de malades atteintes d'hypertrichose commune. Am. Radiol. 11 (1968), 21
51. FUCHS, W. A.: Lymphographie und Tumordiagnostik. Springer-Verl. Berlin-Heidelberg-New York, 1965
52. GANDINI, S. u. E. MONETA: Osservazioni pneumoginecografiche in casi di amenorrea primaria. Ann. Ostet. Ginec. 83 (1961), 555
53. GEBAUER, A.: Das diagnostische Pneumoperitoneum. Georg Thieme Verl. Stuttgart, 1959
54. GERSHAN-COHEN, J. u. M. B. HERMEL: Pelvic pneumoperitoneum. The X-ray appearance of the normal female pelvic organs. Amer. J. Obstet. Gynec. 64 (1952), 184
55. GINGLIGER, A., G. M. GROS u. R. KELLING: Sur les indications de la gynécographie. Strasbourg méd. 9 (1958)
56. GIUDICI, E.: Pneumoginecografia e laparoscopia. Utilità della lor' associazione nella diagnosi della pelvipatie. Minerva Medica, Torino, 1963
57. GREENBERG, E. M.: Gynecography. Amer. J. Obstet. Gynec. 54 (1947), 1081
58. GROS, C. M., R. KELLING u. SCHNITZLER: Contributions à la gynécographie. J. Radiol. Electrol. 38 (1957), 770
59. HAHN, G. A., S. WALLACE, L. JACKSON u. G. DODD: Lymphangiography in gynecology. Amer. J. Obstet. Gynec. 85 (1963), 754
60. HENZL, M.: Beitrag der Pneumopelvigraphie zur Diagnostik der Entwicklungsstörungen der inneren weiblichen Genitalorgane. Thesen der Karls-Univ. Prag, 1960
61. HENZL, M., J. HORSKY u. J. PRESL: Die Bedeutung der Pneumopelvigraphie für die Diagnostik spezifischer Adnexentzündungen. Geburtsh. u. Frauenheilk. 24 (1964), 691
62. HENZL, M., J. HORSKY, J. PRESL u. M. VALENTA: Pneumopelvigraphy of developmental malformations of the female internal genitalia. Acta radiol. (Stockh.)53 (1960), 201
63. HERMAN, P. G., D. L. BENNINGHOFF, J. H. NELSON u. H. Z. MELLIUS: Roentgenanatomy of iliopelvic-aortic lymphatic system. Radiology 80 (1963), 182
64. HERBEAU, J.: La gynécographie dans le diagnostic des tumeurs pelviennes. Lille cancérol. 2 (1955), 177
65. HERBEAU, J., A. LEQUINT u. M. VERHAEGHE: Le bilan de l'extension endopelvienne des tumeurs pelviennes. Lille cancérol 2 (1955), 177
66. HERBEAU, J. u. M. VERHAEGHE: La pelvigraphie gazeuse dite gynécographie. J. Radiol. Electrol. 38 (1957), 803
67. HERBEAU, J., M. VERHAEGHE u. A. LEQUINT: La pelvigraphie gazeuse (gynécographie). Presse méd. 67 (1969) 1
68. HERBEAU, J., M. VERHAEGHE u. A. LEQUINT: La pelvigraphie gazeuse (son intérêt dans le bilan de l'extension endopelvienne des cancers du col utérin). J. Radiol. Electrol. 39 (1958), 1
69. HERBEAU, J., M. VERHAEGHE u. A. LEQUINT: Difficultés d'interprétation des images des tissus mous endopelviens, obtenues par la pelvigraphie gazeuse. J. Radiol. Electrol. 40 (1959), 344
70. HEUGHEBAERT, R., M. THIERY, E. VAN DE VELDE, F. BARBIER, M. KUNNEN u. G. DARDENNE: Bull. Soc. roy. belge Gynéc. Obstet. 34 (1964), 131
71. HOFMANN, D.: Zur diagnostischen Bedeutung der Gynäkographie (Pneumoperitoneum). Zbl. Gynäk. 85 (1963), 1049
72. HORSKY, J., J. PRESL, M. HENZL u. M. VALENTA: Pneumopelvigraphie in der Gynäkologie. Staatl. Gesundheitsverlag Prag, 1961 (tschechisch)
73. HOULNE, P.: Application de la gynécographie dans certains cas de malformation des organes génitaux de la femme. Presse méd. 65 (1957), 1046
74. JUNG, P. u. A. SCHIRMER: Über die Kombination des pneumoperitonealen Röntgenbildes der weiblichen Kleinbeckenorgane mit der Hysterosalpingographie. Acta radiol. 5 (1926), 395
75. KAINDL, F., E. MANNHEIMER, L. PFLEGER-SCHWARZ u. B. THURNER: Lymphangiographie und Lymphadenographie der Extremitäten. Georg Thieme Verl. Stuttgart, 1960
76. KANKELWITZ, B., L. TESCH u. G. BÖCK: Zur Methodik der Chromogenentwicklung von Röntgenaufnahmen. Dtsch. Ges.wesen 23 (1968), 397
77. KOEHLER, P. R., G. T. WOHL u. B. SCHAFFER: Lymphangiography, a survey of its current status. Amer. J. Roentgenol. 91 (1964), 1216
78. LAGARDE, C., A. HUGUES, J. CHAUVERGNE u. G. LAURENS: La pneumopelvigraphie, technique d'examen gynécologique. Masson u. Cie. Paris, 1962
79. LAMARQUE, P., P. BÉTOUILIÈRES, M. PÉLISSIER, P. LEENHARDT u. J. GARY-BOBO: Étude radiologique des organes génitaux internes de la femme par pneumopéritoine. Essai de gynécographie. J. Radiol. Electrol. 35 (1954), 226
80. LA TORETTA, G., F. CATURANI u. M. NAPOLITANO: La pneumopelvigrafia nella diagnostica ginecologica. Arch. ostet. ginec. 65 (1960), 575
81. LE GÉNISSEL, M. u. M. DUPLAN: Pelvigraphie gazeuse et infiltration des paramètres dans les cancers du col utérin. Bull. Algér. Carcinol. 11 (1959), 255
82. LE GÉNISSEL, M., AUBRY u. BARGES: Stéréopelvigraphies gazeuses. J. Radiol. Electrol. 42 (1961), 770
83. LENZI, M.: Tomografia e laporoscopia nello studio della patologia abdominale. 5. Corso intern. Tomografia. Genova, 1963
84. LEQUINT, A.: La pelvigraphie gazeuse. Confrontations radiochirurgicales de 44 cas opérés sur une série de 250. Lille chir. 12 (1957), 109
85. LEQUINT, A.: L'interprétation des clichés de pelvigraphie gazeuse. Lille chir. 12 (1957), 115
86. LEVIN, B., A. C. RAMBAR u. I. J. SHAPIRO: Female pseudo-hemaphorditism. Report of a case proved roentgenologically. Am. J. Roentgenol. 69 (1953), 948
87. LOREY: Über das Einblasen von Luft in die Bauchhöhle als diagnostisches Hilfsmittel bei der röntgenologischen Untersuchung der Bauchorgane. Eppendorfer Festschrift 1914 zit. nach WINTZ u. DYROFF
88. LUNDERQUIST, A.: Pneumopelvigraphy in the early diagnosis of intersexuality. Amer. J. Roentgenol. 103 (1968), 202

89. Mach, S., K., Richter u. G. Lisewski: Über die Aussagekraft der Pneumopelvigraphie in der gynäkologischen Diagnostik. Zbl. Gyn. 89 (1967), 1297

90. Magendie, J.: Progrès en gynécologie (Pneumopelvigraphie et gynécographie). J. Méd. Bordeaux 133 (1956), 1106

91. Magendie, J., J. Reboul, J. Delorme, F. Perrotin u. D. Herpe: Pneumopelvigraphie et gynécographie en gynécologie. Bordeaux chir. 3 (1954), 117

92. Magendie, J., J. P. Secousse u. M. Regnier: Sur l'intérêt de la coelioscopie en gynécologie. J. Méd. Bordeaux 133 (1956), 265

93. Maralli, G. u. F. Galiardi: Il pneumoperitoneo nella diagnosi radiologica delle affezioni ginecologiche. Riv. Ostet. Ginec. prat. 33 (1951), 273

94. Marcozzi, G. u. M. Maurizi-Enrici: Technique et valeur diagnostique de la pelvipneumographie (dite gynécographie). Gaz. int. Med. Chir. 61 (1956), 2076

95. Maxfield, J. R.: Pneumoperitoneum in the study of pelvic structures. J. Amer. Med. Ass. 146 (1951), 920

96. Moneta, E. u. S. Gardini: Possibilità e limiti della pneumopelvigrafia nella diagnostica delle amenorree secondarie Ann. Ost. Ginec. 88 (1961), 909

97. Montes, E. A. M. u. E. P. Gagnati: La pneumopelvigraphie. Technique et importance dans le diagnostic endocrinologique la femme. Prensa méd. 47 (1957), 3423

98. Moulouguet, P., N. Arvay, J. D. Picard u. G. Manlot: La lymphographie: technique, indications et résultats. J. Radiol. Electrol. 42 (1961), 281

99. Nocca, G. F. u. M. Faccini: Il pneumoperitoneo. Parte II: Il pneumoperitoneo nella diagnosi delle peritoniti tuberculari. Arch. Chir. rotop. 22 (1957), 1

100. Ogier, E. u. M. Mainelli: L'impiego della pneumopelvigrafia nella diagnostica ginecologica. Atti soc. Ostet. Ginec. 10 (1961), 307

101. Oliva, L.: La pneumostratiginecografia. Inform. méd. 10 (1955), 410

102. Orndorff, B. H.: Pneumoperitoneum in X-ray diagnosis. Amer. J. Roentgenol. 2 (1919), 265

103. Pelissier, M., L. Heltrando, P. Reynes, J. Voisin u. M. Herbrad: La pneumopelvigraphie. Revue générale après 3 ans de pratique. Rev. franc. Gynéc. 51 (1956), 406

104. Persianinov, L. S., L. Bakuleva, J. M. Gryaznova u. E. M. Volin: La gynécographie gazeuse dans le diagnostic des affections gynécologiques. Akoucherst vo Guinek 6 (1960), 62

105. Peterson, R.: Value of pneumoperitoneal roentgenography in obstetrics and gynecology. J. Amer. Med. Ass. 78 (1922), 397

106. Piernes, A.: Radiologia del ovario poliquistico. Prensa Med. Argent. 42 (1955), 1775

107. Polano, O. u. C. Dietl: Die Diagnostik gynäkologischer Veränderungen im kleinen Becken durch Pneumoperitoneum und Röntgenbild. Münch. med. Wschr. 69 (1922), 1621

108. Radberg, C. u. I. Wickbom: Pelvic angiography and pneumoperitoneum in diagnosis of gynecologic lesions. Acta radiol. 6 (1967), 133

109. Ramos, P., J. Guitarte u. A. Bianchi: La pneumopelvigraphie en gynécologie. Pren. méd. argent. 33 (1946), 2306

110. Rautenberg, E.: Pneumoperitoneale Röntgendiagnostik. Dtsch. med. Wschr. 45 (1919), 203

111. Rautenberg, E.: Fortschritte der pneumoperitonealen Diagnostik. Fortschr. Röntgenstr. 26 (1919), 411

112. Reboul, J., J. Magendie, G. Delorme, D. Herpe u. F. Perrotin: La pneumopelvigraphie en gynécologie. J. Med. Bordeaux 132 (1955), 489

113. Richter, K., S. Mach u. G. Lisewski: Röntgendiagnostik der weiblichen Beckenorgane durch Pneumopelvigraphie. Radiol. diagn. 7 (1966), 431.

114. Richter, K., S. Mach u. G. Lisewski: Die Pneumopelvigraphie in der gynäkologischen Diagnostik. 1. Mitteilung: Methodik und röntgenanatomische Grundlagen. Fortschr. Röntgenstr. 106 (1967), 541; 2. Mitteilung: Differentialdiagnostische Bedeutung, Indikationen und Nebenwirkungen. Fortschr. Röntgenstr. 106 (1967), 822

115. Richter, K., S. Mach u. G. Lisewski: Die Bedeutung der Pneumopelvigraphie für die Diagnostik gynäkologischer Tumoren. 46. Tagung der Deutschen Röntgengesellschaft 1965

116. Richter, K., S. Mach u. G. Lisewski: Die Pneumopelvigraphie in der Röntgendiagnostik der Beckenorgane. 11. Tagung der Österr. Röntgengesellschaft 1967

117. Roux, G., G. Marchal u. G. Candon: La gynécographie, technique et indication. Gynéc. Obstet. 53 (1954), 545

118. Rüttimann, A.: Die Lymphographie in: Lehrb. der Röntgendiagnostik, 6. Aufl., Bd. I, hsg. von Schinz, H. R., W. E. Baensch, W. Frommhold, G. Glauner, E. Uehlinger u. J. Wellauer. Thieme Verl. Stuttgart, 1965

119. Rüttimann, A.: Zur Lymphknotenbeurteilung im Lymphogramm. Radiol. clin. 32 (1963), 456

120. Rüttimann, A. u. Ms. del Buono: Die Lymphographie mit öligem Kontrastmittel. Fortschr. Röntgenstr. 97 (1962), 551

121. Salasc, J., di Meglio u. C. Maimejac: Sur la pelvigraphie gazeuse. Bull. Féd. Soc. Gynéc. Obstét. franc. 11 (1959), 357

122. Schulz, E. u. S. W. Rosen: Gynecography. Technique and interpretation. Amer. J. Roentgenol. 86 (1961), 866

123. Seguy, J., A. Granjon u. J. Bellair: La gynécographie. Bull. Féd. Soc. Gynéc. Obstét. 4 (1952), 672

124. Sieber, F.: Die Lymphographie in der klinischen Praxis. Georg Thieme Verl. Leipzig, 1966

125. Sieber, F., H. Trinkauf u. K. Köhler: Cavographie und Lymphographie bei gynäkologischen Tumoren. Radiol. diagn. 8 (1967), 691

126. Silinková-Malková, E.: Radiol. diagn. 2 (1961), 61

127. Stein, A.: Oxygen peritoneal inflation before X-ray. Ann. Surg. 1919, 70

128. Stein, A. u. W. H. Stuart: Roentgen ray study of abdominal organs following oxygen inflation of peritoneal cavity. Am. J. Roent. 6 (1919), 533

129. Stein, I. F.: Roentgenographic diagnosis in gynecology; pneumoperitoneum. Surg. Gynec. Obst. 42 (1926), 83

130. Stein, I. F.: Eight years experience with roentgen diagnosis in gynecology; pneumoperitoneum and lipiodol in pelvic diagnosis. Am. J. Obst. Gynec. 21 (1931), 671

131. Stein, I. F.: Roentgen diagnosis in gynecology and obstetrics. J. Michigan M. Soc. 30 (1931), 675

132. Stein, I. F.: Pelvic diagnosis by roentgen visualisation. Surg. Gynec. Obst. 55 (1932), 207

133. Stein, I. F.: Oxygen pneumoperitoneum in diagnosis and treatment of tuberculosis of genitalia, intestine and peritoneum. Surg. Gynec. Obst. 58 (1934), 567

134. Stein, I. F.: Why pneumoperitoneum? Radiology 28 (1937), 391

135. Stein, I. F.: Further Studies in infertility and sterility analysis of 200 couples (Max Ballin memorial lecture). Surg. Gynec. Obst. 67 (1938), 731

136. Stein, I. F.: Case of unruptured tubal pregnancy diagnosed by gynecography. Am. J. Obst. Gynec. 43 (1942), 525

137. Stein, I. F.: Gynecographic aid in diagnosis of ectopic pregnancy. Am. J. Obst. Gynec. 43 (1942), 400
138. Stein, I. F.: Gynecography. S. Clin. North. America 23 (1943), 165
139. Stein, I. F.: Bilateral polycystic ovaries; significance in sterility. Am. J. Obst. Gynec. 50 (1945), 385
140. Stein, I. F.: Gynecography in Davis' Gynecology and Obstetrics. Vol. III chapter 3. W. F. Prior, édit., Hagerstown, Maryland, 1955
141. Stein, I. F.: The role of gynecography in the evaluation of the intertile woman. West S. Surg. Obst. Gynec. 66 (1958), 262
142. Stein, I. F.: Gynecography for the diagnosis of female sterility. Internat. J. of Fertil. 4 (1959), 115
143. Stein, I. F.: La gynécographie: apport inestimable au diagnostic de l'état du petit bassin chez la femme. Gynécol. pratique 10 (1959), 397
144. Stein, I. F. u. R. A. Arens: Iodized oil and pneumoperitoneum combined in gynecologic diagnosis; preliminary report. J.A.M.A., 87 (1926), 1299
145. Stein, I. F. u. R. A. Arens: Pneumoperitoneum in gynecology. Radiology 7 (1926), 326
146. Stein, I. F. u. R. A. Arens: Iodized oil and pneumoperitoneum in gynecology; clinical radiological study. Radiology 8 (1927), 494
147. Stein, I. F. u. R. A. Arens: New radiographic table, with description of author's complete equipment for pelvic radiography with iodized oil and pneumoperitoneum. Am. J. Obst. Gynec. 18 (1929), 130
148. Stein, I. F. u. R. A. Arens: Roentgen diagnosis in gynecology; iodized oil and pneumoperitoneum combined. Radiology 12 (1929), 341
149. Stein, I. F. u. R. A. Arens: Visualisation of the pelvic viscera; iodized oil and pneumoperitoneum combined in gynecology. Radiology 15 (1930), 85
150. Stein, I. F. u. M. L. Leventhal: Amenorrhea associated with bilateral polycystic ovaries. Am. J. Obst. Gynec. 29 (1935), 181
151. Stewart, W. H. u. A. Stein: Roentgen ray study of the abdominal organs following oxygen inflation of the peritoneal cavity. Amer. J. Roent. 6 (1919), 533
152. Stuart, C.: Metodiche contrasto-grafiche gassose e technice radiografiche nello studio radiologico della pelvi femminile. Rad. méd. 47 (1961), 975
153. Tardiveau, J. u. J. Legrand: De l'intèrêt de la gynécographie dans le cancer du col utérin. Soc. de Gyn. et d'Obst. de l'Ouest de la France. Presse méd. 65 (1957), 1046
154. Tenti, L.: Implego pratico del craniostato per la pneumoginecografia. Minerve med. 50 (1959, 351
155. Tenti, L., G. F. Nocca u. J. Belli: Pneumoginecografia e laparoscopia: utilità della lor' associazione nella diagnosi delle pelvipatie. Ed. Min. Med. 1963
156. Tenti, E., E. Seassaro, G. F. Nocca u. G. F. Maffioli: Il contributo diagnostico della pneumoginecografia associata alla laparascopia nelle algie genito pelviche aderenziali. Ann. Ostet. Ginec. 86 (1964), 915
157. Tetti, A.: La pneumopelvigrafia: indicazioni e possibilità. Minerva Ginec. 12 (1960), 531; Minerva Med. 51 (1966), 3176
158. Theander, G. u. L. Wehlin: The radiology of pelvic endometriosis. Clin. Radiology 19 (1968), 19
159. Trucchi, O.: L'associazone del pneumoperitoneo pelvico e della pneumocistografia nell' esame radiologico della pariete della vesica urinaria con particolare riguardo alla ricerca delle neoplasie. Radiol. med. 44 (1958), 421
160. Vaglio, N. u. A. Graziani: La ginecografia nella diagnosi delle malformazioni uterine. Arch. Ostet. Ginec. 65 (1960), 145
161. Vallebona, A.: A proposito di ginecografia. Rad. med. 41 (1955), 1014
162. Vallebona, A. u. V. Dogliotti: Contributo alla esplorazione radiologica dell'apparato genitale femminile. Annali di Radiologia e Fisica Medica 11 (1937), 126
163. Vallebona, A. u. V. Dogliotti: L'esplorazione radiologica e stratigrafica dell'apporto genitale femminile col piccolo pneumoperitoneo e con la pneumoperitoneo e con pneumocistografia. Folia demografica gynecologica, vol. 37, fasciocolo 3, 1940
164. van de Velde, E., M. Thiery, R. Heughebaert, M. Kunnen, F. Barbier u. G. Dardenne: La pneumopelvigraphie dans les affections gynécologiques non tumorales. Journ. Belge Radiol. 47 (1964), 363
165. Verhaeghe, M. u. J. Herbeau: La gynécographie dans le diagnostic des tumeurs pelviennes. Bull. Féd. Soc. Gynéc. Obstét. 7 (1955), 546
166. Verhaeghe, M., J. Herbeau u. A. Lequint: La pelvigraphie gazeuse dans le diagnostic des affections utérines et ovariennes. C. R. Soc. Franc. Gynéc. 28 (1958), 451
167. Weber, D.: Über die Bedeutung der Einführung von Sauerstoff resp. Luft in die Bauchhöhle für die experimentelle und diagnostische Röntgenologie. Fortschr. Röntgenstr. 20 (1913), 453
168. Werner, K., W. Bader, D. Buttenberg u. H. Zeitz: Logetronographie in der Röntgenologie. Fortschr. Röntgenstr. 90 (1959), 110
169. Wintz, H. u. A. Dyroff: Das Pneumoperitoneum in der Gynäkologie. G. Thieme Verl. Leipzig, 1924
170. Yung: Radiographica des organes du petit bassin de la femme après pneumoperitoine. Surg. Gynéc. Obstétr. 8 (1923), 329, zit. nach Wintz u. Dyroff
171. Zwaluwenburg, van J. G. u. R. Peterson: Pneumoperitoneum of the pelvis; gynecological studies. A preliminary resport. Am. J. Roent. 8 (1921), 12

Sachverzeichnis

Subject index

Bei Fragen zur Produktsicherheit wenden Sie sich bitte an:
If you have any questions regarding product safety,
please contact:

Walter de Gruyter GmbH
Genthiner Straße 13
10785 Berlin
productsafety@degruyterbrill.com